Caffeine

CAFFEINE

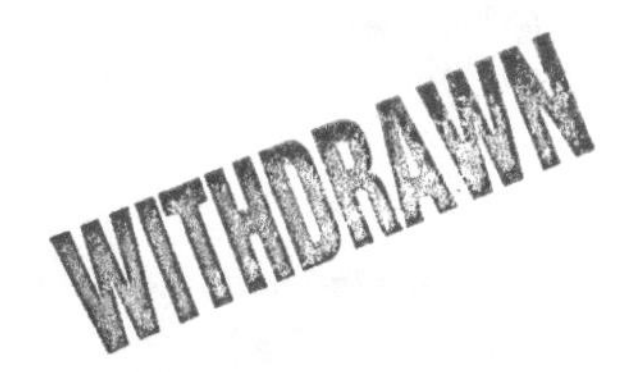

edited by
Gene A. Spiller, Ph.D., D.Sc., FACN
Health Research and Studies Center and Sphera Foundation
Los Altos, California

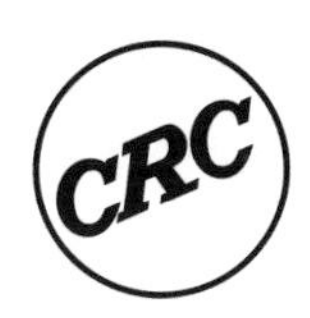

CRC Press
Boca Raton London New York Washington, D.C.

Acquiring Editor: *Harvey Kane*
Project Editor: *Susan Fox*
Cover Design: *Dawn Boyd*
Prepress: *Kevin Luong and Walt Cerny*

Library of Congress Cataloging-in-Publication Data

Catalog record is available from the Library of Congress.

International Standard Book Number 0-8493-2647-8
Printed in the United States of America 2 3 4 5 6 7 8 9 0
Printed on acid-free paper

Preface

Caffeine was conceived for a wide range of readers interested in the effects on human health, nutrition, and physiological function of the methylxanthine beverages and foods—tea, coffee, maté, cola beverages, and cocoa and chocolate products. These products supply one or more of the dietary methylxanthines—caffeine, theobromine and theophylline—and are an integral part of the diet of many people in many countries. The interest in the health effects of both the methylxanthines in isolation and in the products containing them has grown rapidly in recent years.

This comprehensive text gathers in a single volume in-depth information on composition, processing, consumption, health effects, and epidemiological correlations for the methylxanthine beverages and foods and should serve as a useful tool for anyone interested in the methylxanthine–containing products. It briefly covers metabolic and physiological aspects. This design should make this book valuable to physicians, nutritionists, other health professionals, and food scientists.

Chapters 1 and 2 offer an introductory, concise overview of the chemistry and analysis of the methylxanthines. In Chapters 3 through 8, each natural product (tea, coffee, maté, and cocoa and chocolate products) is described. Botany, cultivation, processing, composition, and consumption patterns are covered in detail. The reader can better grasp how the chemical complexity of the methylxanthines makes it important to carefully distinguish between the effects of the methylxanthines in isolation and as part of one of these natural products. The extremely critical and complex question of consumption is discussed in more than one chapter, but is the specific focus of Chapter 9. Chapter 10 covers the basic physiology and biochemistry of caffeine, not with the physiologist or biochemist in mind, but rather the health professional in need of a concise, easy to read overview of these topics. Chapters 11 and 12 focus on the ergogenic, cognitive, and emotional effects of caffeine, while Chapters 13 through 16 deal directly with the health effects of methylxanthines, coffee, or tea and their effects on serum cholesterol, cancer and fibrocystic breast disease, calcium and bone health, and human reproduction. Appendix I lists the caffeine content of various popular cola beverages.

No single book can possibly cover all aspects of the chemistry, consumption, and health effects of the methylxanthines, but I hope that this volume will help a wide variety of readers to better understand coffee, tea, maté, cola beverages, and cocoa and chocolate products and their effects on human health.

Gene A. Spiller, Ph.D.
Los Altos, California

The Editor

Gene Alan Spiller, Ph.D., D.Sc., is the director of the Health Research and Studies Center and of the Sphera Foundation in Los Altos, California.

Dr. Spiller received his first doctorate in chemistry from the University of Milan (Italy), and later a Master's degree and a Ph.D. in nutrition from the University of California at Berkeley. He did additional studies at the Stanford University School of Medicine at Stanford, California. He is a Fellow of the American College of Nutrition, a Certified Nutrition Specialist, and a member of many professional nutrition societies.

In the 1970s, Dr. Spiller was head of Nutritional Physiology at Syntex Research in Palo Alto, California, where he did extensive human and animal research. At the same time he edited many clinical nutrition books. He continued his work in clinical nutrition research and publishing in the 1980s and 1990s, as a consultant and as the director of the Health Research and Studies Center and of the Sphera Foundation in Los Altos, California. Many human clinical studies, reviews, and other publications were the results of this work. Dr. Spiller has carried out clinical studies on the effect of complex whole foods, fiber and high fiber foods such as raisins and whole grains, lipids such as monounsaturated fats, and foods high in fiber such as nuts. Some of his recent research has focused on antioxidants, immunity, and bone density in aging. Since the early 1980s, Dr. Spiller has had a special interest in the health effects of coffee and tea. In addition, he has been a lecturer in nutrition in the San Francisco Bay Area, first at Mills College and currently at Foothill College.

Dr. Spiller is the editor of many clinical nutrition books. Among his multiauthor books are *The Methylxanthine Beverages and Foods: Chemistry, Consumption, and Health Effects* (Alan R. Liss, 1984), *The Mediterranean Diets in Health and Disease* (Van Nostrand Rheinhold, 1991), *CRC Handbook of Fiber in Human Nutrition 2nd Edition* (CRC Press, 1993) and *CRC Handbook of Lipids in Human Nutrition* (CRC Press, 1996).

Contributors

Joan L. Apgar, B.A.
Food Science & Technology
Hershey Foods Corporation
Hershey, PA 17033-0805

Douglas A. Balentine, Ph.D.
Lipton
Englewood Cliffs, NJ 07632

Bonnie Bruce, Dr.P.H., M.P.H., R.D.
Health Research and Studies Center and Sphera Foundation
Los Altos, CA 94023-0338

Christopher Gardner, Ph.D.
Stanford University Medical School
Center for Research in Disease Prevention
Palo Alto, CA 94304

Harold N. Graham, Ph.D.
Lipton (retired)
Englewood, NJ 07632

Matthew E. Harbowy
Lipton
Englewood, NJ 07632

David Lee Hoffman
Silk Road Teas
Lagunitas, CA 94938

W. Jeffrey Hurst
Food Science & Technology
Hershey Foods Corporation
Hershey, PA 17033-0805

Roland J. Lamarine, H.S.D.
Department of Health and Community Services
California State University
Chico, CA 95929-0505

Lisbet S. Lundsberg, Ph.D.
Perinatal Epidemiology Unit
Yale University School of Medicine
New Haven, CT 06511

Robert A. Martin, Jr., Ph.D.
Food Science & Technology
Hershey Foods Corporation
Hershey, PA 17033-0805

Barry D. Smith, Ph.D.
Department of Psychology
University of Maryland
College Park, MD 20742

Gene A. Spiller, D.Sc., Ph.D.
Health Research and Studies Center and Sphera Foundation
Los Altos, CA 94023-0338

Monica Alton Spiller, M.Sc.
Alton Spiller, Inc.
Los Altos, CA 94023-0696

Stanley M. Tarka, Jr., Ph.D.
Food Science & Technology
Hershey Foods Corporation
Hershey, PA 17033-0805

Kenneth Tola
Department of Psychology
University of Maryland
College Park, MD 20742

Myron Winick, M.D.
R. R. Williams Professor of Nutrition (Emeritus)
Columbia University
College of Physicians and Surgeons

Acknowledgments

The editor gratefully acknowledges Mr. William F. Shannon, Contracts Manager at John Wiley & Sons, Inc., whose efforts in obtaining reversion of the copyright of *The Methylxanthine Beverages and Foods* (Alan R. Liss, 1984) from John Wiley & Sons to Dr. Gene Spiller enabled us to produce this volume. Thanks also to Rosemary Schmele for assistance in various phases of the editing process and in coordinating the final manuscript.

Dedication

To Drs. Denis Burkitt and Hugh Trowell, who have given me a unique perception of the correlation of health and disease with food, and to Drs. John Farquhar and David Jenkins, who always inspire me with their work on the relation of diet to chronic diseases.

TABLE OF CONTENTS

Chapter 1

INTRODUCTION TO THE CHEMISTRY, ISOLATION, AND BIOSYNTHESIS OF METHYLXANTHINES

Stanley M. Tarka, Jr and W. Jeffrey Hurst

CONTENTS

0-8493-2647-8/98/$0.00+$.50

I. INTRODUCTION

The methylxanthines of interest are caffeine (1,3,7-trimethylxanthine), theophylline (1,3-dimethylxanthine), and theobromine (3,7-dimethylxanthine) and they occur in coffee, tea, maté, cocoa products, and cola beverages. This chapter is an introduction to their chemistry, isolation, and biosynthesis. While the class of methylxanthines is large and comprised of more members than these three, this chapter will essentially be limited to caffeine, theobromine, and theophylline.

Purine is the parent heterocyclic compound of the methylxanthines, which are often referred to as the purine alkaloids.[1–7] Purine is also the parent compound of some of the base constituents of the nucleotides, which in turn are part of the nucleic acids RNA and DNA. Thus, it appears that the purine alkaloids have similar precursors to nucleic acids.

II. PHYSICAL AND CHEMICAL PROPERTIES OF THE METHYLXANTHINES

A. Organoleptic Properties

Caffeine, as an example methylxanthine, is a colorless powder at room temperature; it is odorless but does have a slightly bitter taste.[8]

B. Melting and Sublimation Temperatures

The trimethylated xanthine, caffeine, sublimes at 1800°C, which is a lower temperature of sublimation than theobromine.[10] Temperatures of melting and sublimation are given in Table 1.

C. Solution Formation

Solubility values are distinctive for caffeine, theobromine, and theophylline (see Table 2). Caffeine dissolves well in boiling water, but at room temperature chloroform is one of the best solvents. Theobromine is generally much less soluble than caffeine but it will dissolve readily in aqueous acids and alkalis. Theophylline is intermediate between caffeine and theobromine in its ability to form solutions. A series of studies were conducted by Hockfield[17] and Gilkey,[18] who, after comparing the solubility rates of the xanthine alkaloids, determined that the methylxanthines in which both heterocyclic nitrogen atoms in the ring are methylated (caffeine and theophylline) display a much greater solubility in polar solvents than those with at least one unmethylated nitrogen atom (theobromine).

TABLE 1

Melting and Sublimation Temperatures for Methylxanthines

Compound	Sublimation point (°C)	Melting point (°C)
Caffeine	180[8]	236.5 under pressure[8]
	178[9]	238[9]
	178[7]	235 anhydrous[7]
Theobromine	290–295[9]	357[9]
	290[7]	330 sealed tube[7]
Theophylline	—	270–274[9]
	269–272[7]	

TABLE 2

Solubility Values for Methylxanthines

Solvent	Caffeine (%)	Theobromine (%)	Theophylline (%)
Water, 150°C	1.3[8]		
Water	2.2[9]	0.005[9]	0.83[9]
Water, 400°C	4.6[8]		
Water, hot		Soluble[9]	
Water, 800°C	18.2[9]		
Water, boiling	66.7[9]	0.67[9]	
Ether	0.3[8]	Almost insol.[9]	Sparingly sol.[9]
	0.2[9]		
Alcohol	1.2[8]	1.25[9]	
	1.5[9]		
Alcohol, 600°C	4.5[9]		
95% Alcohol	0.045[9]		
Ethyl acetate	2.5[8]		
Chloroform	13.0[8]	Almost insol.[9]	0.91[9]
	18.2[9]		
Acetone	2.0[9]		
Benzene	1.0[9]	Almost insol.[9]	
Benzene, boiling	4.5[9]		
Pyrrole	Freely sol.[9]		
Tetrahydrofuran and 4% water	Freely sol.[9]		
Petroleum ether	Sparingly sol.[9]		
Carbon tetrachloride		Almost insol.[9]	

These studies indicate that intermolecular hydrogen bonding between lactam systems in the nonmethylated alkaloids is responsible for these differences. The findings indicate a difference between the enthalpies of theobromine, which would be expected to form a dimer, and those of caffeine and theophylline, whose structures would preclude dimerization, is approximately that of one hydrogen bond per molecule.

D. Ultraviolet and Infrared Absorption

The methylxanthines show useful strong ultraviolet (UV) absorption between 250 and 280 nm.[11] The spectra for the methylxanthines are very similar and only when one uses techniques such as derivative spectroscopy can substantial differences be seen. In addition to the UV absorption, the methylxanthines also exhibit strong infrared (IR) spectra which can provide critical information about these compounds.

E. Complex Formation

In aqueous solution, caffeine associates to form at least a dimer and probably a polymer;[12] the molecules are arranged in a stack.[13] Caffeine will also associate with purines and pyrimidines either as the free bases or as their nucleosides.[13] Caffeine crystallizes from water as a monohydrate [9].

Chlorogenic acid forms a 1:1 complex with caffeine, which can be crystallized from aqueous alcohol and yields very little free caffeine on extraction with chloroform. Other compounds with which caffeine will complex in this way include isoeugenol, coumarin, indole-acetic acid, and anthocyanidin. The basis for this selection was the requirement for a substituted aromatic ring and a conjugated double bond in forming such a complex. This kind of complex does modify the physiological effects of caffeine.[14] Complex formation will also increase the apparent aqueous solubility of caffeine in the presence of alkali benzoates, cinnamates, citrates, and salicylates.[9]

A description of the physical properties and behavior of caffeine in its aqueous solution was published in 1980 by Both and Commenga.[15]

Where the complexing agent is phenolic, the pH must be such that the phenol is undissociated; usually such complexes form at a pH below 6. Free caffeine concentrations are increased above pH 6.[14]

The methylxanthines vary in their ability to form certain metal complexes. For example, theophylline will complex with both copper and silver whereas caffeine will not.[16] The interpretation of this is that the metal ion forms a pentacyclic complex involving the phenolic 0 at C-6 and N at 7.[16]

F. Acidic and Basic Equilibria

The acidic and basic equilibrium constants Ka and Kb are given in Table 3.

Caffeine behaves as a very feeble base and reacts with acids; the salts produced are very readily hydrolysed.[9]

Evidence for the formation of protonated caffeine can be seen in the changed UV spectrum for caffeine at pH 0.[14]

Theobromine and theophylline are weakly amphoteric and behave more distinctly as acids or bases than caffeine does. This is evident from the ease with which theobromine and theophylline will dissolve in aqueous acids and bases; they are only sparingly soluble in pure water.[9]

TABLE 3

Acidic (Ka) and Basic (Kb) Equilibrium Constants Expressed as pKa and pKb

Compound	pKa	pKb
Caffeine, 19°C	14.2	
Caffeine, 250°C	14 (approx.)	
Theobromine, 180°C	10.0	13.9
Theophylline, 25°C	8.8	13.7

III. ISOLATION OF THE METHYLXANTHINES

A possible task facing the scientist is the isolation of the methylxanthine compounds from plant material. Use can be made of the solubility values given in Table 2 and the pKa and the pKb values in Table 3 in designing an isolation scheme for each individual methylxanthine. There are two possible approaches to this task,[19] one involving aqueous extraction and the other involving an organic solvent extraction. These methods are not without problems since the extract is usually contaminated with various organic and inorganic compounds. If extraction with organic compounds is desired, and the plant has a large amount of lipid, then a preliminary extraction with petroleum ether or hexane might be followed by extraction with a solvent such as methanol. The methanolic extract can be concentrated to a small volume and acidified to pH 2. It is possible to steam-distill the extract and refrigerate the distillate. After 24 h, a clear liquid can be decanted and filtered through activated charcoal or a similar filter aid. The aqueous solution can be made basic with ammonium hydroxide or sodium carbonate, which may cause precipitation of the basic compounds. A further step would involve the extraction of the basic solution with chloroform. The chloroform would contain the methylxanthines and could be readily removed.

Another scheme for methylxanthine isolation involves the extraction of the dried ground plant with 10% ammonium hydroxide:chloroform (1:10). A large proportion of the extraction mixture is used, relative to the sample, to ensure complete extraction of any theobromine. Caffeine and theophylline will be extracted easily under these conditions.[20] After removing water from the organic layer, filtration, and solvent removal, any methylxanthines present will be in the residue together with some impurities. An approach to finally isolating these methylxanthines from this residue would involve redissolving the residue in a dilute acid with subsequent filtering and reprecipitation. Other possible avenues to explore would be thin-layer chromatography, column chromatography, or fractional recrystallization.

Recently, solid phase extraction (SPE) has been used to isolate members of this class of compounds. No solid phase support has been used exclusively and both hydrophobic- and hydrophilic-based solid phase extraction columns have been used for this assay.

These procedures outlined are not all-encompassing and should serve only as guidelines. Additionally, the end use of the extract (i.e., biochemical studies, analytical methodology, toxicological studies) will have a large effect on the required purity of the final product. Some uses need only water extraction while others need a more rigorous clean-up procedure with methods outlined in Chapter 3.

IV. BIOSYNTHESIS OF THE METHYLXANTHINES

A. In Coffee

Roberts and Waller[21] and Looser et al.[22] have outlined the biosynthesis of caffeine in coffee. Looser et al.[22] propose a pathway for biosynthesis starting with the "purine pool" via nucleic acids through 7-methylguanylic acid, 7-methylguanosine, 7-methylxanthosine, 7-methylxanthine, 3,7-dimethylxanthine (theobromine), and then to 1,3,7-trimethylxanthine (caffeine). Their studies determined intermediates to 7-methylxanthosine. The later work of Roberts and Waller[21] provides further reinforcement of this proposal. Schulthess and Baumann[23] examined caffeine biosynthesis in suspension cultured coffee cells. In that study, suspension-cultured coffee cells were subjected to various conditions such as photoperiod (13 h in a growth chamber), 1 mM adenine, 0.1 to 10 mM ethephon, or to the combination of both adenine and ethephon. Concentration of purine bases, nucleosides, nucleotides, and purine alkaloids (PA; i.e., 7-methylxanthine, theobromine, and caffeine) were measured by HPLC. In the dark, both adenine and ethephon drastically stimulated overall PA formation by a factor of 4 and 7, respectively. Their simultaneous application resulted in an additional increase yielding a stimulation factor of 11. Under the photoperiod, caffeine formation was, as compared to the control in the dark, enhanced by a factor of 21 without affecting theobromine and 7-methylxanthine pools; additional stimulation by ethephon was not possible. Conversely to light and ethephon, which had no effect on the accumulation of primary purine metabolites, adenine feeding resulted in persistently enlarged pools of nucleosides (xanthosine, guanosine, inosine) and 7-glucopyranosyladenine. 7-Methylxanthosine, the postulated precursor of 7-methylxanthine in caffeine biosynthesis, could not be detected under any conditions at any time. Since no other methylated purine was found, it is not yet feasible to discard the 7-methylxanthosine hypothesis.

Mazzafera[24] described studies on the isolation and purification of the N-terminal sequence of S-adenosyl-L-methionine:theobromine 1-N-methyltransferase (STM), the enzyme responsible for the methylation of theobromine leading to caffeine formation in coffee. STM was purified from developing endosperms of immature fruits by DEAE-cellulose, hydrophobic interaction, and affinity chromatography, using S-adenosyl-L-homocysteine as a ligand. The enzyme showed apparent Mr of 54,000 and approximately 60,000 determined by gel filtration and SDS-PAGE, respectively. A pH of 5.1 and 4.8 was obtained by liquid chromatofocusing and by isoelectrofocusing in PAGE, respectively. Using theobromine as substrate, the Km value for S-adenosyl-L-methionine was 10 μM, being competitively inhibited by S-adenosyl-L-homocysteine (Ki = 4.6 μM). STM is a bifunctional enzyme because it also methylated 7-methylxanthine, the immediate precursor of theobromine in the caffeine biosynthesis pathway. The specific activity of STM with 7-methylxanthine was approximately 55% of that determined with theobromine. Km values obtained for theobromine and 7-methylxanthine were 0.196 and 0.496 mM, respectively. STM was also purified from leaves using the same procedures used for endosperms, plus an additional chromatography step on a Mono Q column; theobromine was used as substrate. The N-terminal sequence for the first 20 amino acids was obtained for STM purified from endosperms. No similarities were found with other methyltransferase sequences or other known proteins.

The metabolism of purine nucleotides and purine alkaloids (e.g., caffeine and theobromine) in tea and coffee plants is reviewed by Suzuki et al.[25] Purine metabolism in these plants is similar to that in other plants that do not contain caffeine; however, tea and coffee plants have purine nucleotides, including those produced directly by purine biosynthesis de novo, as effective precursors of caffeine. Xanthosine is the first methyl acceptor from S-adenosylmethionine in caffeine biosynthesis, and is also metabolized by a purine degradation pathway via xanthine. The regulation of purine alkaloid biosynthesis remains elusive, but the activity of the 3 N-methyltransferases is considered. Production and accumulation of the alkaloids are associated with the developmental stage of tissues (i.e., leaves, flowers, fruits, and seeds) and with seasonal changes, especially in tea grown in temperate climates. The metabolism (especially biosynthesis) of purine alkaloids differs among *Camellia* spp. In *Coffea* plants and in cultured cells, the rate of caffeine synthesis and turnover (i.e., biodegradation and/or biotransformation to xanthine or to methyluric acids) differs markedly among species. Ecological roles of the alkaloids have been reported, but their physiological significance in tea and coffee plants remains uncertain.

Coffea arabica is one of the plant species that has been widely studied with attention largely being given to its secondary products, caffeine and other purine alkaloids. The biosynthesis and significance of these alkaloids for the plant are elucidated and presented in a paper by Presnosil et al.[26] Tissue cell culture and fundamental aspects of cell growth and alkaloid productivity are also discussed. The feasibility of *Coffea* cultivation in cell suspension has recently attracted the interest of many researchers. Although this cultivation is not of commercial interest, *Coffea* is especially suitable as a model cell line for reaction engineering studies because the purine alkaloids are well-characterized and readily released in culture medium.

B. In Tea

Several studies have investigated the biosynthesis of caffeine in tea. The results of a study by Suzuki and Takahashi[27–30] suggest a pathway for caffeine biosynthesis in tea from 7-methylxanthine to theobromine and then to caffeine. Additionally they suggest that theophylline is synthesized from 1-methylxanthine. Another study by Ogutuga and Northcote[31] proposes a pathway through 7-methylxanthosine to theobromine followed by caffeine.

Much research has centered on identifying the source of the purine ring in caffeine. Two possible sources are likely: methylated nucleotides in the nucleotide pool and methylated nucleotides in nucleic acids. Extensive experimental work by Suzuki and Takahashi[27–30] proposes a scheme whereby caffeine is synthesized from methylated purines in the nucleotide pool via 7-methylxanthosine and theobromine. Information relating to the formation of 7-methylxanthine from nucleotides in the nucleotide pool is sparse. They also provide data that demonstrate that theophylline is synthesized from 1-methyladenylic acid through 1-methylxanthine as postulated by Ogutuga and Northcote.[31]

The conversion of purine nucleosides and nucleotides to caffeine in tea plants was investigated by Negishi et al.[32] and involved feeding -1-4C-labeled adenosine, inosine, xanthosine, and guanosine to excised tea shoots. The radioactivity of -1-4C-labeled adenosine, inosine and guanosine was detected in caffeine after 24 h incubation; radioactivity of -1-4C-labelled xanthosine was incorporated into caffeine via 7-methylxanthosine, 7-methylxanthine, and theobromine. The activity of enzymes involved in the conversion of nucleosides in cell-free extracts of tea leaves was also measured. Enzyme activity was detected in the reaction from guanosine to xanthosine but not from inosine to xanthosine. The rate of phosphorylation in cell-free extracts of purine nucleosides to their respective nucleotides was adenosine greater than inosine, guanosine greater than xanthosine. It is concluded that the pathway leading to the formation of xanthosine from adenine nucleotides in caffeine biosynthesis is via AMP.

Seasonal variations in the metabolic fate of adenine nucleotides prelabelled with [8—1-4C]adenine were examined in leaf disks prepared at 1-month intervals, over the course of 1 year, from the shoots of tea plants (*Camellia sinensis* L. cv. Yabukita) which were growing under natural field conditions by Fujimori et al.[33] Incorporation of radioactivity into nucleic acids and catabolites of purine nucleotides was found throughout the experimental period, but incorporation into theobromine and caffeine was found only in the young leaves harvested from April to June. Methylation of xanthosine, 7-methylxanthine, and theobromine was catalyzed by gel-filtered leaf extracts from young shoots (April to June), but the reactions could not be detected in extracts from leaves in which no synthesis of caffeine was observed *in vivo*. By contrast, the activity of 5-phosphoribosyl-1-pyrophosphate synthetase was still found in leaves harvested in July and August.

C. In Cacao

While caffeine biosynthesis in coffee and tea has been reasonably well investigated, little information is available about the biosynthetic pathways of methylxanthines in cacao. Published studies[34, 35] have established the presence of 7-methylxanthine and adenine in cocoa. Since both coffee and tea exhibit similar pathways where theobromine is a direct precursor for caffeine, it is reasonable to assume that a similar mechanism is possible in cacao.

REFERENCES

1. Nakanishi, K., Goto, T., Ito, S., Natori, S., and Nozoe, S., Eds., *Natural Products Chemistry*, Vol. II, Academic Press, New York, 1979.
2. Pelletier, S.W., Ed., *Chemistry of the Alkaloids*, Van Nostrand Reinhold Co., New York, 1978.
3. Robinson, T., *Alkaloids*, WH Freeman and Co., San Francisco, 1968.
4. Hesse, M. *Alkaloid Chemistry*, Wiley Interscience, New York, 1978.
5. Acheson, R.A., *An Introduction to the Chemistry of Heterocyclic Compounds*, Interscience, New York,1960.
6. Barker, R., *Organic Chemistry of Biological Compounds*, Prentice Hall, Englewood Cliffs, NJ, 1978.
7. Tarka, S.M. Jr.,The toxicology of cocoa and methylxanthines: A review of the literature, *CRC Crit. Rev. Toxicol.* 9,275,1982.
8. Vitzthum, O.G., Chemie und Arbeitung des Kaffees, in Eichler, 0., Ed., *Kaffee und Coffeine*, Springer-Verlag, Heidelberg, 1976.

9. Windholz. M,, Bundavari, S., Stroumtsos, L., Fertig, M., Eds., *The Merck Index*, 9th ed., Merck and Co, Rahway, 1976.
10. Dean, J.A. Ed., *Lange's Handbook of Chemistry*, McGraw-Hill, New York, 1978.
11. Tu, A.T. and Reinosa, J.A., The interaction of silver ion with guanosine, guanosine monophosphate and related compounds: Determination of possible sites of complexing, *Biochemistry*, 5,3375,1966.
12. Ts'o, P.O.P., Melvin, I.S., and Olson, A.C., Interaction and association of bases and nucleosides in aqueous solution, *J. Chem. Soc.*, 85,1289,1963.
13. Thakkar, A.L., Self association of caffeine in aqueous solution: IH nuclear magnetic resonance study, *J. Chem. Soc. Chem. Commun.*, 9,524,1970.
14. Sondheimer, E., Covitz, F., and Marquisee, M.J., Association of naturally occurring compounds, the chlorogenic acid-caffcine complex, *Arch. Biochem. Biophys.*, 93,63,1961.
15. Both, H. and Commenga, H.K., Physical properties and behavior of caffeine in aqueous solution, *9th Int. Sci. Colloq. Coffee*, 1980.
16. Tu, A.T., Friedrich CG: Interaction of copper ion with guanosine and related compounds, *Biochemistry*, 7,4367,1968.
17. Hockfield, H.S., Fullom, C.L., Roper, G.C., Sheeley, R.M., Hurst, W.J., Martin, R.A., Thermochemical investigations of the dimerization of theobromine, 14 *MARM*, 1982.
18. Gilkey, R., Sheeley, R.M., Hurst, W.J., Martin, R.A. Dimerization of xanthine alkaloids as an explanation of extreme solublity differences, 16 *MARM*, 1984.
19. Manske, R.H.F. and Holmes, H.F., Eds., *The Alkaloids: Chemistry and Physiology*, Academic Press, New York, 1950.
20. Jalal, M.A.F. and Collin, H.A., Estimation of caffeine, theophylline and theobromine in plant material, *New Phytol.*, 76,277,1976.
21. Roberts, M.F. and Waller, G.R., N-methyltransferases and 7-methyl-N9-nucleoside hydrolase activity in *Coffea arabica* and the biosynthesis of caffeine, *Phytochemistry*, 18,451,1979.
22. Looser, E., Baumann, T.W., and Warner, H., The biosynthesis of caffeine in the coffee plant, *Phytochemistry*, 13,2515,1974.
23. Schulthess, B.H. and Baumann, T.W., Stimulation of caffeine biosynthesis in suspension cultured coffee cells and the in-situ existence of 7-methylxanthosine, *Phytochemistry*, 38,1381,1995.
24. Mazzafera, P, Wingsle, G., Olsson, O., Sandberg, G., S-adensoyl-L-methionine: theobromine 1-N-methyltranferase, a enzyme catalyzing the synthesis of caffeine in coffee Phytochemistry 37:1577 1994
25. Suzuki,, T., Ashihara, H., Waller G.R.., Purine and purine alkaloid metabolism in Camellia and Coffea plant, *Phytochemistry*, 31,2575,1992
26. Prenosil, J.E., Hegglin, M., Baumann, T.W., Frischkneechtt, P.M., Kappeler, A.W., Brodeliuss,P., and Haldimann,D., Purine alkaloid producing cell cultures; fundamental aspects and possible applications in biotechnology, *Enzyme Microbial. Technol.*, 9,450,1987.
27. Suzuki, T. and Takahashi, E., Biosynthesis of caffeine by tea-leaf extracts, *Biochemistry*, 146,87,1975.
28. Suzuki, T. and Takahashi, E., Further investigation of the biosynthesis of caffeine in tea plants, *Biochemistry*, 160,81,1976a.
29. Suzuki, T. and Takahashi, E., Caffeine biosynthesis in *Camellia sinensis, Phytochemistry*, 15,1235,1976b.
30. Suzuki, T. and Takahashi, E., Metabolism of methionine and biosynthesis of caffeine in tea plant, *Biochemistry*, 160,171,1976c.

31. Ogutuga, D.B.A. and Northcote, D.H., Biosynthesis of caffeine in tea callus tissue, *Biochemistry,* 117,715,1970.
32. Negishi, O., Ozzawa,T., and Imagawa, H., Biosynthesis of caffeine from purine nucleotides in tea plant, *Bioscience, Biotechnology , and Biochemistry,* 56,499,1992
33. Fujimori, N., Suzuki, T., and Ashihara, H., Seasonal variations in biosynthetic capacity for the synthesis of caffeine in tea leave, *Phytochemistry,* 30,2245,1991
34. Aleo, M.D., Sheeley, R.M., Hurst, W.J., and Martin, R.A., The identification of 7-methylxanthine in cocoa products, *J. Liquid Chromatogr.,* 5,939,1982.
35. Keifer, B.A., Sheeley, R.M., Hurst, W.J., and Martin, R.A.,Identification of adenine in cocoa products, *J. Liquid Chromatogr.,* 6,927,1983.

Chapter 2

ANALYTICAL METHODS FOR QUANTITATION OF METHYLXANTHINES

W. Jeffrey Hurst, Robert A. Martin, Jr., and Stanley M. Tarka, Jr.

CONTENTS

0-8493-2647-8/98/$0.00+$.50

I. INTRODUCTION

The analysis of the methylxanthines (caffeine, theobromine, and theophylline) is important in the areas of nutrition and clinical chemistry. These three compounds compose the majority of the alkaloids present in coffee, tea, cocoa, cola nuts, and guarana.

This chapter on analysis of methylxanthines is divided into three sections: historical methods, current analytical methods for foods, and current methods for biological samples which can include plasma, blood, urine, cell extracts, and other potential samples of biological significance.

This chapter will provide an introduction to each of the technologies described and the use of the specific technique for analysis of samples. It will also provide additional references for other samples and recommendations for further reading on a specific technique.

A. Ultraviolet Spectroscopy

The most basic method for the determination of the methylxanthines is ultraviolet (UV) spectroscopy. In fact, many of the HPLC detectors that will be mentioned use spectroscopic methods of detection. The sample must be totally dissolved and particle-free prior to final analysis. Samples containing more than one component can necessitate the use of extensive clean-up procedures, a judicious choice of wavelength, the use of derivative spectroscopy, or some other mathematical manipulation to arrive at a final analytical measurement. A recent book by Wilson has a chapter on the analysis of foods using UV spectroscopy and can be used as a suitable reference for those interested in learning more about this topic.[1]

B. Thin-Layer Chromatography

Thin-layer chromatography (TLC)[2] has become a valuable tool for the qualitative and semi-quantitative analysis of various organic and inorganic compounds. It has found large use in many laboratories and in a wide number of industries, although it does not seem to possess the accuracy, precision, and reliability of modern gas chromatography (GC) or high-performance liquid chromatography (HPLC). The growth of high-performance TLC (HPTLC) in the past few years has seen improved resolution and speed. Quantitation is accomplished through instrumental means. However, the cost of instrumental determination can approach that of GC or HPLC. Another TLC variant that has seen increased use and interest includes radial chromatography, in which the sample to be separated is spotted in the middle of a circular plate. It is then separated as a series of concentric rings. TLC serves a useful purpose since it is easy to use, can use relatively inexpensive equipment, and can be used with a large variety of matrices.

C. Gas Chromatography

Gas chromatography (GC) is an extremely popular analytical tool due to its speed, versatility, precision, and reliability. It has the ability to separate complex mixtures through the use of a large number of detectors that can be coupled to a unit. In addition to the classical electron-capture detector, flame-ionization detector, or thermal-conduction detector, many GCs are now routinely coupled to a mass spectrometer (MS). The costs of MS interfaces for GC have dropped substantially and they have become extremely easy to use so their use is becoming almost routine in many laboratories. Additionally, there are more specialized detectors available for use with GC such as the Hall electrolytic conductivity detector or the photoionization detector. GC can be used to analyze volatile and semi-volatile organic and organometallic compounds; it is possible to convert nonvolatile compounds into volatile derivatives and use temperature programming of the system. If one does not have access to an MS detector, then derivatives can be formed. General ones for the analysis of methylxanthines are BSTFA (N,O-bis-trimethylsilyltrifluoroacetamide), TMSDEA (trimethylsilyidiethylamine), and triphenylmethyl ammonium hydroxide which are used as derivatizing agents. BSTFA is an extremely powerful trimethylsilylating reagent since it is a highly volatile compound and produces a volatile product. TMSDEA is a basic trimethylsilylating agent used for the derivatization of low molecular weight acids and amino acids;[3, 4] it can trimethylsilylate four functional groups: amino, carboxyl, hydroxyl, and thiol. The reaction by-product, diethylamine, is extremely volatile and can be removed easily. It is not within the scope of this document to describe the uses of GC in the analytical laboratory in great detail but there are a number of excellent references available on the topic.

D. High-Performance Liquid Chromatography

High-performance liquid chromatography (HPLC) is probably one of the most important instrumental methods in analytical chemistry and continues to grow at a rapid rate. HPLC can be used to analyze volatile and nonvolatile organic compounds as well as inorganic compounds. It is an extremely versatile technique that is rapid, accurate, and precise. In addition, there are a large number of detectors that can be used in analysis. In the analysis of methylxanthines, the UV detector has seen the widest usage but newer variants of this detector such as the photodiode array (PDA) detector are seeing increasing usage. The PDA allows one to develop a three-dimensional profile of the data with data being displayed on time, wavelength, and absorbance axes. Once these data are available, then absorbance spectra can be obtained for the compounds of interest and these can then be mathematically manipulated much as one uses standard UV data. Electrochemical detectors and mass spectrometers have been used for this determination. As in the case of the GC, MS detectors for HPLC have become less difficult to use and less expensive. There are four interface types available: thermospray (TSP), particle beam, electrospray (ESI), and atmospheric pressure chemical ionization (APCI) . Each has its own advantages and will not be discussed in great detail. Particular applications of this type of detector are described in the appropriate section of this chapter. New developments include microbore column technology and capillary column technology. This development allows for increased sensitivity with decreased solvent consumption of 90 to 95% but can make instrument modifications necessary since standard HPLC pumping systems and detectors are not suitable for these low flow rates and attendant problems. The standard 4-mm ID HPLC is being replaced by 2- and 3-mm ID columns since they can be used with standard HPLC equipment with no loss of performance while cutting solvent consumption by 60 to 75%.

E. Capillary Electrophoresis

Capillary electrophoresis (CE) was introduced to the analytical community in the mid-1980s and at that time only a few laboratory manufactured units were available but as the technique became better accepted, many commercial vendors developed instruments to serve this growing market. CE has become an orthogonal technique to HPLC and offers some distinct advantages for the analyst including superior resolution, reduced solvent consumption, and the ability to use extremely small sample volumes compared to HPLC. For example, a day's operation using a capillary electrophoresis unit may generate 10 ml of solvent which is primarily comprised of buffer. The standard detector for CE is UV and ranges from fixed wavelength to PDA, depending on the sophistication of the instrumentation. There are other detectors used in CE and recently an MS interface has been introduced that offers some interesting possibilities for methylxanthine analysis. As CE evolves, one expects the database on methylxanthine analysis to grow.

II. HISTORICAL METHODS FOR THE DETERMINATION OF METHYLXANTHINES

There are numerous methods in the literature for the determination of caffeine, theobromine, and theophylline in food matrices, including coffee, tea, and cocoa. Until recently, methods have emphasized the determination of the major methylxanthines in a commodity, for example, caffeine in coffee or theobromine in cocoa. Present methods range from being specific for one of the compounds in a single matrix to being an all-encompassing assay of major and minor methylxanthines in food products.

Historically, the determination of methylxanthines was usually accomplished by spectrophotometric, gravimetric, Kjeldahl, or titrimetric methods. In many early methods, both caffeine and theobromine were extracted either into hot aqueous or hot alkaline solution and then transferred to an organic solvent such as chloroform. It was necessary to do a preliminary separation of this extract since, in addition to the extraction of the methylxanthines, amino acids, tannins, and carbohydrates were also extracted, which interfered with the final measurement. In the case of cocoa, it was usually necessary to pre-extract the commodity with a solvent such as hexane or petroleum ether to eliminate interferences due to fat. The preliminary separation might also have involved the precipitation of the impurities with compounds such as magnesium oxide (MgO). In an AOAC collaborative study[5,6] on the determination of caffeine in nonalcoholic beverages, a column chromatographic procedure was used to isolate the caffeine. It involved the use of two Celite 545 columns mounted in series, with a chloroform elution solvent. Caffeine was then measured at 276 nm against the chloroform blank. A 1948 paper by Moores and Campbell[7] on the determination of theobromine and caffeine in cocoa materials proposed an extraction with hot water in the presence of MgO. The extract was clarified with zinc acetate-potassium ferrocyanide reagents with the theobromine absorbed onto a column of Fuller's earth and selectively eluted with sodium hydroxide. Theobromine was then determined by a titrimetric method. The zinc acetate-potassium ferrocyanide solution was made alkaline and the caffeine was extracted with chloroform and measured by a Kjeldahl nitrogen determination.

Similar methods with modifications such as the one by Schutz et al.[8] have been in use for over 20 years. In 1968, Ferren and Shane[9] published a paper on the differential spectrometric determination of caffeine in soluble coffee and drug combinations. It had the advantage of eliminating a preliminary separation that was required by the earlier method. While the method was successful for coffee, it was not as successful in the determination of caffeine in acetaminophen/phenacetin/caffeine tablets. They proposed that phenacetin was a limiting factor. The official AOAC methods for these methylxanthines in coffee and tea still involve similar methods.[10]

Other methods have involved compleximetric titration, nephelometry, potentiometric titration, and gravimetric methods. In 1981, a paper by Mayanna and Jayaram[11] outlined the determination of caffeine in a wide variety of products including pharmaceuticals and food products using sodium N-chloro-p-toluene-sulphonamide (chloramine-T) in a titrimetric procedure.

III. CURRENT ANALYTICAL METHODS FOR THE DETERMINATION OF METHYLXANTHINES IN FOODS

A. Ultraviolet Spectroscopy

In the determination of methylxanthines by UV spectroscopy in foods, it is necessary to separate out the large number of substances that potentially interfere. Chromatographic techniques are the most conveniently used for the final separation of methylxanthines, so that they can be determined by UV, without interference. Cepeda[12] described a method for the determination of caffeine in coffee which is based on grinding the sample, preparation of an infusion under specified conditions, clarification of the infusion with light MgO, filtration, acidification of the filtrate to pH 4, clean-up on a C-18 Sep Pak C18, and elution with ethanol with determination of caffeine by spectrometry at 272 nm. Tests showed this method to be rapid, simple and reliable. Recovery is approximately 100%; coefficient of variation is less than 0.5%. The Morton & Stubb method and the second derivative method were used to overcome background interference. Data are given for caffeine concentration in five samples each of green coffee and natural roasted coffee, determined by this method and the AOAC Micro Bailey-Andrew method; results by the two methods did not differ significantly.

Li[13] developed a method for the individual determination of caffeine and theobromine in cocoa beans. Cocoa bean samples are ground as finely as possible (less than 0.5-mm diameter particles), the powder is boiled in water for 5 min, basic lead acetate solution is added as a clarifying agent, the solution is filtered to remove the precipitate and sodium hydrogencarbonate is added to remove unreacted lead ions. Caffeine is extracted from the resultant clear solution (pH regulated at 12.5 to 12.7 with NaOH) using chloroform, with theobromine remaining in the aqueous solution. Caffeine is determined by UV spectrophotometry at 275.9 nm and theobromine in the aqueous solution is measured at 272.7 nm. Average contents of theobromine, caffeine, and total alkaloids found in five samples (1 g) of cocoa powder were 14.439, 2.316, and 16.76 mg, respectively. Relative standard deviations were 0.57 to 0.69%. Recoveries of the alkaloids from mixtures of pure theobromine and caffeine were 98.8 to 102.2%.

A method for spectrophotometric measurement of caffeine, furfural, and tannins in "Licor cafe" (coffee liqueur) is described by Lage.[14] The method involves separation of furfural by steam distillation and selective extraction of caffeine from the residue by chloroform in an alkaline medium. This step is followed by UV spectrophotometric or colorimetric detention of furfural. Caffeine and tannic acid are determined by UV spectrophotometry. Tables are provided of the sensitivity of the furfural colorimetric reaction and percent recovery of furfural, tannic acid, and caffeine by spectrophotometry. In six coffee samples, caffeine concentration ranged from non-detectable to 980 mg/l, tannic acid ranged from 22.1 to 902 mg/l, and furfural ranged from 4.32 to 46.5 mg/l.[20] Trigonelline and caffeine are separated fully by a Sephadex G 15 column (1.65×40 cm). Polyamide adsorbs almost all polyphenolics which influence UV absorption spectrophotometry. Chromatography is carried out with distilled water on a single column packed with 3.2 g of polyamide placed on Sephadex G 15. The eluate is monitored at 270 and 300 nm. Quantification is achieved from the difference between the absorbances of the two peaks corresponding to trigonelline and caffeine on the elution chromatogram.

A simple paper chromatographic method for qualitative and quantitative analysis of alkaloids in cocoa is reported in a paper by Sjoeberg.[15] It includes paper chromatographic extraction in which a sample applied directly to the strip baseline was moistened with dilute NH3 solution (12.5%) for ascending chromatography, fats were first removed by chromatographing the paper with light petroleum for about 1.5 h, the paper was then chromatographed with n-butanol saturated with NH3 for 1.5-2 h, repeated after drying, and the dried strip observed under UV light (254 nm) to locate the alkaloids. The marked bands were cut out, eluted in diluted NH3 solution (1%) and alkaloids determined from their UV absorption spectra; absorption maximum of theobromine and caffeine were at 274 and 275 nm, respectively. Results of analysis of cocoa powders compared well with those obtained using HPLC. Analysis of other cocoa products, e.g., cocoa powders with milk and sugar added or chocolate products, suggested that the method should be applicable to cocoa-containing foods in general. It also stated that caffeine could be determined in foods such as coffee, tea, and cola drinks, requiring only a single short chromatographic run for rapid separation of caffeine alone.

The amount of coffee in beverages was determined by a method based on the relationship between the concentration of coffee in the beverage and optical density of a solution of the beverage at 270 to 300 nm.[16] Caffeine, chlorogenic acid, and beverage from natural ground coffee showed intensive absorption in the UV region between 270 and 290 nm; maximum absorption of caffeine was at 273 nm, and maximum absorption of coffee beverage was at 280 nm. Since the content of caffeine in coffee varies largely according to variety, and the chlorogenic acid content is dependent on the method of roasting, a standard sample from a known amount of a given coffee must be prepared as a reference standard. When analyzing beverages containing milks, the proteins must be removed by precipitation with trichloroacetic acid, and the fats by means of extraction with benzene before analysis.

B. Thin-Layer Chromatography

TLC offers an ability to analyze a large number of samples with reasonably good separation of the methylxanthines at a relatively low cost. TLC is now applied to a variety of food systems. Table 1 outlines a group of typical systems for the separation of methylxanthines.[17] Table 2 outlines possible spray reagents for the detection of the various methylxanthines.[17] For example, Senanayake and Wijesekera[18] outlined a TLC method for estimating caffeine, theobromine, and theophylline using silica gel plates and a solvent for the sample containing n-butanol:acetic acid (3:1); the eluting solvent was chloroform:carbon tetrachloride:methanol (8:5:1). The method was relatively simple, accurate, and convenient. The final measurement was accomplished by the measurement of the spot area, which somewhat limited the range of this method.

Jalal and Collin[19] used paper chromatography and TLC to determine caffeine in both coffee and tea, and theobromine in tea. Their TLC method used cellulose plates that were developed with butanol:hydrochloric acid:water (I 00: 1 1:28) for 4 h. The spots were eluted from the plates with ammonium hydroxide and measured spectrophotometrically against a blank at 272 nm for caffeine and 274 nm for theobromine.

Subsequent to removal of fats by extraction with petroleum ether, and processing with ammonia, alkaloids of maté, cola, and cocoa were isolated by extraction with CHCl3, and separated by thin layer chromatography. On UV irradiation, the alkaloids showed dark spots on a light fluorescent

TABLE 1.

Typical Thin-Layer Chromatography (TLC) Systems for Theobromine and Caffeine Determinations

Support	Eluting solvents
Silica gel G buffered pH 1.8	Chloroform:ethanol (9:1)
	Acetone:chloroform:n-butanol:ammonium hydroxide (3:3:4:1)
	Benzene:acetone (3:7)
Silica gel GF254	Chloroform:ethanol:formic acid (88:10:2)

Note: Benzene and chloroform are suspected carcinogens. Perhaps they could be replaced by toluene and methylene chloride, respectively, with some modification of the proportions used.

From Anon, *Dyeing Reagents for Thin Layer and Paper Chromatography*, E. Merck, Rahway, NJ, 1975. With permission.

TABLE 2

Visualizing Reagents for TLC

Component	Visualizing agent
Caffeine	Chloraminc-T
Xanthine derivatives	Iron (111) chloride followed by iodine
Purines	Silver nitrate followed by sodium dichromate
Purines, pyrimidines	Fluorescein
Purines	Silver nitrate followed by bromophenol blue

From Anon, *Dyeing Reagents for Thin Layer and Paper Chromatography*, E. Merck, Rahway, NJ, 1975. With permission.

background. Maté, cola, and cocoa contained respectively 71 to 74, 48 to 52, and 1000 to 2500 mg theobromine/100 g and 1 to 1.1, 5.1 to 5.3, and 0.20 to 0.22 mg theophylline/100 g. Recovery rates of added theobromine and theophylline ranged from 94 to 102%.[20]

Caffeine was extracted from ficw varieties of roasted coffee beans and was determined in parallel by (1) measurement of spot area after thin layer chromatography on silica gel GF plates (development with chloroform/cyclohexane/glacial acetic acid, 8:2:1, visualization in UV light), and (2) Kjeldahl N determination. Caffeine contents by (1) and (2), respectively, in the five varieties analyzed were (percent in DM): Santos lave 0, 1.10, and 1.12; Java Robusta 3, 1.19, and 1.22; Camerun Robusta 2, 1.16, and 1.19; Mocca 2, 1.21, and 1.26; Guatemala 0, 1.18, and 1.20. (1) is considered slightly less accurate than (2) but rather easier and more rapid.[21]

C. Gas Chromatography

GC has seen wide use in food analysis but has not seen a large following in the determination of the nonvolatile alkaloids in foods when compared to HPLC. The 13th edition of the *AOAC Methods of Analysis*[22] lists a GC method for the determination of caffeine in coffee or tea using a thermionic KCI detector with a glass column 6 ft × 4 mm i.d. packed with 10% DC-200 on 80 to 100-mesh Gas Chrom Q.

A GC method for determination of caffeine in beverages using a non-polar DB-1 column (5 m × 0.53 mm) with splitless direct injection and FID is described.[23] Direct quantitative analysis of caffeine in beverages is carried out without any sample pretreatment and lauryl alcohol is used as an internal standard. The detection limit was 4 to 8 p.p.m. Recovery studies were performed using tea, coffee, and cola beverage, each fortified with caffeine at 100, 50, and 25 mug; recoveries were 94.0 to 100.6% with coeff. of variation less than 6.5%. Using a chloroform extraction method for comparison, recoveries were 84.5 to 87.6% with coefficient of variation less than 6.4%. Results indicate that the direct injection method gave better results than the chloroform extraction method and it was concluded that the direct injection method was suitable for quantitation of caffeine in beverages. Twenty-four samples of tea, coffee, and cola beverage were analyzed by the direct injection method. Caffeine contents were: 83 to 128 p.p.m. for green tea; 40 to 70 p.p.m. for oolong tea; 36 to 51 p.p.m. for black tea; 321 to 493 p.p.m. for coffee; and 28 to 92 p.p.m. for cola beverages.

Determination of caffeine in soft drinks was undertaken using the aerosol alkali flame ionization detector.[24] Soft drinks studied were Coke, Diet Coke, Pepsi, Diet Pepsi, Dr. Pepper, and Mountain Dew. A sample clean-up and concentration procedure is employed followed by GC separation with alkali flame ionization detection. Results showed that Coke, Diet Coke, Pepsi, Diet Pepsi, Dr. Pepper, and Mountain Dew contained 41 ± 2, 52 ± 2, 43 ± 4, 35 ± 9, 46 ± 6, and 60 ± 15 mg caffeine per 355-ml serving. These values compared favorably with levels reported in the literature.

Solid extracts of (1) alfalfa and (2) red clover (used in food flavorings) were examined by GC/MS. 389 of 450 detected components were identified in (1), vs. 210 of 309 components detected in (2). In both extracts, predominant compounds identified were: esters (1) 105, (2) 55; acids (1) 42, (2) 31; alcohols (1) 34, (2) 31; and hydrocarbons (1) 28, (2) 14. Many other compounds were also found, including cannabinol, caffeine, scopolamine, isocoumarin, phenylpentadienal, phenylhexadiene, and nepetalactone.[25]

Capillary GC was used to obtain high resolution profiles of 27 organic acids, caffeine, and sucrose in dimethylsulphoxide extracts of roast and ground coffees in a 60-min analysis.[26] A shortened procedure is also reported for quantitative detection of 5-caffeoylquinic (5-CQA) and quinic (QA) acids and sucrose; ng detection limits were achieved. Major commercial brands of caffeinated and decaffeinated coffee produced under different roasting conditions could be distinguished based on their 5-CQA and sucrose contents and the QA:5-CQA ratio.

Theobromine was determined by GC in various foods (bitter chocolate, milk chocolate, chocolate cake, cocoa powder, chocolate milk), and results are given in graphs and tables.[27] Homogenized samples were boiled in alkaline aqueous media, then fat was extracted with n-hexane. The aqueous layer was acidified with diluted HCl and NaCl was added. Theobromine was extracted from this treated aqueous solution with dichloromethane and the extract was evaporated to dryness. The residue was redissolved in dichloromethane containing an internal standard. GC analysis was performed on a column packed with 1% cyclohexane dimethanol succinate on Gaschrom Q, with FID. Average recoveries were 99 to 101%, coefficient of variation was less than 3% and the limit of detection for theobromine in foods was about 0.005%.

D. High-Performance Liquid Chromatography

HPLC allows a quantitative determination with relatively simple extractions. In many cases, extraction only involves a heating of the commodity with water, followed by filtration and injection onto an HPLC column. In the determination of caffeine, theobromine, and theophylline in cocoa, coffee, or tea, as well as in other foods, there is scarcely a month that passes without a new paper on this assay. Kreiser and Martin provide typical conditions for analysis.[28] In their studies, samples were extracted in boiling water and filtered prior to injection onto the HPLC column. The HPLC conditions used a Bondapak reversed phase column and a mobile phase of water:methanol:acetic acid (74:25: 1) with detection at 280 nm. This method is accurate, precise, and conserves time. It has also been adopted by the AOAC as an official method for the determination of theobromine and caffeine in cocoa beans and chocolate products.[29]

Zoumas et al.[30] presented work on the use of this method in the determination of caffeine and theobromine in various chocolate-containing products, while Blauch and Tarka[31] reported the use of a similar method for the determination of caffeine and theobromine in various beverages containing these methylxanthines.

A simple method for simultaneous determination of five types of catechins, i.e., epigallocatechin (EGC), epigallocatechin gallate (EGCg), epicatechin (EC), epicatechin gallate (ECg), and catechin (C), and three types of methylxanthines, i.e., theobromine (TB), theophylline (TP), and caffeine (CA), in tea and tea-containing foods by semi-micro HPLC was developed.[32] Samples were extracted with 40% aqueous ethanol and cleaned up using a Sep pak C18 cartridge. Extracts were chromatographed on a semi-micro size Inertsil ODS-2 column, with a mobile phase of methanol:water:0.2M phosphate buffer pH 3.0 (12:33:5) and UV detection at 207 nm. Recoveries from common grade green tea (sencha) and foods containing finely ground green tea (maccha ice cream, maccha senbei [Japanese cracker], maccha jelly) and candy containing oolong tea extract were (%): EGC, 90.9 to 120.4; EGCg, 91.8 to 117.3; EC, 91.2 to 96.7; ECg, 83.2 to 104.3; C, 90.2 to 101.6; TB, 53.0 to 106.4; TP, 74.6 to 101.6; and CA, 88.4 to 98.8. Detection limits were 0.1 mug/g for each compound

A French Standard, which corresponds to ISO 10095 issued in 1992, specifies a method for determination of caffeine in green or roasted coffee or in coffee extracts (decaffeinated or not).[33] Caffeine is extracted with water at 90°C in the presence of MgO. The extract is filtered, then cleaned-up on a mini-column packed with a silica phenyl group derivative, and analyzed by HPLC on a C18 column with a methanol/water (30:70) mobile phase and a UV detector operating at 254 to 280 nm.

A method for determining the caffeine content of regular and decaffinated green and roasted coffee beans and of regular and decaffeinated coffee extract powders, using HPLC, is specified in a British Standard Instruction.[34] Caffeine is extracted from the sample with water at 90°C in the presence of magnesium oxide. The mixture is filtered and an aliquot purified on a silica microcolumn modified with phenyl groups. The caffeine content is then determined by HPLC with UV detection.[35]

A method for determining aspartame, acesulfam-K, saccharin, caffeine, sorbic acid, and benzoic acid in foods is described[36] based on clarification of the sample with Carrez reagents, and analysis by HPLC on a Superspher RP-select B 4 mum column with 0.02M phosphate buffer/acetonitrile (90:10) mobile phase and UV detection. A theophylline internal standard is used. Methods of sample preparation for various product types (soft drinks, sweetener preparations, juices, milk shakes, quarg products, yoghurt products, and delicatessen salads) are described. Mean recoveries were: aspartame 96%; acesulfam-K 103.4%; saccharin 106.1%; and caffeine 97.1% (no recovery data given for benzoic or sorbic acid). Detection limits for standard solutions were (mg/l): aspartame 0.2; benzoic acid 0.02; sorbic acid 0.09; and acesulfam-K, saccharin, theophylline, and caffeine 0.004. Detection limits in foods are higher, generally in the range 0.5 to 1 mg/kg.

HPLC was applied to analysis of caffeine, trigonelline, nicotinic acid, and sucrose in Arabica and Robusta coffees.[37] Green and roasted coffee samples were used in this study, and degradation of sucrose and trigonelline, with formation of nicotinic acid, was followed during roasting. Caffeine did not undergo significant degradation, with only 5.4% being lost under severe roasting. Sucrose was degraded rapidly during processing, light roasting producing a 97% loss and dark roasting degrading it completely. Loss of trigonelline was strongly dependent on degree of roasting, being higher in the Robusta coffee. Trigonelline degradation was associated with nicotinic acid formation both in the Arabica and Robusta coffees as a consequence of roasting. Trigonelline and sucrose were determined simultaneously by partition chromatography and detection with the mass detector. Detection of caffeine was carried out using reversed phase chromatography and nicotinic acid by ion-pair reversed phase chromatography. Detection in both cases was achieved using a UV detector at 272 or 254 nm, respectively. HPLC showed adequate precision and accuracy for routine analyses. In addition, the methods used were more rapid and simple than traditional procedures. HPLC appears to be a suitable technique for quality control in the coffee industry, and for fundamental investigation of the mechanisms involved in the roasting process.

This chapter describes use of solid-surface room temperature phosphorimetry (SSRTP) as a detection technique in the liquid chromatographic (LC) analysis of caffeine, theophylline, and theobromine. Measurements were made in a continuous mode, using a 2-nebulizer automatic system for SSRTP analysis (previously optimized for LC detection). Use of SSRTP and UV absorption detection was compared under identical experimental conditions.[38]

Application of HPLC-MS to the analysis of a black tea liquor was studied in a paper by Bailey;[39] a great deal of useful information could be obtained without sample pretreatment. A tea liquor was applied to a wide-pore HPLC column connected to a mass spectrometer by a VG Plasmaspray interface. Pseudo-molecular ions were obtained from the flavanols, flavanol gallates, chlorogenic acids, 4-coumarylquinic acids, and caffeine, but the flavanol glycosides were extensively fragmented by the interface. Fragments were obtained from unresolved polymer that supported its previous designation as a flavanol polymer.

HPLC with thermospray MS was reported by Hurst et al.[40] where residues from an archeological site were analyzed for caffeine and theobromine using reversed phase HPLC coupled to a thermospray MS interface. Samples were extracted in water and separated on a reversed phase column. The presence of theobromine in this sample was confirmed by monitoring the MH+ ion at 181 for theobromine.

E. Capillary Electrophoresis

As was indicated, there have not been a large number of publications on the CE analysis of methylxanthines in food systems. Analusis published a method using a 20-mm Borate buffer at pH 9.6 and UV detection at 254 nm and +22 kV applied voltage.[41] Samples were diluted and prepared for analysis by filtration and analyzed using free solution electrophoresis (FSE). Analysis time was less than 10 min and the results favorably compared literature and HPLC data. A ThermoSeparation Products Application Note described the analysis of caffeine and other components in a sample of diet cola. The method used a fused silica capillary with a buffer of 20 mM phosphate at pH 2 and an applied voltage of +30 kV. The detection system used was a scanning detector with wavelengths of 200 to 300 nm.[42]

F. Other Analytical Methods

The various methods that have been outlined in the previous sections are not exclusive and other analytical methods have been used for the determination of methylxanthines in food systems. One of the most widely used methods for food analysis is flow injection analysis (FIA). In a study by Numata,[43] a flow injection analysis method for the determination of hypoxanthine in meat was described.

IV. CURRENT METHODS FOR THE DETERMINATION OF METHYLXANTHINES IN THE BIOLOGICAL FLUIDS

Analytical studies in clinical chemistry relating to the determination of methylxanthines are concentrated in two areas. The first of these involves the analysis of various ethical pharmaceuticals. The second area involves the analysis of various body fluids for methylxanthines and their metabolites.

In the clinical area, the largest share of analytical methods development and publication has centered on the determination of theophylline in various body fluids, since theophylline is used as a bronchodilator in asthma. Monitoring serum theophylline levels is much more helpful than monitoring dosage levels.[44] Interest in the assay of other methylxanthines and their metabolites has been on the increase, as evidenced by the citations in the literature with a focus on the analysis of various xanthines and methylxanthines.

A. Ultraviolet Spectroscopy

Ultraviolet spectroscopy is used in many clinical laboratories due to its ease of operation and availability. A classical method for theophylline determination in plasma is the one of Schack and Waxler.[45] The original method had interferences from phenobarbitol and various xanthine derivatives such as theobromine.[46] The modification of the method by Jatlow[47] eliminated the interferences from barbituates but included the various xanthine interferences. In 1978, Bailey[48] published a study on "Drug Interferences in the Ultraviolet Spectrophotometric Analysis of Plasma Theophylline". In his study, he evaluated 45 common drugs as interferences in the UV assay and concluded that 18 of the drugs interfered with the basic method as well as Jatlow's modification. Fourteen drugs were found to give positive interferences, while four gave negative ones. He further stated that drug interferences do exist and that they are recognizable by nongaussian peaks, but the identity of the interfering compounds is hard to determine. A study by Gupta and Lundberg[49] used differential UV analysis but required a large sample volume (5 ml) and was relatively insensitive. It should be noted that a 3-ml sample can be required for UV methods but smaller volumes can be used with microsampling accessories available on some UV instrumentation.

B. Thin-Layer Chromatography

As was the case in food commodity-related systems, TLC is a powerful tool that is extremely useful for screening large numbers of samples. It is also useful for obtaining qualitative information about a substance or group of substances (see Tables 1 and 2). Recently, Salvadori and colleagues published a study in which TLC was used as a screening tool for the determination of caffeine, theobrmine, and theophylline in samples of horse urine after the horses had ingested guarana powder.[50]

C. Gas Chromatography

GC continues to have a great deal of use in clinical analysis. The literature contains a number of citations on the use of GC for the determination of theophylline in body fluids,[51–53] but now it is possible to selectively determine not only theophylline in the presence of barbiturates, but also caffeine, theobromine, and other xanthine derivatives. The GC methods in the literature are used as a final determination step after extraction with organic solvents. It is, however, necessary to form a derivative of the methylxanthine, to use a flame-ionization (FID) or electron capture detector, and to use an internal standard. Pranskevich et al.[54] used isothermal GC on a 3% SP2250-DB with an FID. This procedure involves the mixture of sample, internal standard, and chloroform in a culture tube. After centrifugation, the aqueous layer is discarded and the chloroform layer is dried under nitrogen. Five milliliters toluene are added in addition to ammonium hydroxide. The mixture is again centrifuged, the toluene layer is discarded, and the aqueous phase evaporated to dryness. Derivatization uses an 8:1 mixture of N-N′-dimethylacetamide and 2.4% tetramethylammonium hydroxide in methanol. The derivatizing agent, iodobutane, is added and then the solution is mixed. The method is specific for theophylline and presents excellent data.

As in the case in the analysis of food samples, the introduction of relatively inexpensive MS detectors for GC has had a substantial impact on the determination of methylxanthines by GC. For example, in 1990, Benchekroun published a paper in which a GC-MS method for the quantitation of tri-, di-, and monmethylxanthines and uric acid from hepatocyte incubation media was described.[55] The method described allows for the measurement of the concentration of 14 methylxanthines and methyluric acid metabolites of methylxanthines. In other studies, GC-MS has also been used. Two examples from the recent literature are studies by Simek and Lartigue-Mattei, respectively.[56,57] In the first case, GC-MS using an ion trap detector was used to provide confirmatory data to support a microbore HPLC technique. TMS derivatives of the compounds of interest were formed and separated on a 25 m DB-% column directly coupled to the ion trap detector. In the second example, allopurinol, oxypurinol, hypoxanthine, and xanthine were assayed simultaneously using GC-MS.

D. High-Performance Liquid Chromatography

HPLC has seen meteoric rise in its use as a tool in the area of methylxantbine and xanthine derivative analysis. In the determination of theophylline in plasma, the method outlined by Peng et al.[58] requires no extraction and only a dilution with acetonitrile prior to analysis. In the method of Sommadossi et al.,[59] samples are extracted with chloroform:hexane (7:3) prior to analysis. Another method by Soldin and Hill[60] extracts serum with a mixture of chloroform:isopropanol (95:5) prior to analysis. Similar methods or variations appear throughout the literature. In many of the studies, 8-chlorotheophylline is used as an internal standard.[61] Detection modes range from fixed-wavelength UV and variable UV to electrochemical. Separation modes range from normal phase and reverse phase to ion-pairing. There is also a large amount of literature on the HPLC separation of purines or xanthines, using a wide variety of supports, that have not yet been applied to either food systems or body fluids but obviously should work well. The literature is full of separations on xanthines and methylxanthines in various biological systems.

HPLC coupled to MS was used for the determination of dimethyl xanthine metabolites in plasma.[62] There have also been a number of methods published on the use of HPLC with a PDA detector. In 1996, Mei published a method for the determination of adenosine, inosine, hypoxanthine, xanthine, and uric acid in microdialysis samples using microbore column HPLC with a PDA detector.[63] In this method, samples were directly injected onto the HPLC without the need for any additional sample treatment.

Hieda et al. determined theophylline, theobromine, and caffeine in human plasma and urine by gradient capillary HPLC with frit fast atom bombardment (FAB) mass spectrometry with 7-ethyl theophylline as the internal standard.[64]

E. Capillary Electrophoresis

As CE evolves, there are a growing number of applications of this technology in the analysis of various biological fluids. Recently Hyotylainen et al.[65] published a method for the determination of morphine analogs, caffeine, and amphetamine in biological fluids by CE. Both capillary zone electrophoresis (CZE) and micellar electrokinetic capillary chromatography (MEKC) were evaluated with detection at 200 and 220 nm were investigated for analytes in human serum and urine. Glycine buffer containing sodium lauryl sulfate (pH 10.5) was used for the MEKC separations with a final analysis time of 18 min.

F. Other Analytical Techniques

The determination of theophylline in plasma can also be accomplished by various immunoassay techniques.[66, 67] Theophylline was also determined by a polarization fluoroimmunoassays but found to have a caffeine interference.[68]. In a more research oriented application, the interaction of caffeine with L-tryptophan was studied using !h NMR with the results indicating that caffeine interacted with tryptophan in a 1:1 molar ratio through parallel stacking.[69]

V. SUMMARY

The methylxanthines can be determined in foods and biological systems by the chromatographic methods of TLC, GC, HPLC, or CE. Ultraviolet spectroscopy following a separation procedure can also be used. More recently, immunoassay methods have been developed. There is no single best method; the analyst must balance the features of each assay with the final requirements for data precision and reproducibility.

REFERENCES

1. Wilson, R.H., Ed., *Spectroscopic Techniques for Food Analysis,* VCH, New York, 1994,

2. Stahl, E., Ed., *Thin Layer Chromatography,* Springer-Verlag, New York, 1970.
3. Knapp, D.R., *Handbook of Analytical Derivatization Reactions,* Wiley Interscience, New York, 1979.
4. Hawk, G.L. and Little, J.N., *Derivatization in Gas and Liquid Chromatography in Zymark Sample Preparation Program (SPF CT 1 103),* Zymark Corporation, Hopkinton, MA, 1982.
5. Johnson, A.J., Collaborative study of a method for the determination of caffeine in non-alcoholic beverages, *JAOAC,* 50,857,1967.
6. Levine, J., Determination of caffeine in coffee products, beverages and pharmaceuticals, *JAOAC,* 45,254,1962.
7. Moores, R.G. and Campbell, H.A., Determination of theobromine and caffeine in cocoa materials, *Anal. Chem.,* 20,40,1948.
8. Schutz, G.P., Prinsen, A.J., and Pater, A., The spectrophotometric determination of caffeine and theobromine in cocoa and cocoa products, *Rev. Int. Choc.,* 25,7,1970.
9. Ferren, W.P. and Shane, N.A., Differential spectrophotometric determination of caffeine in soluble coffee and drug combinations, *JAOAC,* 51,573,1968.
10. Horwitz, W., Ed., Coffee and tea, spectrophotometric and chromatographic methods, in *Official Methods of Analysis of AOAC,* 13th ed., AOAC, Washington, D.C, 1980, p 234.
11. Mayanna, S.M. and Jayaram, B., Determination of caffeine using N-chloro-p-toluene-sulfonamide, *Analyst,* 106,729,19811
12. Cepeda, A., Paseiro, P., Simal, J., and Rodriguez, J.L., Determination of caffeine by UV spectrometry in various types of coffee: green coffee and natural roasted coffee, *Anales de Bromatologia,* 42,241,1990.
13. Li, S., Berger, J., Hartland, S., UV spectrophotometric determination of theobromine and caffeine in cocoa beans, *Analytica Chimica Acta,* 232,409,1990.
14. Lage, M.A., Simal, J., Yanez, T., Analytical methods applied to coffee liqueur. III. Determination of furfural, caffeine and tannic substances, *Tecnicas de Laboratorio,* 12,204,1989
15. Sjoeberg, A.M. and Rajama, J., Simple method for the determination of alkaloids in cocoa using paper chromatography and UV spectrometry, *J. Chromatography,* 295,291,1984.
16. Maksimets, V.P., Kravchenko, E.F., Osinskaya, L.I., and Fetisova, M.M., Determination of the amount of coffee in beverages, *Izvestiya Vysshikh Uchebnykh Zavedenii, Pishchevaya Tekhnologiya,* No. 3,1121982.
17. Anon, *Dyeing Reagents for Thin Layer and Paper Chromatography,* E. Merck, Rahway, NJ, 1975.
18. Senanayake, U.M. and Wijesekera, R.O.B., A rapid micro method for the separation, identification and estimation of the purine bases, *J. Chrom.,* 32,75,1968.
19. Jalal, M.F.F. and Collin, A., Estimation of caffeine, theophylline and theobromine in plant material, *New Phytot.,* 76,277,1976.
20. Franzke, C.L., Grunert, K.S., and Griehl, H., Estimation and contents of theobromine and theophylline in mate, cola and cocoa. *Zeitschrift fuer Lebensmitteluntersuchung und Forschung,* 139,85,1969
21. Washuettl, J., Bancher, E., and Riederer, P., A new thin-layer chromatographic method for determination of caffeine in roasted coffee beans, *Zeitschrift fuer Lebensmitteluntersuchung und Forschung,* 143,253,1970.
22. Horwitz, W., Ed., Coffee and tea, GLC method, in *Official Methods of Analysis of AOAC,* 13th ed., AOAC, Washington, D.C., 1980, p 234.
23. Mei, L.W. and Min, H.L., Simple and rapid method for the determination of caffeine in beverages, *J. Chinese Agricultural Chem. Soc.,* 33,114,1995
24. Conte, E.D. and Barry, E.F., Gas chromatographic determination of caffeine in beverages by alkali aerosol flame ionization detection, *Microchem. J.,* 48,372,1993.

25. Volatile constituents in alfalfa and red clover extracts, in *Flavors and Fragrances: A World Perspective*, Lawrence, B. M. et al., Eds., Conference. Washington, D.C., 16-20 Nov. 1986, Elsevier Science Publishers, Amsterdam, The Netherlands, 1988.
26. Lage, M.A., Simal, J., and Yanez, T., Analytical methods applied to coffee liqueur. III. Determination of furfural, caffeine and tannic substances, *Tecnicas de Laboratorio*, 12,204,1989.
27. Ishida, H., Sekine, H., Kimura, S., and Sekiya, S., Gas chromatographic determination of theobromine in foods, J. Food Hygienic Soc. Jpn., 27(1),75,1986.
28. Kreiser, W.R. and Martin, R.A. Jr., High pressure liquid chromatographic determination of theobromine and caffeine in cocoa and chocolate products, *JAOAC*, 61,1424,1978.
29 Horwitz, W., Ed., Cocoa bean and its products, HPLC method, in *Official Methods of Analysis of AOAC*, 13th ed., AOAC, Washington, D.C., 1980, p 382.
30. Zoumas, B.L., Kreiser, W.R., and Martin, R.A. Jr., Theobromine and caffeine content of chocolate products, *J. Food. Sci.*, 45,314,1980.
31. Blauch, J. and Tarka, S.M. Jr., HPLC determination of caffeine and theobromine in coffee, tea and instant hot cocoa mixes, *J. Food. Sci.*, 48,745,1983.
32. Terada, H., Suzuki, A., Tanaka, H., and Yamamoto, K., Determination of catechins and methylxanthines in foods by semi-micro HPLC, J. Food Hygienic Soc. Jpn., 33(4),347,1992
33. Coffee. Determination of the caffeine content, HPLC method, Association Francaise de Normalisation French Standard, France, NF ISO 10095, 1992.
35. Methods of test for coffee and coffee products. Part 12. Coffee: determination of caffeine content (routine method by HPLC), British Standards Institution, United Kingdom, British-Standard, BS 5752:Part 12, 1992.
36. Hagenauer-Hener, U., Frank, C., Hener, U., Mosandl, A., Determination of aspartame, acesulfam-K, saccharin, caffeine, sorbic acid and benzoic acid in foods by HPLC. Bestimmung von Aspartam, Acesulfam-K, Saccharin, Coffein, Sorbinsaeure und Benzoesaeure in Lebensmitteln mittels HPLC Deutsche-Lebensmittel-Rundschau, 86(11),348-351,1990.
37. Trugo, L.C. and Macrae, R., Application of high performance liquid chromatography to the analysis of some non-volatile coffee components, *Archivos Latinoamericanos de Nutricion*, 39(1),96,1989.
38. Campiglia, A.D., Laserna, J.J., Berthod, A., and Winefordner, J.D., Solid-surface room-temperature phosphorimetric detection of caffeine, theophylline and theobromine in liquid chromatography, *Anal. Chim. Acta*, 244(2),215,1991.
39. Bailey, R.G., Nursten, H.E., and McDowell, I., J. Sci. Food Agriculture., 66(2),203-208,1994.
40. Hurst, W.J., Martin, R.A. Jr, Tarka, S.M. Jr. and Hall, G.D., Authentication of cocoa in maya vessels using high performance liquid chromatographic techniques, *J. Chromatography*, 466,279,1989.
41. Hurst, W.J. and Martin, R.A. Jr, The quantitative determination of caffeine in beverages using capillary electrophoresis analysis, 21,389-91,1993.
42. ThermoSeparation Products Application Note UN92-4 , ThermoSeparation Products; San Jose, CA, 1992
43. Numata, M., Funazaki, N., Ito, S., Asano, Y., and Yano, Y., Flow injection analysis for hypoxanthine in meat with dissolved oxygen detector and enzyme reactor, *Talanta*, 43,2053,1996.
44. Jacobs, M.H., Senior, R.M., and Kessler, W.R., Clincial experience with theophylline: Relationship between dosage, serum concentration and toxicity, *JAMA*, 235,1983,1976.

45. Schack, J.A. and Waxler, S.H., Ultraviolet spectrophotometric method for the determination of theophylline and theobromine in blood and tissues, *J. Pharmacol. Exp. Ther.*, 97,283,1949.
46. Matheson, L.E., Bighley, L., and Hendeles, L., Drug interferences with the Schack and Waxler plasma theophylline assay, Am. J. Hosp. Pharmacol., 34,496,1977.
47. Jatlow, P., Ultraviolet spectrophotometry of theophylline in plasma in the presence of barbiturates, *Clin. Chem.*, 21,1518,1975.
48. Bailey, D.N., Evaluation of drug interferences in the ultraviolet spectrophotometric analysis of plasma theophylline, *J. Anal. Toxicol.*, 2,94,1978.
49. Gupta, R.C. and Lundberg, G.D., Qualitative determination of theophylline in blood by differential spectrophotometry, *Anal Chem.*, 45,2402,1973.
50. Salvadori, M.C., Rieser, E.M., Ribeiro Neto, L.M., and Nascimmento, E.S., Determination of xanthines by high performance liquid chromatography and thin layer chromatography in horse urine after ingestion of Guarana powder, *Analyst*, 119,2701,1994
51. Johnson, G.F., Dechtiaruk, W.A., and Solomon, H.M., Gas chromatographic determination of theophylline in human serum and saliva, *Clin. Chem.*, 21,144,1975.
52. Chrzanowski, F.A., Niebergall, P.J., and Nikelly, J.G., Gas chromatographic analysis of theophylline in human serum, *Biochem. Med.*, 11,26,1974.
53 Greeley, D.H., New approach to derivatization and gas chromatographic analysis of barbiturates, *Clin. Chem.*, 20,192,1974.
54. Pranskevich, C.A., Swihart, J.I., and Thoma, J.J., Serum theophylline determination.by isothermal gas-liquid chromatography on 3% SP2250-DB, *J. Anal. Toxicol.*, 2,3,1978.
55. Benchekroun, Y., Desage, M., Ribon, B., and Brazier, J.L., Gas chromatographic-mass spectrometric quantition of tri-, di- and monomethylxanthines and uric acid from hepatocyte incubation media, *J. Chromatogr.*, 532,261,1990.
56. Simek, P., Jegorov, A., and Dusbabek, F., Determination of purine bases and nucleosides by conventional and microbore high performance chromatography and gas chromatography with an ion trap detector, *J. Chromatogr.*, 679,1951,1994.
57. Lartigue-Mattei, C., Chabard, J.L., Ristori, J.M., Bussiere, J.L., Bargnoux, H., Petit, J., and Berger, J.A., Kinetics of allopurinol and it's metabolite oxypurinol after oral administration of allopurinol alone or associated with benzbromarone in man. Simultaneous assay of hypoxanthine and xanthine by gas chromatography-mass spectrometry, *Fund. Clin. Pharm.*, 5,621,1991.
58. Peng, G.W., Gadalia, M.A.F., and Chiou, W.L., High performance liquid chromatographic determination of theophylline in plasma, *Clin. Chem.*, 24,357,1978.
59. Sommadossi, J.P., Aubert, C., Cano, J.P., Durand, A., and Viala, A., Determination of theophylline in plasma by high performance liquid chromatography, *J Liquid Chromatogr.*, 4,97,1981.
60. Soldin, S.J. and Hill, J.G., A rapid micro method for measuring theophylline in serum by reversed phase high performance liquid chromatography, *Clin. Biochem.*, 10,74,1977.
61. Hill, R.E., Retention behavior of a bonded reversed phase in high performance liquid chromatographic assay of serum theophylline, *J. Chromatogr.*, 135,419,1977.
62. Midha, K.K., Sved, S., Hossie, R.D., and McGilveray, I.J., High performance liquid chromatographic and mass spectrometric identification of dimethylxanthine metabolites of caffeine in human plasma, *Biomed. Mass. Spectrom.*, 4,172,1977.
63. Mei, D.A., Gross, G.J., and Nithipatikom, K., Simultaneous determination of adenosine, inosine, hypoxanthine, xanthine and uric acid in microdialysis samples using microbore column liquid chromatography with diode array detection, *Analyt. Biochem.*, 238,34,1996.

64. Hieda, Y., Kashimura, S., Hara, K., and Kageura, M., Highly sensitive and rapid determination of theophylline, theobromine and caffeine in human plasma and urine by high performance liquid chromatography frit fast atom bombardment spectrometry, *J. Chromatogr.*, 667,241,1995
65. Hyotylainen, T., Siren, H., and Riekkola, M.L., Determination of morphine analogues, caffeine and amphetamine in biological fluids by capillary electrophoresis with the marker technique, *J, Chromatogr.*, 735,439,1996
66. Koup, J.R. and Brodsky, B., Comparison of homogeneous enzyme immunoassay and high pressure liquid chromatography for the determination of theophylline concentration in serum, *Am. Rev. Respir. Dis.*, 117,1135,1978.
67. Oellerich, M., Klupmann, W.R., Beneking, M., Sybrecht, G.W., Staib, A.H., and Schuster, R., Determination of theophylline in serum by nonisotopic immunoassays (EMIT, SLFIA, NIIA) and HPLC-CA comparative study, *Fresenius Z. Anal. Chem.*, 311,355,1982.
68. Tibi, L. and Burnett, D., Interference by caffeine in polarization immunoassays for theophylline, *Ann. Clin. Biochem.*, 291 1994.
69. Nishio, J., Yonetani, I., Iwamoto, E., Tokura, S.,Tagahara, K., and Sugiura, M., Interaction of caffeine with l-tryptophan: study of 1H nuclear magnetic resonance spectroscopy, *J. Pharm. Sci.*, 79,14,1990.

Chapter 3

Tea: The Plant and Its Manufacture; Chemistry and Consumption of the Beverage

Douglas A. Balentine, Matthew E. Harbowy, and Harold N. Graham

CONTENTS

0-8493-2647-8/98/$0.00+$.50

I. INTRODUCTION

Tea is second only to water in worldwide consumption. Annual production of about 1.8 million T of dry leaf provides world per capita consumption of 40 L of beverage (Table 1).[1] The scientific interest in tea is due in part to the unusual chemical composition of its leaf and the complex series of reactions that occur when these components are converted to those found in commercial dry tea. Many of the reaction products interact with caffeine, modifying flavor and contributing to the technical problems of tea processing, as will be shown later.

"Tea", in this work, refers only to the plant *Camellia sinensis*, its leaves, and the extracts and infusions thereof. Leaf, bark, stem, root, or flower extracts of scores of other plants are also sold as "teas", creating confusion. An important reason for the consumption of these other "teas", a.k.a. "herbal teas" or "tisanes", is their lack of methylxanthines, unlike beverages prepared from *Camellia sinensis* which are naturally rich in these substances, especially caffeine.

TABLE 1

Consumption Data for Tea, 1993–1995

	kg/pop	Cups/d
U.S.	0.34	0.43
Canada	0.47	0.59
Belgium & Lux.	0.12	0.15
Czechoslovakia	0.15	0.19
Denmark	0.38	0.48
France	0.21	0.26
Germany Fed. Rep.	0.21	0.26
Ireland	3.16	3.95
Italy	0.09	0.11
Netherlands	0.54	0.68
Poland	0.87	1.09
Sweden	0.33	0.41
Switzerland	0.27	0.34
U.K.	2.53	3.17
USSR/CIS	0.63	0.79
Chile	0.97	1.21
Afghanistan	1.67	2.09
Hong Kong	1.48	1.85
India	0.63	0.79
Iran	1.32	1.65
Japan	1.03	1.29
Kuwait	2.52	3.15
Pakistan	0.92	1.15
Saudi Arabia	0.82	1.03
Sri Lanka	1.29	1.61
Syria	1.55	1.94
Thailand	0.01	0.01
Algeria	0.23	0.29
Egypt	1.04	1.30
Kenya	0.46	0.58
Morocco	1.24	1.55
S. Africa[a]	0.49	0.61
Sudan	0.35	0.44
Tanzania	0.12	0.15
Australia	0.95	1.19

[a] Including Botswana, Lesotho, Namibia, and Swaziland.

Note: Formula for cups per day: (kg/year × 1000)/352 = grams per day/2.27 = cups per day. 2.27 is the assumption of tea leaves used per cup. Kilograms per population is the average consumption per head of total population. All data is based on imported and (where applicable) locally produced tea.

II. OCCURRENCE AND HISTORY

Camellia sinensis is native to the southern portion of the People's Republic of China and parts of India, Burma, Thailand, Laos, and Vietnam.[2] The earliest authenticated description of tea and its preparation as a brewed beverage is that by the Chinese scholar Kuo P'o in the year 350 A.D.[3] An earlier account attributed to the legendary Emperor Shen Nong in 2737 B.C. is taken from the Shen Nong Ben Cao Jing compiled ca. 22-250 A.D. The taste and stimulative properties of brewed tea led to its use in treating tumors, abscesses, bladder ailments, lethargy, and several other conditions.[4]

Kuo P'o refers to the cultivation of the plant, indicating early domestication. Tea was first described as an article of trade in the fifth century and soon thereafter as a nonmedical beverage.

A definitive, three-volume work summarizing the horticulture and manufacture of tea was written by Lu Yu at the request of tea merchants in 780 A.D in China. The "Ch'a Ching", or "Tea Book", codified all tea-related materials and practices, including descriptions of implements used in its preparation and serving.

The spread of tea to Japan probably occurred during the introduction of Buddhism in the seventh century. Tea cultivation began in the eighth century, but tea consumption did not become a permanent and widespread fixture of Japanese life until the thirteenth century.[5]

Tea was introduced into Europe by Dutch traders who brought it to the Netherlands from China and Japan in 1610. Its popularity grew slowly amid vigorous claims of its beneficial effects and counterclaims concerning its dangers. In 1657, tea was sold for the first time in England where it gradually achieved popularity in the existing coffee houses and eventually became the national drink.[6] Tea consumption spread throughout Europe in the seventeenth century.

Tea was introduced into America by the Dutch at New Amsterdam ca. 1650 and was later sold in the Colonies by the British. In Boston, tea came to symbolize British rule, which may account for the development of the United States as a nation of coffee drinkers.[6]

Lucrative, expanding tea trade with China became a world monopoly of the East India Company. When the treaty between Britain and China expired in 1833, location of alternate tea sources became desirable. All attempts to cultivate the relatively superior Chinese varieties in India failed. However, local cultivation of the Assam variety indigenous to northeast India was promising, and eventually allowed tea production in India to flourish. India became one of the foremost tea growing areas of the world,[7] only recently being surpassed in export by Kenya.

Sri Lanka (Ceylon) was an important coffee-growing country until a leaf disease decimated crop production. In the 1880s, tea cultivation was substituted for that of coffee, and Sri Lanka has been another of the world's major tea producers ever since.[7]

Production of tea in the Georgian region of the USSR began on a large scale in 1892 in the warmer areas near the Black and Caspian Seas.[8] The dissolution of the former Soviet Union and the Chernobyl nuclear accident have contributed significantly to the decline of tea production in the region. Regional production is one tenth that in the early 1980s.

Tea was introduced by the Dutch into Indonesia with seed that originated in China and Japan. As was characteristic of tropical areas, the industry developed only after replacement of planting stock with Assam varieties in 1878.[9]

More recently, the cultivation of tea has spread to other Asian countries such as Turkey, Iran, Taiwan, Bangladesh, Malaysia, and Vietnam.

The most significant spread of tea cultivation to new areas has been the establishment of large acreage in Africa. The first successful plantings took place in Malawi around 1900, but Kenya has become the prime producer of the continent though tea was not introduced until 1925. Tea is now cultivated in Tanzania, South Africa, and other areas.[10]

In South America, Argentina has become a major producer after introduction of the crop in 1946. Brazil, Ecuador, and Peru have smaller industries.[11]

The first tea plantings in Papua, New Guinea were carried out in 1962 and a thriving industry now exists. Australia has a small experimental program started in 1960.

Although efforts to grow tea commercially in the United States date from ca. 1800 with several sporadic attempts in the southeast, the only sustained effort was carried out in Summerville, South Carolina. An estate was established in 1893 that eventually encompassed about 40 ha, and currently produces the only packaged tea grown in the United States.

III. BOTANY

A. Classification

The botanical designation of the tea plant as *Camellia sinensis* did not come about easily. The plant was originally named in 1753 by Linnaeus as Thea sinensis. He also recognized a separate *Camellia* genus. Later, he split the tea specie into *Thea viridis* and *Thea bohea*. Succeeding taxonomic efforts added to the confusion but eventually it was recognized that the separation of the genera *Thea* and *Camellia* was not useful and the generic name *Camellia* was applied to both. Since 1958 all tea is considered a single species, with several specified varieties including *var sinensis, var assamica,* and *var irrawadensis.*[13]

Var. *sinesis,* usually referred to as China-type tea, grows to a height of 4 to 6 m if unattended and produces a very large number of vertical stems. The leaf is generally erect in co-formation and 7 to 12 cm in length. It is dark green, smooth with a matte surface and without a well-defined apex. The plant is relatively resistant to cold and is, therefore, the variety found in the more temperate producing regions such as China, Japan, the Soviet Union, Turkey, Iran, and the northern, higher altitude growing areas of India. It is known to produce delicately flavored tea when grown at high altitudes under the proper conditions. Var. *sinesis* can tolerate brief cold periods, but average minimum temperatures below -5°C are decidedly detrimental to the plant.

Var. *assamica* grows to a greater height (12 to 15 m unattended) and bears large elliptical leaves up to 25 cm in length with a marked apex. The leaf is pendent and glossy. *Assamica* exhibits much less cold resistance and survived at high altitudes only very close to the equator. In general, it is a much higher-yielding plant than *sinensis* and produces a less delicately flavored beverage. There is some evidence that another *Camellia* specie, *irrawadiensis,* was hybridized with var. *assamica* to produce the uniquely flavored Darjeeling tea. In fact, hybridization of tea varieties has occurred to a very great extent, obscuring the identification of the original tea plant as to both varietal form and geographic origin.

Several investigators have not accepted the concept of a single specie and make a strong case for two distinct species with a third type referred to variously as tran-ninh type, or as the subspecie *lasiocalyx* of *C. assamica.*[14] This contention is based on significant leaf differences at the cellular level, flower morphology, and chemical differences in leaf components.[15]

B. Root System

Plants grown from seed have a long tap root that puts out strong, lateral extension roots in a variety of distribution patterns. These, in turn, produce the feeding roots that are usually confined to a shallow soil layer. Besides serving to absorb water and nutrients, the feeding roots develop small starch granules that become important food sources, especially during incidents of defoliation.[16] Vegetatively propagated plants do not develop tap roots.

C. Flowers

Tea flowers are globular, about 3 to 5 cm in diameter, white, and delicately fragrant. They are borne in the axils of scale leaves (small leaves that do not develop further) and may occur singly or in small clusters. There are five to seven petals and an equal number of sepals. The flowers are mostly self-sterile and are produced in cycles corresponding to leaf growth, and require 9 to 12 months to form mature, round seed pods 1 to 1.5 cm in diameter. The tea plant is not generally allowed to flower during production cycles, with only a small number of the plants allowed to go to seed production to maintain seed stock.

D. Leaves

The leaf is the commercially significant portion of the tea plant. Its general shape and size have already been described. A cross-section of the leaf shows a thick, waxy cuticle on both surfaces that coats a layer of rectangular epidermal cells. Below the upper layer, there are one or two layers of regularly arranged rectangular palisade cells, the long axes of which are at right angles to the leaf surface. Below the palisades cells are layers of irregular, loosely arranged cells constituting the spongy mesophyll. The somata are on the lower leaf surface.

E. Leaf Growth

Tea leaf growth occurs in a definite and distinctive cycle.[17] A typical cycle begins with the formation of a small (5 mm) leaf bud that swells but does not break for a considerable time. Eventually a scale leaf is formed from the bud and then a second scale leaf. This is followed by the production of a slightly larger growth known as fish-leaf. Further development of the bud results in the formation of normal leaves, known as the flush, which constitutes the commerically useful portion of the tea plant. Four or five such leaves are produced at intervals of a few days. Internodal distances become progressively longer and the leaves are distributed in a spiral around the stem. The cycle is then repeated with the formation of another leaf bud and a new dormant period. As will be discussed later, the leaf cycle determines the plucking cycle as well as other agricultural practices.

IV. AGRICULTURE

A. Requirements

The tea plant is not especially fastidious with regard to soil conditions, but certain criteria must be met. Good drainage is essential, since water-logging impedes growth markedly. Soil pH should be maintained on the acid side. Values of pH 4.5 to 5.5 appear to be optimal although under some conditions tea can be satisfactorily grown at higher levels of alkalinity. It is probable that the decreased availability of aluminum at higher pH values is a limited factor.[18] Soils of virtually all origins and a wide variety of textures are generally tolerated.

Rainfall is an important criterion of climatic suitability, but precise requirements cannot be stated since its distribution pattern, atmospheric humidity, temperature, and altitude all affect plant requirements. If drainage is adequate, there does not seem to be an upper limit since tea is grown successfully in some parts of Sri Lanka where rainfall exceeds 500cm/yr.[19] Long periods of drought are harmful, but are mitigated to some extent by high atmospheric humidity and lower temperatures.

Some aspects of temperature limitations have already been discussed with regard to cold sensitivity. Mean monthly temperature maxima over 30°C usually result in such low atmospheric humidity that normal growth is impeded.

Dormant periods that are brought about by lower temperatures or decreased rainfall are generally beneficial with regard to quality, but not if excessively prolonged. One of the major tea-growing areas of the world is Assam, where a dormant period of several months results from the flow of cool air from the Himalayas. The Darjeeling area, known for its teas of very high quality, is affected in the same way. Similarly, tea in parts of Japan and China and in the Soviet Union, Iran, and Turkey go through a dormant period during winter.

B. Propagation

1. Seed

Most existing tea has been grown from seed. Tea estates have traditionally included areas given over to the growth of seed producing plants. These are generously spaced (250 per ha for Assam varieties) and allowed to grow to heights of 3 to 5 m.[20] Seed pods are usually gathered from the ground at frequent intervals during the producing season and planted in well-prepared soil in protected nurseries. Germination takes place in 3 to 4 weeks. Seedlings are protected from hot sun by light shade. Water is provided but drainage must be adequate to prevent waterlogging. Seedlings produce several flushes and may reach a height of 75 cm during the nursery stage.

Selection and hybridization are the techniques employed for maintaining and improving the qualities of planting material based on seed. Varieties that have become stabilized through breeding programs are designated as specific *jats*, but a field of a single *jat* still displays a considerable degree of heterogeneity with regard to leaf color, texture, and yield.

The most important criteria for selection of breeding plants are quality, yield, and resistance to cold, drought, and the various pests of the area. Seed tea plants have a long economic life and there are known instances of plants over 100 years old.

2. Vegetative Propagation

The tea plant is easily and efficiently propagated by making use of leaf cuttings. This provides the opportunity to produce several hundred genetically identical plants at one time from a single elected plant, followed by the rapid multiplication of the clone in subsequent years.

This technique has now become the most prevalent method for replacing inefficient plants or for establishing new stands of tea. A large number of clones have been produced by the various tea research institutes of the world and by individual estates. Vegetative propagation has resulted in the development of very high-yielding plants especially well adapted to the local conditions of growth. All plants of a single clone will perform identically under uniform growing conditions.

Cuttings consisting of one or two leaves are usually rooted in plastic sleeves filled with an appropriate rooting medium. The sleeves are cared for in a nursery with the same precautions exercised as for seedlings. Callus development occurs in a few weeks, rooting begins in 6 to 8 weeks, and shoot growth is substantial in 4 to 5 months.[21]

The absence of a tap root in vegetatively propagated tea might conceivably represent a hazard during extended drought periods, but there is no documented evidence of such preferential damage to clonal tea. Biological identity also affords the possibility for widescale destruction as a result of the appearance of new or modified disease or insect attack. The use of several clones on an estate minimizes the possibility of catastrophic destruction. Another approach, which is becoming prevalent in East Africa, is the use of biclonal seed, i.e., seed derived from the hybridization of two selected clones.

C. Field Establishment

Cuttings or seedlings are transplanted to the prepared fields at a suitable time, depending on climatic conditions. A plant density of about 13,000/ha is achieved by planting in rows that are 1.2 to 1.5 m apart with plant spacings of 60 to 75 cm within a row. More dense planting will result in faster ground cover and higher yields in the earlier years but at the increased cost incurred for developing more plants.

Fertilization is carried out to replenish soils and to maintain desirable pH levels. Nitrogen is usually applied in an acidic form. Minor element requirements have been studied. Copper availability is important, as it affects leaf processing, as will be shown later.

Pruning is required during the early growth of the plant in order to encourage spreading. Mature tea is pruned according to a schedule based on growing conditions. This is necessary to maintain the plant in the vegetative stage in order to stimulate young shoot growth and to keep the height of the bush controlled for efficient plucking. There is a wide range of pruning techniques in effect, not always based on sound physiological data.[22]

Pesticides are used in accordance with local conditions. Fungal diseases affecting roots are treated by removal and burning of infected plants. It is especially useful prophylactically in nurseries and when establishing new plantings. Fungal leaf diseases are prevalent and usually treated with copper sprays.

A large variety of insects, mites, and soil nematodes also infest tea. Pesticide usage is now well controlled so that only materials approved by the U.S. FDA are generally employed.

Irrigation is generally not required for mature tea. It has been shown, however, that under conditions of prolonged drought it can be helpful.[23]

The desirability of partial shade on tea estates has been a controversial subject. Desirable effects include temperature moderation at the leaf surface, which decreases low-humidity stress, and an increased yield of chlorophyll, amino acid, and caffeine production. The undesirable effects include decreased photosynthetic activity and competition for water and solid nutrients by the shade tree employed. In general, the trend has been toward the elimination of shade in most black-tea growing areas. Green tea products benefit from the additional chlorophyll and amino acid production caused by shading, and tea used for production of green tea is generally shaded for some duration of time.

D. Plucking

The objective of plucking is to optimize, to the greatest extent possible, yield, quality, cost, and future productivity. As previously described, "flush" is the new growth of leaf after a short dormant period. Traditional tea phraseology refers to "two and a bud" as the desirable plucking standard for maximizing quality. This encompasses the immature leaf bud and the two leaves below it on a flushing shoot. Hand plucking is the norm and frequently, for economic reasons, includes material beyond the second leaf in that three or four leaves and a bud are often plucked.

Plucking cycles should correspond to flush development, which is regulated by climatic factors. If too short, they represent inefficient use of labor. If too long, older leaf accumulates, which should be removed so as not to diminish productivity or quality. On most tea estates, plucking labor represents half of the employed staff. A single worker will usually pluck 20 to 25 kg of fresh leaf per day.

E. Mechanical Harvesting

Where labor costs are relatively high, some form of mechanical plucking is utilized. This may range from the simple use of scissors to large self-propelled harvesters that straddle the tea hedge row and pluck to a uniform height. Mechanical harvesting is not practical on the steep slopes that exist in many tea growing areas or where labor is abundant, and is therefore not in common practice.

V. COMPOSITION OF TEA

A. Composition of Fresh Leaf

Tea leaf, in common with all plant leaf matter, contains the full complement of genetic material, enzymes, biochemical intermediates, carbohydrates, protein, lipids, and structural elements normally associated with plant growth and photosynthesis. In addition, tea leaf is distinguished by its remarkable content of methylxathines and polyphenols. These two groups of compounds are predominantly responsible for those unique properties of tea that account for its popularity as a beverage. It must be noted that the chemical composition of tea leaf varies with climatic condi-

TABLE 2

Composition of Fresh Green Leaf

Components	% of dry weight
Flavanols	25.0
Flavonols and flavonol glyosides	3.0
Polyphenolic acids and depsides	5.0
Other polyphenols	3.0
Caffeine	3.0
Theobromine	0.2
Amino Acids	4.0
Organic acids	0.5
Monsaccharides	4.0
Polysaccharides	13.0
Cellulose	7.0
Protein	15.0
Lignin	6.0
Lipids	3.0
Chlorophyll and other pigments	0.5
Ash	5.0
Volatiles	0.1

tions, season, position on the flushing shoot, cultural practices, and, above all, with the clone or *jat* being examined. Compositional data must therefore be considered as valid only for a particular sample. A representative analysis of fresh leaf flush is presented in Table 2. Comprehensive reviews including additional data are available.[24–29]

Compositional data refering to fresh leaf are based on dry-leaf solids, since leaf moisture varies from 75 to 80%. Detailed consideration will be given to those components and their precursors that characterize teas as a beverage and are, therefore, of special interest.

B. Methylxanthines

1. Caffeine

The range of caffeine levels in the tea plant is affected by all of the parameters that bring about variation in plant composition. Nitrogen application in fertilizers can increase caffeine by as much as 40%. Seasonal variations, leaf position on the cutting, and genetic origin show similar effects. For instance, var. *sinensis* is slightly lower in caffeine than var. *assamica*.

It must also be recognized that a serving of tea beverage is based on the incomplete extraction of a relatively small amount of tea leaf. Extraction of caffeine during brewing and its quantitative occurrence in tea beverages will be considered later. The weighted average caffeine level for tea sold in the U.S. is approximately 3%[30, 31] on a dry-weight leaf basis.

2. Theobromine

Theobromine levels in tea are considerably lower than those of caffeine. Little has been reported with regard to effect of variation in cultural procedures. Values range in manufactured tea from 0.16 to 0.20%[32, 33] on a dry-weight leaf basis.

3. Theophylline

Theophylline levels in tea are less than 0.04% on a dry-weight leaf basis. Little is known about the causes of variation in experimental reports, and may be attributed to experimental error or degradation of caffeine as a result of experimental procedure. One report did not detect theophylline in a variety of commercially available tea extractions.[32]

4. Biosynthesis

Caffeine had been thought to be principally synthesized during the withering stage of freshly plucked tea leaves,[34] although it is probably synthesized throughout the life of the plant. Caffeine is most likely synthesized from adenine nucleotides, the dominant free purine forms in tea.[35] Adenosine is a major product of RNA metabolism in tea.[36] Adenosine is converted to adenine,[37] and through hypoxanthine (or inosine) to xanthine (or xanthosine), from which xanthosine is the starting branch of caffeine biosynthesis.[38] Guanosine is also converted to xanthosine, but plays an apparently minor role in caffeine biosynthesis.[38] Xanthosine is methylated at the 7-position[39] to 7-methyl xanthosine. 7-Methyl xanthosine is then hydrolyzed to 7-methyl xanthine,[40] which is subsequently methylated to theobromine and caffeine.[41, 42] The final methylation can be terminated, as found in *var. irrawadiensis*.[43] Figure 1 illustrates the mechanism of formation of theobromine and caffeine in the tea plant.

C. Polyphenols

1. Tea Flavanols (catechins)

As indicated in Table 2, the polyphenols constitute the most abundant group of compounds in tea leaf. Of these, the *epi-* form of the catechin group of flavanols predominate. Their structure is shown in Figure 2.

All tea leaf is characterized by high catechin levels. The relative proportions of the various catechins present affect the course of oxidation and the nature of the final beverage will be shown. Total catechin level varies between 20 and 30% of the dry matter of fresh leaf.

The catechins are soluble in water, colorless, and possess an astringent taste. They are easily oxidized and form complexes with many other substances including the methylxanthines.[44] Epigallocatechin gallate is the

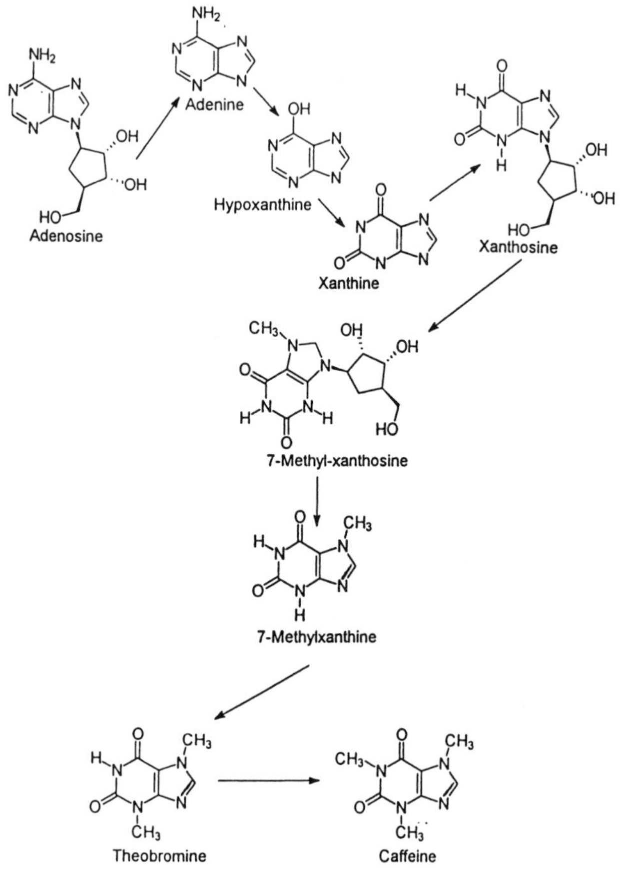

FIGURE 1
Biosynthesis of caffeine in tea.

major tea polyphenol, constituting 12% or more of fresh leaf solids. The quality of tea is correlated with the catechin levels of the fresh leaf, which decrease with leaf age.[45, 46] The proportion of flavanol in the gallate ester form also decreases with leaf age.[47] The catechins occur in the cytoplasmic vacuoles of the palisade cells. They play the most significant role of any group of substances during the course of manufacture of finished tea.

The pathways for the *de novo* biosynthesis of flavonoids in both soft and woody plants have been generally elucidated and reviewed in detail elsewhere.[48, 49] Similar pathways for biosynthesis are used by a wide variety of plant species. The regulation and control of these pathways in tea and the nature of the enzymes involved in synthesis in tea have not been studied exhaustively.

		R_1	R_2
Epicatechin	EC	H	H
Epicatechin Gallate	ECG	Gallate	H
Epigallocatechin	EGC	H	OH
Epigallocatechin Gallate	EGCG	Gallate	OH

		R_1	R_2
Afzelechin		H	H
Catechin	C	OH	H
Gallocatechin	GC	OH	OH

FIGURE 2
The tea flavanols.

2. Flavonols and Glycosides

These substances are present in small amounts in tea leaf but there is little quantitative data on their occurrence. Figure 3 shows the structure of several of these that have been identified. They occur both as free flavonols and glycosides.[24] They may enter into the oxidative reactions that take place during tea manufacture.[50]

3. Gallic Acid

Gallic acid is present in tea leaf and is a known reactant during the complex enzymatic and organochemical reactions that occur when tea components are oxidized.[51] The gallic and quinic acids originate via the shikimate/arogenate pathway. The key enzymes in shikimic acid biosyn-

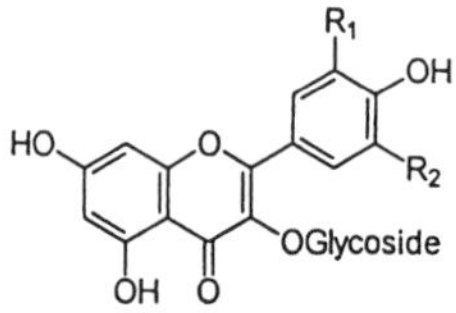

		R_1	R_2
Kaempferol Glycoside	KaG	H	H
Quercitin Glycoside	QuG	OH	H
Myricitin Glycoside	MyG	OH	OH

FIGURE 3
The tea flavonol glycosides.

thesis have been detected in tea.[52] Carbohydrates play an important role, presumably as a precursor to shikimic acid, since radiolabels from both *myo*-inositol and glucose are incorporated into catechins.[53] Gallic acid and quinic acid play key roles in forming esters with various polyphenols. Gallic acid is a key component of tannins and gives the catechins their tannin-like qualities, although tannic acids are not present in tea.

D. Enzymes

In addition to all of the expected enzyme systems present in leaf tissue, fresh tea leaves contain a high level of polyphenol oxidase that catalyzes the oxidation of the catechins by atmospheric oxygen. Tea polyphenol oxidase exists as series of copper-containing (0.32%) isoenzymes. The major component has a molecular weight of about 144,000.[54] The enzyme is concentrated in the leaf epidermis.[55] Soil copper deficiency is sometimes responsible for inadequate oxidation during processing.[56]

5-Dehydroshikimate reductase and phenylalanine ammonia lyase mediate reactions involved in the synthesis of the polyphenols and are therefore key components of tea leaf.[24]

Peroxidase is found in tea leaf and has been recently recognized to play a role in the catechin oxidation system and in the further oxidation of the initial components produced.[57]

There are also enzymes present that participate in the formation of many of the several hundred volatile compounds found in tea aroma. The important enzyme systems responsible for the biosynthesis for the methylxanthines have already been mentioned.

E. Amino Acids

Aside from the usual amino acids, tea leaf contains a unique substance known as theanine (5-N-ethylglutamine).[58] It usually accounts for more than 50% of the free amino acid fraction of tea leaf. Many of the amino acids of tea are involved in aroma formation.[59]

F. Carotenoids

Carotenoids are present at low levels in tea leaf.[60] Neoxanthin, violaxanthin, lutein, and B-carotene are the major components of this group. They enter into reactions that lead to aroma formation.[61]

G. Minerals

Potassium accounts for 40% of the total mineral matter. Tea leaf is relatively rich in fluoride[62] and is a significant accumulator of aluminum and manganese.[63]

H. Volatile Components

A very large number of volatile substances have been identified in fresh tea leaf.[64] Substances present at the highest levels include the ubiquitous leaf aldehyde, trans-2-hexenal, and leaf alcohol, *cis*-3-hexenol. Both arise from *cis*-3-hexenal, which is biosynthesized from linoleic acid in leaf as a result of enzymic splitting.[65]

The components of fresh leaf aroma have not been studied as thoroughly as those of manufactured tea but the biogenesis of several groups of substances has been extensively investigated.[66] A significant fraction of aroma components exists as glycoside derivitives, released by glucosidases in the leaf during withering and fermentation.[28]

VI. MANUFACTURING

A. Introduction

The conversion of freshly harvested green leaf to products of commerce is carried out in factories on large tea estates. When tea is grown on small plots, manufacturing is effected at centralized facilities. The three major types of tea manufacturing result in the production of green tea, black tea, and oolong tea.

Aside from China, Japan, North Africa, and the Middle East, most tea is consumed as black tea, which is produced by promoting the enzymic oxidation of tea flavanols. For the production of green tea, inactivation of the tea enzyme system by rapid firing is carried out to prevent flavanol oxidation. Oolong tea is produced when leaf is fired after being partially oxidized by a gentle fermentation process.

The detailed processing that must be carried out to produce tea suitable for shipment and beverages will be described after consideration of the chemical changes that occur when green-leaf flavanols are oxidized.

B. Chemistry of Tea Oxidation

1. Introduction

Tea oxidation is generally referred to as "fermentation" because of the erroneous early conception of black tea production as a microbial process.[66] Not until 1901 was there recognition of the process as one dependent on an enzymically catalyzed oxidation.[67] This step and further reactions result in the conversion of the colorless flavanols to a complex mixture of orange-yellow to red-brown substances and an increase in the amount and variety of volatile compounds. Extract of oxidized leaf is amber-colored and less astringent than the light yellow-green extract of fresh leaf and the flavor profile is considerably more complex.

2. Flavanol Oxidation

The initial oxidation of the flavanol components of fresh leaf to quinone structures through the mediation of tea polyphenol oxidase is the essential driving force in the production of black tea. While each of the catechins is oxidizable by this route, epigallocatechin and its galloyl ester are preferentially oxidized.[68] Subsequent reactions of the flavonoid substances are largely nonenzymic.

3. Theaflavin Formation

The oxygen-consuming reaction between a quinone derived from a simple catechin and a quinone derived from a gallocatechin results in the formation of a theaflavin. These compounds possess the benztropolone group that is based on a seven-membered ring. Figure 4 illustrates the formation of theaflavins.

Each of the four theaflavins theoretically are derived from the reactions the quinones of epicatechin or its gallate with those of epigallocatechin or its gallate has been identified in black tea and its structure authenticated.[50]

Theaflavins are orange-red substances that contribute significantly to the desirable appearance of black tea beverage. They can by quantitatively detected in tea by means of their intense absorption spectra.[69]

Although theaflavin content is considered to be an important criterion of black tea quality, it does not exceed 2% of final product (dry leaf) weight

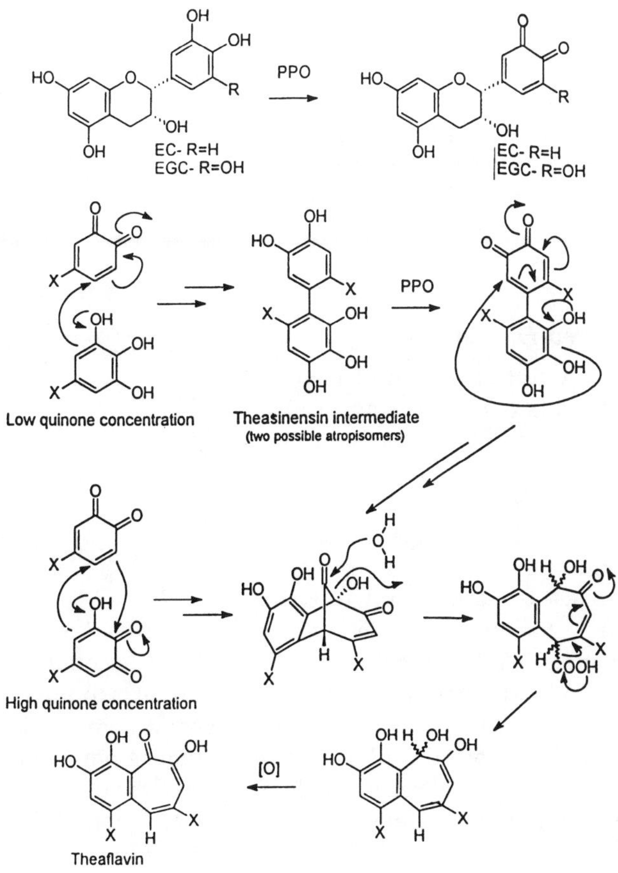

FIGURE 4
Biosynthesis of theaflavin.

and therefore only accounts for 10%, at the most, of the original catechin content of the leaf.

Theaflavin content increases initially as the oxidation process proceeds but falls off rapidly on prolonged oxidation. The mechanism for its further reaction in the oxidizing leaf system is not definitely known.

4. Bisflavanol Formation

Bisflavanols are the compounds formed by the coupling of the quinones produced by the oxidation of epigallocatechin and epigallocatechin gallate.[50] The three predicted bisflavanols have been found and characterized in black tea. They are illustrated in Figure 5. They occur only in very small quantities in black tea, presumably because of high reactivity. Re-

FIGURE 5
Bisflavonols (theasinesins).

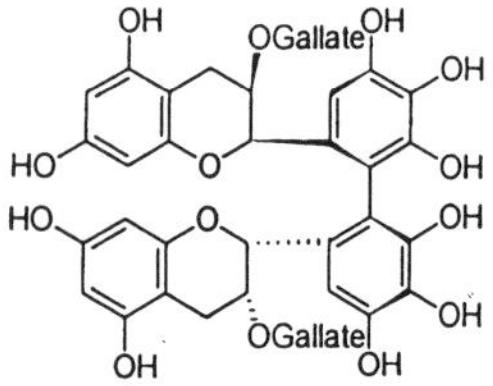

Bisflavonol A, or Theasinensin A

Theasinensin F

cent discovery of a 3-3 coupling product of epigallocatechin and epicatechin in oolong tea has led to the broader classification of these compounds as theasinensins.[70]

5. Thearubigen Formation

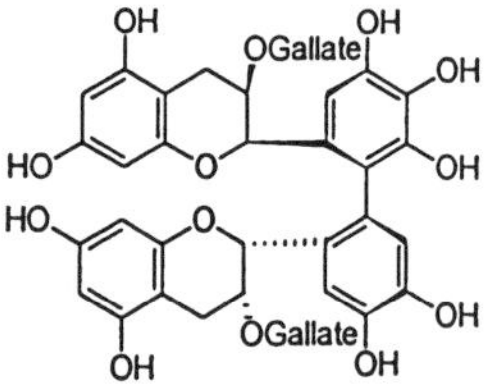

A large proportion of the hot-water extractable solids obtained from black tea is derived from tea flavanols but is not accounted for by the known oxidation products previously described. Approximately 15% of the original fresh-leaf flavanol fraction is recoverable from black tea, and about 10% is identifiable in the form of theaflavins and bisflavanols. While some flavanol material may become tightly bound to the insoluble portion of the leaf, the major amount is found in a complex mixture of only partially resolved substances known as thearubigens because of their red-brown color. The thearubigens have not been completely chemically characterized partly because of the difficulties encountered in their separation. Molecular weight determinations have yielded results ranging from less than 1,000 to over 40,000.[71] These differences may occur because of the tendency of the compounds to condense on prolonged holding in solution.[25]

Small amounts of cyanadin and delphinidin have been detected by acid hydrolysis of the thearubigen mass.[72] These compounds are the anthocyanin analogs of epicatechin and epigallocatechin. Development of HPLC techniques for separation of the tea polyphenols[73–75] have added little to the understanding of the mass balance of the thearubigens, although two new minor uncharacterized fractions have been identified, termed theafulvins[76] and theacitrins.[77]

Theaflavin levels decrease during prolonged oxidation of tea leaf. It is assumed that these compounds enter into reaction with catechin quinones and become part of the thearubigen complex.[71] In addition, it is possible that chlorogenic acid, theogallin, and the flavonol glycosides are also oxidized by the quinones and become included in the thearubigen fraction. Because of the ambiguous nature of the thearubigens, the term "thearubigen" has lost significance as a chemically unique class of compounds and the categorization is more correctly referred to as "unknown polyphenols". Thearubigen should be considered a sensory parameter, useful in qualitative assesment of the progress of tea fermentation.

C. Black Tea Manufacturing

1. Withering

All steps in black tea manufacturing are designed to expedite the oxidation of the tea flavanols and to control the reaction so that the end products are optimized with respect to flavor as well as to leaf and beverage appearance.

Fresh leaf is brought to the factory with a few hours of harvesting. Careful handling prevents bruising and allows for the dissipation of heat generated by continuing respiration. It is then subjected to a withering step to reduce leaf moisture from 75-80% to 55-65%. Withered leaf is flaccid and can be worked further without excessive fracture.

Leaf is spread in 8 to 10 cm layers on nylon netting occupying a high proportion of total factory space. Warm air from the tea-drying ovens is usually circulated across the beds to facilitate evaporation.

More modern and efficient systems utilize troughs in which beds of tea up to 30 cm in depth can be withered by a forced flow of warm air. Withering time is reduced by these techniques.

Depending on the system used and the prevailing weather conditions, the withering process takes 6 to 18 h. It is now recognized that significant chemical changes begin at this step. Cell membranes become more permeable and there are increases in the caffeine, amino acid, and organic acid levels. These processes are independent of water loss and have been referred to as "chemical withering".[78] The increase in caffeine level during the withering process can exceed 20%.[31] Caffeine formation is independent of moisture loss but proportional to withering time. Low withering temperature (13°C) decreases caffeine formation as does high temperature (35°C).

The end point of withering is usually determined by experienced observation of leaf texture or sometimes by checking the weight loss of an isolated portion of leaf.

2. Rolling

The "rolling" or leaf maceration step is carried out in order to disrupt cell structure and allow contact between tea flavanols and tea polyphenol oxidase. The physical condition of the leaf mass must also facilitate oxygen availability.

Orthodox rolling takes place on a rotating circular table 1 to 1.3 m in diameter that is equipped with battens. A circular sleeve with an attached pressure cap rotates eccentrically above the table. Withered leaf is charged into the sleeve and is cut and squeezed by the roller action until it is adequately twisted and reduced in size. Rolled leaf has a coating of leaf juices on the surface and a moist, fluffy texture.

The orthodox roller is being supplanted in many areas by more efficient maceration equipment. The McTear Rotovane consists of a varied cylinder equipped with a rotorshaft so that leaf is cut as it is propelled through the equipment. A pressure cap at the end determines dwell time and degree of maceration.

Rotorvaned leaf is usually further cut in a CTC (crush, tear, curl) machine, which is made up of two closely spaced grooved rollers rotating at different velocities. After leaf passes through this equipment, it is more finely divided than that processed by orthodox rolling.

The Lawrie Tea Processor (LTP) is used in Africa to macerate lightly withered leaf. A hammer mill, in which final particle size can be controlled by degree of wither and adjustment of the tungsten-carbide-tipped beaters, is essential.

It is desirable to prevent leaf temperature from rising above 35°C during the maceration process to preserve quality.

3. Fermentation

The oxidative process actually starts with the onset of maceration of withered leaf. At the end of the rolling process leaf is allowed to oxidize in 5 to 8 cm beds on trays in another fermentation room. It is desirable to keep temperatures below 30°C. Oxidation at 15 to 20°C is said to improve flavor.[79] High humidity prevents surface drying and consequent retardation of oxidation.

Oxidation time depends on the temperature, degree of maceration, degree of wither, and the type of tea to be produced. It ranges from 45 min to 3 h. Completion is judged by the change in color (green to copper) and the aroma that develops. The decision is entrusted to the process supervisor, generally known as the "tea maker". In some areas there is growing use of more highly controlled oxidation systems. These may consist of metal mesh belt conveyors. In a few instances, the moving fermentation belts are enclosed, allowing for control of temperature, air flow, and humidity.

The known changes in polyphenolic material have already been noted. Fermentation also results in slight loss of extractable caffeine. Decreases of 5 to 7% have been observed.[31] Higher-than-normal fermentation times and temperatures accelerate this effect. The fate of caffeine made unavailable during fermentation is not definitely known. It has been demonstrated that caffeine interacts with polyphenols,[80,81] so it is likely that the alkaloid becomes complexed with the most insoluble thearubigen fractions that do not become part of the beverage.[31]

4. Firing

The fermentation step is terminated by firing. It is usually accomplished by passing trays of fermented leaf through a hot-air dryer in a countercurrent mode. The drying process takes about 20 min and its control is crucial to product quality. Smoky teas such as Lapsang Souchong are produced by introducing controlled amounts of smoke from the woodburning during this step.

During firing, enzyme systems are inactivated after a brief period of reaction acceleration. Organochemical changes take place and the moisture level of the leaf is reduced to 2 to 3%. A noticeable effect of firing is the change of color brought by the transformation of chlorophyll to pheophytin, which imparts the desired black color to the dried product. Much of the characteristic black tea aroma is generated during firing. Some low-boiling fresh leaf volatiles are lost but many new components are generated.[64] Firing results in the loss of small amounts of caffeine through sublimation.[31]

5. Grading

Fired leaf is subjected to several grading steps. The tea is separated into particle size grades by passing it over a series of oscillating screens. Some of the most common black tea grades produced include (in descending particle size order): orange pekoe (OP), pekoe, broken orange pekoe (BOP), broken orange pekoe fannings (BOPF), fannings, and dust.

Stalk is removed by the use of electrostatic separators. The process is effective because of the higher moisture level of stalk as compared to leaf after emergence from the drier. Fiber and dust can be eliminated by winnowing.

6. Black Tea Production

More than 75% of world tea production is black tea.

7. Marketing

About half of the world black tea production is sold through auctions. These take place weekly during the producing season in the manufacturing countries. Major auctions are held in Mombasa, Cochin, Calcutta, Columbo, and Jakarta. In addition, large quantities of tea are sold in London auctions as bulked lots in Rotterdam, and through private or government sales in several countries.

In the U.S., 440 tea bags (or servings) are obtained from 1 kg. Costs of shipment, blending, packaging, and marketing must be added on to raw material cost.

TABLE 3

Composition of Green and Black Tea Solids

	Green Tea (%)	Black Tea (%)
Catechins	30	9
Theaflavins		4
Simple polyphenols	2	3
Flavonols	2	1
Other polyphenols	6	23
Theanine	3	3
Amino acids	3	3
Peptides/proteins	6	6
Organic acids	2	2
Sugars	7	7
Other carbohydrates	4	4
Lipids	3	3
Caffeine	3	3
Other methylxanthines	<1	<1
Potassium	5	5
Other minerals/ash	5	5
Aroma	Trace	Trace

VII. BLACK TEA BEVERAGE

A. Composition

There is no exact black tea beverage composition because of variability in starting material, manufacturing process, and preparation. Data based on the extractable solids present in the beverage for black and green tea is shown in Table 3.

B. Black Tea Aroma

The aroma of black tea has been investigated in considerably greater depth than that of fresh leaf. Over 300 compounds have been positively identified in this small fraction.[28] None of these alone or in simple mixtures is reminiscent of tea aroma.

The origin of many of the components of black tea aroma has been studied. Aldehydes are produced by catechin quinone oxidation of amino acids. Enzymic oxidation of carotenoids during manufacture generates ionones and their secondary oxidation products such as theaspirone and dihydroactinidolide. Oxidation of linoleic acid is responsible for the formation of *trans*-2-hexenal.[82]

It has been suggested that enzymic reaction of leucine during processing could lead to the formation of desirable aroma components and that these reactions would be varied during periods of climatic stress when the best flavor is actually produced.[83] During firing, additional compounds are formed as many others decrease. Pyrazines, pyridines, and quinolines are formed at this stage.[84] At all steps of the manufacturing process, the relative proportions of the various aroma components change as fresh tea aroma is converted to black tea aroma.

C. Preparation

Tea beverage is generally prepared by infusing one part of manufactured leaf in about 100 parts of hot water. In the U.S., tea bags represent the most prevalent form of presentation. Approximately 93% of black tea leaf sold at the retail level in the U.S. is packaged in bags. Cup-sized bags are packed at 200/lb or 2.27 g per bag. A larger "family size" tea bag containing 1/4 oz. or 7.09 g is in increasing use. Food service bags containing 1 oz. or 28.35 g of tea are used to make up 1 gal of beverage. Packaged black tea is sold in a variety of sizes. The rise in popularity in the U.S. of small gourmet coffee stores along with the increase in consumtion of meals outside the home has led naturally to an upspringing of small tea shops selling packaged gourmet teas, either blended or from single estates.

A proper tea bag paper is essential to the preparation of a good beverage. The paper must retain fine tea dust particles, and yet allow for efficient fluid transfer into and out of the bag. It is essential that the paper and other substances in contact with the infusion impart no taste.

Tea bag paper is generally made from a mixture of wood cellulose (30 to 40%) and abaca fiber (60 to 70%). The latter is derived from the plant *Musa texitilis* grown in Madagascar and the Philippines.

Extraction rate is determined by the water:tea ratio, temperature, particle, size, and bag geometry. Table 4 shows the relationships among extraction time, total beverage solids, and beverage caffeine levels when 180 ml of boiling water is poured onto a standard tea bag in a cup covered during the brewing period.

Caffeine is extracted at about the same rate as the remainder of the beverage solids as shown by the proportion of caffeine in the extracted solids. Replication of data is difficult unless small steps in the brewing procedure are precisely controlled. There is much conflicting data in the literature,[32, 85-87] but the brewing results shown above are consistent with the known composition of tea and its extraction characteristics.

TABLE 4

Production Variable Effect on Caffeine

Variable	Caffeine (% of dry wt.) Low	High
Nitrogen application	2.22	3.19
Leaf position	4.00	5.13
Season	1.5	3.5

There is also confusion in the literature concerning theobromine and theophylline levels in tea beverage. The most reliable data indicate 0.16 to 0.20% theobromine and no theophylline in black tea.[32, 88] Assuming the same level of extraction as for caffeine, 3 to 4 mg of theobromine is to be expected in an average cup of tea.

The kinetics of tea extraction have been studied in detail.[89, 90] Rates for caffeine, theaflavin, and thearubigen extraction have been determined. It has been demonstrated that extraction is not a transport-controlled process. Temperature and time are the rate-limiting variables.

D. Consumption Patterns

In the U.S., most black tea leaf[79] is used for iced tea preparation. This is made from a hot infusion or by extraction over a period of many hours at ambient temperature. The latter product is sometimes referred to as "sun tea" and consists of a relatively dilute beverage. Sugar and lemon are common additives.

Hot tea accounts for 35% of black tea leaf use in the U.S. It is most popular in the Northeast, where milk is a frequently used additive.

E. Quality

1. Terminology

A unique lexicon of descriptors for tea has been built up over the years in the tea trade. By its use, the tea-buyer and the tea-taster communicate quality parameters to guide the purchase, blending, and quality control of tea. Some terms in common use include brisk, bright, dull, flat, green, harsh, plain, pungent, quality, and soft.[91]

It should be noted that the terms do not necessarily correspond to their normal connotation, e.g., "quality" refers primarily to the presence of a desirable aroma fraction. Some terms that characterize black tea, as compared to green tea, include "quality", "color", "strength", and "briskness".

2. Role of Theaflavin

The significance of the theaflavin level in black tea with regard to beverage color and taste has been recognized.[69] It has been shown that for African teas there is a good correlation of theaflavin level with value.[79] Processing and storage conditions have been studied to find techniques for maximizing and retaining theaflavin levels.

Maintenance of fermentation temperature at 15°C increases theaflavin levels whereas higher temperatures vary for thearubigen formation. Teas fermented at 15°C bring higher prices than those manufactured at 25°C or

35°C.[79] Higher temperatures also accelerate a decline in polyphenolase activity, whereas peroxidase activity remains high. This favors thearubigen formation at the expense of theaflavin.[92]

Theaflavin levels are enhanced and teas are valued at higher prices when fermentation is carried out at lower (4.5 to 4.8) pH values.[93]

Black tea quality as determined by theaflavin levels is also affected by storage conditions. Low temperatures, low moisture levels, and low oxygen availability retard theaflavin loss. Residual peroxidase activity, which accelerates theaflavin loss on storage, is diminished by acid treatment during fermentation.[94]

3. Role of Caffeine

Extractable caffeine levels increase on storage, presumably because of decomplexation from theaflavins as the latter decrease. Since caffeine binding with thearubigens is weaker than that with theaflavins, more caffeine may become available.[94] An increase in "free" caffeine may be responsible for decreased value because of the bitterness imparted to the beverage. Caffeine in combination with the normal tea complement of oxidized polyphenolic matter does not exhibit bitterness.[95]

Black tea taste is primarily a function of the polyphenols, caffeine, and aroma components. Astringency, an important characteristic of the organoleptic sensation, has been described as consisting of a "tangy" and a "nontangy" component.[95]

The combination of caffeine with the oxidation products of gallated flavanols produces the characteristic described as "tangy astringency", probably equivalent to the term "briskness" applied by professional tea-tasters.

The complex between caffeine and oxidized polyphenolic matter is also responsible for the phenomenon known as "creaming", or the precipitation of material from a strong black tea infusion as it cools. Tea cream consists primarily of caffeine and theaflavin gallate but also theobromine, thearubigens, catechins gallate, gallic acid, and several other components. Removal of caffeine from black tea infusions prevents the formation of cream.[80] Caffeine causes the precipitation of theaflavins and gallated catechins. Hydrogen bonding is responsible for the formation of the insoluble agglomerates.[67, 96] Cream formation is generally considered to be a desirable attribute for traditional black tea use but is a disadvantage in iced tea and instant tea.

4. Black Tea Varieties

Assam and Kenyan teas are described as being strong, thick, colory, and are not known for outstanding aroma due to the preponderance of the

CTC processing technique which results in high yield and good color but small leaf size. Keemun teas from China are also noted for their colory brew. China varieties and China-Assam hybrids when grown at high altitudes often produce highly desirable aromas such as those characteristic of Darjeeling tea from North India. High-grown Sri Lanka teas from the Uva, Dimbula, and Nuwara Eliya areas are also flavorful. The Yunnan region of China produces a wide variety of teas due to the wide variety of gene stock in the region and are typically noted for a peppery flavor.

VII. GREEN TEA

A. Manufacturing

Green tea processing is designed to achieve a dry product exhibiting the desirable twisted leaf appearance, but without flavanol oxidation. This is accomplished by carrying out rapid enzyme inactivation either with steam in a rotating cylinder as practiced in Japan or with dry heat as practiced in the People's Republic of China. The inactivated tea is cooled, rolled partially dried, rerolled, and then completely dried.

Because of the presence of unoxidized catechins, green tea beverage is yellow-green in color and more astringent than black tea. While many of the components of black-tea aroma are represented in green tea, their relative proportions differ.

B. Varieties

Some varieties of green tea including the following: Sencha — the most widely drunk grade of green tea in Japan; Gyokuro — the most prized grade of Japanese tea (grown under shade); Matcha — the ceremonial green tea, the beverage is a suspension of finely ground leaf; Gunpowder — a small compact pellet of Chinese green tea; and Pi-lo-Chun — a small-leaved Chinese tea made from the first spring flush.

C. Composition

Plant varieties used for green tea production usually have higher amino acid levels and lower catechin levels than those used for making black tea. Caffeine levels are slightly lower except in the finest grades,[85] with variations attributed to shading and leaf processing.

E. Quality

Green tea quality is dependent to a large extent on amino acid levels, especially that of theanine.[97] Ascorbic acid content, although very low, also correlates positively with quality. Free reducing sugars and catechin gallates show a negative correlation.[98] Caffeine levels do not have much effect on quality.

IX. OTHER TEAS

A. Oolong Tea

Oolong tea is only partially oxidized, so that its appearance and chemical composition is somewhat intermediate between that of green and black tea. It is manufactured primarily in the People's Republic of China and in Taiwan.

B. Brick Tea

Tea is compressed into a molded brick in part of the Soviet Union and China. Portions of the bricks are broken off for use and are sometimes cooked with butter or other fats.[26]

C. Flavored Teas

Earl Grey tea is flavored with the peel oil of bergamot, a citrus fruit, which is added by spraying onto black tea before final packaging. Other flavors may also be applied to black tea by spraying onto the leaves, incorporation of flowers into the blend, or by addition of encapsulated flavor crystals. Other common flavored teas include Rose Congou and Lychee.

Jasmine flowers are sometimes added to manufactured green tea in the country of origin and they impart characteristic floral notes.

Lapsang Souchong tea is a Chinese black tea flavored during firing by the use of smoky woods such as pine. These smoky teas are commonly added to blends of other black teas to create "Russian Caravan" blends.

Stabilized flavors in a solid form are also used to prepare a variety of flavored teas. Orange and spice, lemon, cinnamon, mint, blackberry, apple, cherry, and almond flavored products are marketed.

Pu-Erh tea is produced in Yunnan Province by the action of microbiological fermentation on green tea. Noted for its 'earthy' flavor, it is often processed into cakes, such as Tuo-cha or bowl-shaped tea.

X. INSTANT TEA

Instant tea is the water-soluble extract of tea leaf usually marketed as a powder, either pure or as a part of flavored mixes. Most instant tea is manufactured in the U.S. It is also manufactured in a few tea-growing countries where the starting material may be fermented leaf that has not been dried.

When starting with dried tea, extraction may be carried out in columns[99] or kettles.[100] In order to extract a high proportion of the soluble components with a minimum amount of water, a countercurrent extraction mode is utilized. Extractable solids yields of 25 to 35% can be obtained. Spent leaf can be treated at high temperatures to further increase yield.[99] Extract is separated from spent leaf by centrifugation.

It is desirable to isolate and preserve aroma. This may be accomplished by low-pressure steam treatment in columns before solids extraction[101] or by vacuum-stripping the extract.[102] The aroma fraction may be further concentrated.

The aqueous extract is usually vacuum-concentrated although freeze concentration has been described.[103]

The concentrated aroma fraction is added back to the tea solids concentrate before drying. It is possible to freeze-dry the product but it is generally spray-dried with some loss of volatiles. Drying conditions are chosen to conserve aroma as much as possible and produce a low-density product.[104]

Instant tea produced as described above will dissolve completely in hot water but not in cold water, as the caffeine-polyphenol complexes are insoluble under those conditions. Since virtually all instant tea manufacture in the U.S. is for iced tea preparation, process modification is required. This initial extract may be cooled to 5 to 10°C and the cold water insoluble material or "cream" be allowed to precipitate. Under these conditions, 20 to 35% of the extract solids may be separated by centrifugation. The supernatant solids will reconstitute in cold water after concentration and drying.[105] It is also possible to process the cream to make a portion of it compatible with the product and thereby retain the caffeine and some polyphenolic components that are present in this fraction.[106] Commercial use of the enzyme Tannase, which removes gallic acid from gallated tea polyphenols[107] and reduces cream formation[108] can be used to reduce cream losses and manufacture instant teas retaining more of the natural polyphenol content.

Instant tea is also marketed with lemon flavor and with flavor and sweetener. The latter may be sugar, saccharin, or aspartame.

The caffeine content of instant teas manufactured in the U.S. averages about 5%. When prepared as an iced beverage at 0.3% solids, 200 ml of beverage provides 30 mg of caffeine.

XII. PHYSIOLOGICAL EFFECTS

A. Introduction

From the time of its earliest usage, beneficial physiological properties have been attributed to tea. It is probable that the pleasant stimulating effects of a moderate amount of caffeine, unaccompanied by substances that cause adverse gastrointestinal side effects, are responsible for the feeling of well-being that has characterized tea consumption as described even in the oldest writings. In addition, the pleasant mouth feel brought about by mild astringency and rapid flavor release also adds to its satisfying nature as a beverage.

As indicated previously, the average caffeine level of a cup of tea prepared by adding 180 ml of boiling water to a tea bag and brewing for 2 to 3 min is about 30 mg. This amount of caffeine appears to provoke minimal symptoms or irritability.

Caffeine contained in tea beverage is absorbed at about the same rate as caffeine in coffee, cola drinks, or in pure water. Data to support this conclusion was obtained in a human feeding experiment.[109] The theory that complexation of caffeine with the polyphenolic material in tea retards absorption[110, 111] is not borne out.

The physiological effects of tea that are caused by caffeine alone will not be discussed further in this chapter.

B. Vitamins

No significant quantity of the macronutrients nor of the vitamins for which U.S. Recommended Dietary Allowance (RDA) have been established can be obtained from the consumption of a cup of tea.[110] The water-soluble B vitamins present are easily extractable. Eight percent extractability for a representative black tea blend is assumed.[110]

Vitamin C (ascorbic acid) is present in green tea but only traces are found in black tea.[112] Five cups of Japanese green tea provide 25 to 30% of the RDA.

Although there are physiologically significant quantities of vitamin E (tocopherol) and vitamin K (phylloquinone) in black tea, their extractability is not adequately known.[110]

C. Minerals

The minerals that might be significant to human nutrition are probably confined to potassium and fluoride. While levels vary according to soil fertilization regimens, tea generally provides about 60 to 70 mg of potassium per cup. Fluoride levels also vary with soil conditions. In general, tea provides 0.10 to 0.12 mg of fluoride per cup. Aluminum in tea is not easily extracted so that the beverage only provides about 0.4 mg per cup. Manganese, the other element that is preferentially accumulated by the tea plant, is extracted to the extent of 0.1 to .3 mg per cup.[110]

D. Polyphenols

The antioxidant activity of tea polyphenols[113] is associated with epidemiological evidence that tea is an anti-carcinogenic[114] and anti-cardiovascular disease[115] agent. Work on investigating the biochemical and mechanistic action of tea polyphenols in the prevention of diseases is in progress, but there is good evidence in animal models that tea prevents the carcinogenicity of cigarette smoke,[116] inhibits nitrosamine formation,[117] and UV-light induced tumor formation.[118]

XII. CONCLUSIONS

There are many factors responsible for the unusual popularity of tea as a beverage. These are agricultural and economic as well as organoleptic and perceptual.

Once established, tea is not a very difficult crop to maintain. Some varieties withstand cold weather fairly well and this allows for a widespread growing area but with a primary requirement for adequate water. Tea can be successfully cultivated by the use of unsophisticated techniques, but also by the use of highly mechanized procedures. It is, therefore, viable in a wide diversity of economics. Tea is among the least expensive of beverages and can usually be provided at less than $0.03 per serving.

The unique chemical composition of the beverage components brought about by the unusual and reactive chemical storehouse that makes up young tea leaf is largely responsible for its properties.

The organoleptic properties of black tea depend to a considerable extent on the astringency resulting from the interaction of caffeine with the oxidized galloyl ester of the flavanols. The aroma components of black tea also constitute a unique flavor profile that blends well with the taste of the nonvolatile materials. The caffeine provides a moderate level of stimulation, which adds further to the appeal of the beverage, although tea has been shown to provide relaxation as well as revival of character.[119]

Tea provides a broad spectrum of flavor experience: there is a considerable degree of diversity in the flavor of different varieties; green tea and oolong tea provided very different taste sensations from those of black tea; flavorants and other additives allow for still greater variety; tea is appreciated both as a hot and a cold beverage.

The composition of tea varies greatly depending on all of the factors that generally affect crops. It is therefore difficult to standardize on a uniform product when investigating or describing tea. In addition, analytical techniques are often difficult to carry out in the presence of the large quantity of oxidized polyphenols that result from black tea manufacturing. Standardized analytical methods and procedures for beverage preparation are highly desirable to maximize the value of investigations. The designation of some teas as standards might also be useful.

Better knowledge of the physiological and health-promoting properties of tea could be obtained by more complete understanding of the chemistry of the mass of oxidized phenolic material, commonly known as thearubigens but better classified as unknown polyphenols. This increased understanding could also be applied to quality improvement. As these compounds become more completely characterized and their organoleptic properties better defined, further modification of black tea manufacture to favor the accumulation of the most desirable substances becomes a possibility. Similar information with regard to the significance of the volatile components might be utilized in a like manner.

The sensitivity of tea production to research has already been demonstrated by the successful process modifications carried out to increase theaflavin levels and value. There is a limit to what can be accomplished to the confining environment of fermenting leaf. For black instant tea production, the conversion of fresh leaf components to those present in black tea might be better accomplished outside of the leaf. This could allow for more highly directed reaction pathways to bring about the formation of the most desirable end-products. Enzymic and chemical techniques could also be used.

REFERENCES

1. *Annual Bulletin of Statistics.* London: International Tea Committee, p. 123, 1995.
2. Harler, C. R., *The Culture and Marketing Of Tea.* 3rd ed. London: Oxford Unversity, p. 4, 1963.
3. Shalleck, J., *Tea.* New York: Viking, p. 7, 1981.
4. Woodward N. H., *Teas of the World.* New York: McMillian, Ch. 1, 1980.
5. Woodward N. H., *Teas of the World.* New York: McMillian, Ch. 2, 1980.
6. Quimme P., *The Signet Book of Coffee and Tea.* New York: New American Library, Ch. 8, 1976.
7. Woodward N. H., *Teas of the World.* New York: McMillian, Ch. 6, 1980.
8. Harler, C. R., *The Culture and Marketing Of Tea.* 3rd ed. London: Oxford Unversity, Ch. 14, 1963.
9. Harler, C. R., *The Culture and Marketing Of Tea.* 3rd ed. London: Oxford Unversity, Ch. 13, 1963.
10. Harler, C. R., *The Culture and Marketing Of Tea.* 3rd ed. London: Oxford Unversity, Ch. 15, 1963.
11. Harler, C. R., *The Culture and Marketing Of Tea.* 3rd ed. London: Oxford Unversity, p. 41, 1963.
12. Mitchell, G. F., *The Cultivation and Manufacture of Tea In The United States.* Bull 234, USDA Bureau of Plan Industry, 1912.
13. Eden, T., *Tea.* 3rd ed. London: Longman, p. 16, 1976.
14. Barua, P. K., Classifcation of the Tea Plant. *Two and a Bud,* 10:3, 1963.
15. Roberts, E. A. H., Wight W., Wood D. J., Paper Chromatography as an aid to the taxnomomy of *Thea chamellias. New Physiol.,* 57:211, 1958.
16. Eden, T., *Tea.* 3rd ed. London: Longman, p. 17, 1976.
17. Bond, T. E. T., Studies in the vegetative growth and anatomy of the tea plan. Part I. *Bot. Ann. Lond New Ser.,* 6:607, 1942. Part II 9:1183, 1945.
18. Chenery E. M., A preliminary study of aluminum and the tea bush. *Plant Soil,* 6: 174, 1955.
19. Eden, T., *Tea.* 3rd ed. London: Longman, p. 9, 1976.
20. Eden, T., *Tea.* 3rd ed. London: Longman, p. 26, 1976.
21. Harler, C. R., *The Culture and Marketing Of Tea.* 3rd ed. London: Oxford Unversity, p. 19, 1963.
22. Harler, C. R., The Culture and Marketing Of Tea. 3rd ed. London: Oxford Unversity, p. 53, 150, 190, 1963.
23. Carr, M. K. V. and Carr, S., *Water and the Tea Plant.* Tea Res. Inst. East Africa, 1971.
24. Wickremashinghe, R. I., Tea. In Chickester C.D., Mrak, E. M., and Stewart, G. F., Eds., *Advances In Food Research.* New York: Academic Press, p. 22, 1978.
25. Sanderson, G. W., The chemistry of tea and tea manufacturing. In Runeckles V. C. and Tso T. C., Eds., *Recent Advances In Phytochemistry.* New York: Academic Press, p. 247, 1972.
26. Bokuchava, M. A. and Skobeleva, N. I., The biochemistry and technology of tea manufacture. *CRC Crit Rev. Food Sci. Nutr.,* 12:303, 1980.
27. Robertson, A., *Tea — Cultivation to Consumption,* Willson and Clifford, Eds., pp. 555-602. Chapman and Hall, London, 1992.
28. Robinson, J.M. and Owuor, P.O., *Tea — Cultivation to Consumption,* Willson and Clifford, Eds., pp. 603-648. Chapman and Hall, London 1992
29. Pintauro, N.D., *Tea and Soluble Tea Products Manufacture.* Noyes Data Corporation, Park Ridge, NJ, 1977.
30. Cloughley, J. B., Factors influencing the caffeine content of black tea: Part 1 — The effect of field variables. *Food Chem.,* 9:69, 1982.

31. Cloughley, J. B., Factors influencing the caffeine content of black tea: Part 2 — The effect of production variables. *Food Chem.*, 10:25, 1983.
32. Hicks, M. B. Hsieh, Y.-H., Bell, L. N., Tea Preparation and its influence on Methylxanthine Concentration. *Food Res. Int.*, 29, 325-330, 1996.
33. Jalal, M. A. F., Collin, H. A., Estimation of caffeine, theophylline and theobromine in plant material. *New Phytol.*, 76: 277, 1976.
34. Roberts, G. R., Sanderson, G. W. *J. Sci. Food Agric.* 17:182-188, 1966.
35. Takino, Y., Imagawa, H., Shishido, K. *Nippon Shokuhin Kogyo Gakkaishi*, 19: 213-218,1972.
36. Imagawa, H., Takino, Y., and Shimizu, M. *Nippon Shokuhin Kogyo Gakkashi* 23: 138-144, 1976.
37. Imagawa, O., Yamano, H., Inoue, K., and Takino, Y. *Agric. Biol. Chem.* 43: 2337-2342, 1979.
38. Negishi, O., Ozawa, T., and Imagawa, H. *Biosci. Biotech. Biochem.* 56: 499-503, 1992.
39. Negishi, O., Ozawa, T., and Imagawa, H. *Agric. Biol. Chem.* 49: 887-890, 1985.
40. Negishi, O., Ozawa, T., and Imagawa, H. *Agric. Biol. Chem.* 52: 169-175, 1988.
41. Suzuki, T., Takahashi, E., *Biochem. J.* 146: 87-96, 1975.
42. Suzuki, T. and Takahashi, E. *Phytochem.*, 15: 1235-1240, 1976.
43. Roberts, E. A. H., Wight, W., Wood, D. J. *New Phytologist* 57: 211-225, 1958.
44. Roberts, E. A. H., Economic Importantance of Flavonoid Substances: Tea Fermentation. In Geissman, T. A., Ed., *The Chemistry of Flavonoid Components.* New York: Macmillian, p. 468, 1962.
45. Nakagawa, M., Anan, T., and Ishima, N., The relation of green tea taste with its chemical make-up. *Bull Nat. Res. Inst. Tea*, 17:69, 1981.
46. Wickremasinghe, R. L. and Perera, K. P. W. C., Factores affecting quality, strength and color of black tea liquors. *J. Natl. Sci. Council Sri Lanka*, 1:111, 1973.
47. Bhatia, I. S. and Ullah, M. R., Polypheols of tea IV, Qualitative and quantitative study of the polyphenols of different organs and some cultivated varieties of tea plant. *J Sci. Food Agric.*, 19:535, 1968.
48. Jain, J. C. and Takeo, T. *Food Biochem.* 8: 243-279, 1984.
49. Heller, W. and Forkmann, G. *The Flavonoids: Advances in Research since 1986.* Harborne, J. B., Ed., Chapman and Hall, London. 1994. pp. 499-536.
50. Takino, Y., Reddish orange pigments of black tea structure and oxidative formation from catechins. *JARQ*, 12:94, 1978.
51. Berkowitz, J. E., Coggon, P., and Sanderson, G. W., Formation of epitheaflavic acid and its transofrmation to thearubigens during tea fermentation. *Phytochemistry*, 10:2271, 1971.
52. Saijo, R. and Takeo, T. *Agric. Biol. Chem.* 43: 1427-1432, 1979.
53. Wang, C. and Huang, Y. *Zhongguo Kexue Jishu Daxue Xuebao*, 17: 469-474, 1987.
54. Gregory, R. P. F. and Bendal, D. S., The purification and some properties of polyphenol oxidase from tea. *Biochem. J*, 101:569, 1966.
55. Wickremasinghe, R. L., Roberts, G., and Perara, B. P. M., Localization of the polyphenol oxidase of tea leaf. *Tea Q*, 38:309, 1967.
56. Harler, C. R., *The Culture and Marketing Of Tea.* 3rd ed. London: Oxford Unversity, p. 49, 1963.
57. Dix, M. A., Fairley, C. J., Millin, D. J., and Swaine, D., Fermentation of tea in aqueous suspension. Influence of tea peroxidase. *J. Sci. Food Gric.*, 32:920, 1981.
58. Sabato, J., Studies of the chemical constitutents of tea. III. On a new amide-Theanine. *Agri. Chem. Soc. Jpn.*, 23:262, 1950.
59. Sanderson, G. W., Biochemistry of tea fermentation: Conversion of aminoa cids to black tea aroma constituents. *J. Food Sci.*, 35:160, 1970.
60. Venkatakrishna, S., Premachandra, B. R., and Cama, H. R., Distribution of carotenoid pigments in tea leaves. *Tea Q*, 47:28, 1977.

61. Sanderson, G. W. and Graham, H.N., On the formation of black tea aroma. *J. Agri. Chem.*, 21:576, 1973.
62. Elivin-Lewis, M., Vitali, M., and Kopjas, T., Anticariogenic potential of commerical teas. *J. Prev. Dent.*, 6:273, 1980.
63. Eden, T., *Tea.* 3rd ed. London: Longman, p. 153, 1976.
64. Yaminishi, T., Tea, coffee, cocoa and other beverages. In Teranishi, R., Flath, R. A., and Sugisawa, H., Eds., *Flavor Research: Recent Advances.* New York: Dekker, 1981, p. 231.
65. Hatanaka, A. and Kajiwara, T., Occurrence of *trans*-3-hexenal in *Thea sinensis* leaves. *Z. Naturforeshung*, 36:755, 1981.
66. Bajaj, H. L., Genesis of volatile constituents of tea. *Riv. Ital.*, 61:123, 1979.
67. Aso, D. On the role of xoidase in the preparation of commerical tea. *Bull. Coll. Agri. Tokyo Imp. Univ.*, 4:225, 1901.
68. Roberts, E. A. H., The phenolic substances of manufactured tea. II. Their origin as enzymic oxidation products in fermentaiton. *J. Sci. Food Agri.*, 9:212, 1958.
69. Roberts, E. A. H. and Smith, R. F., "Spectrophotometric measurements of theaflavins and thearubigens in black tea liquors in assessments of quality in teas. *Analyst (Lond)*, 86:94, 1961.
70. Nonaka, G., Kawahara, O., and Nishioka, I. *Chem. Pharm. Bull.* 31: 3906-3914, 1983.
71. Millin, D. J. and Rustidge, D. W., Tea manufacture. *Proc. Biochem.*, 2:9, 1967.
72. Brown, A. G., Eyton, W. B., Holmes, A., and Ollis, W. D., The Identification of the thearubigens as polymeric proanthoxyanadins. *Phytochemistry*, 8:2333, 1969.
73. Ozawa, T., Separation of the components in black tea infusion by chromatography on Toyopearl. *Agric. Biol. Chem.*, 46:1079, 1982.
74. Opie, S. C., Clifford, M. N., and Robertson, A. *J. Sci. Food Agric.* 67: 501-505, 1995.
75. Wedzicha, B. L., Lo, M. F., and Donovan, T. J. 1990. *J. Chrom.*, 505: 357-364
76. Bailey, R. G., Nursten, H. E., and McDowell, I. *J. Sci. Food Agric.* 59: 365-375, 1992.
77. Powell, C., Clifford, M. N., Opie, S. C., and Gibson, C. L. From What's in a Cuppa? Recent Advances in the Chemistry and Biochemistry of Tea. *Sci Conference Papers Series, London,* No. 0027, 1994, 18 pp.
78. Sanderson, G. W., The theory of withering in tea manufacture. *Tea Q.*, 35:146, 1964.
79. Cloughley, J. B., The effect of fermentation temperature on the quality parameters and price evaluation of Central African black teas. *J. Sci. Food Agri.*, 31:911, 1980.
80. Smith, R. I., Studies on the formation and composition of cream in tea infusion. *J. Sci. Food Agri.*, 19:530, 1966.
81. Collier, P. D., Mallows, R., and Thomas, P. E., Interactions between theaflavins, flavanols, and caffeine. *Proc. Phytochem. Soc.*, 11:867, 1972.
82. Dev Choudhury, M. N., Chemistry of tea flavor. In Atal, C. K. and Kapur, B. M., Eds., *Cultivation and Utilization of Aromatic Plants.* Jammu-Tawi Council of Science and Industrial Research (India), 1982, p. 715.
83. Wickrremasinghe, R. L., The mechanism of operaiton of climatiic factors in the biogenesis of tea flavor. *Phytochemistry*, 13:2057, 1974.
84. Vitzthum, O. G., Werkoff, P., and Hubert, P., New volatile constituents of black tea aroma. *J. Agri. Food Chem.*, 23:999, 1975.
85. Bunker, M. L. and McWilliams, M., Caffeine content of common beverages. *J. Am. Diet Assoc.*, 74:28, 1979.
86. Gilbert, G. M., Marshman, J. A., Schwieder, M., and Berg, R., Caffeine content of beverages as consumed. *Can. Med. Assoc. J.*, 114:205, 1976.
87. Burg, A. W., Effects of caffeine on the human system. *Tea Coffee J.*, 147:40, 1975.

88. Sontag, G., Kral, K., Bestimmung von Coffein, Theobromine and Theophyllin in Tee, Koffee and Getranken durch Hochdrucksflussigkeits chromatographie mit electrochemischem Detektor. *Microchim. Acta*, II:39, 1980.
89. Spiro, M. and Siddique, S., Kinetics and equilibria of tea infusion. Kinetics of extraction of theaflavins, thearubigens and caffeine from Koonsong Broken Pekoe. *J. Sci. Food Agri.*, 32:1135, 1981.
90. Spiro, M. and Jago, D. S., Kinetics and equilibria of tea infusion. *J. Chem. Soc. Faraday, Trans I*, 78:295, 1982.
91. Black Tea — Vocabulary. International Organization for Standards, No. 60, p. 78, 1982.
92. Cloughley, J. B., The effect of temperature on enzyme activity during the fermentation phase of black tea manufacture. *J. Sci. Food Agri.*, 31:920, 1980.
93. Cloughley, J. B. and Ellis, R. T., The effect of pH modification during fermentation on the quality parameters of Central African black teas. *J. Sci. Food Agric.*, 31:924, 1980.
94. Cloughley, J. B., Storage deterioration in Central African tea: Changes in chemcial composition, sensory characteristics and price evaluation. *J. Sci. Food Agri.*, 32:1213, 1981.
95. Sanderson, G. W., Ranadive, A. S., Eisenberg, L.S. Farrell, F. J., Simons R., Manley, C. H., and Coggon, P., Contribution of polyphenolic compounds to the taste of tea. In Charalambous, G. and Katz, I., Eds., Sulfur and Nitrogen Compounds in Food Flavors. Washington, D.C.: ACS Symp, 26, 14, 1976.
96. Harbowy, M. and Balentine, D., U.S. Patent #5532012.
97. Nakagwa, M., Relationship between chemical constituents and the taste of green tea. *Tea Res. J. (Jpn)*, 40:1, 1973.
98. Nakagawa, M., Anan, T., and Iwasa, K., The difference of flavor and chemical constituents in spring and summer green teas. *Study Tea*, 53:74, 1977.
99. Mishkin, A. R., Marsh, W. C., Fobes, WA. W., and Ohler, J. L., Extraction process. U.S. Pat. 3,451,823, June 24, 1969.
100. Seltzer, E. and Saporito, F. A., Method of producing a tea extract. U.S. Pat. 2,902,368, Sept, 1959.
101. Continuous manufacture of powdered extracts from vegetable material. Br. Pat 946, 346, Jan. 8, 1964.
102. Seltzer, E. and Saporito, F. A., Method of making a tea extract. U.S. Pat. 2,927,860, Mar. 8, 1960.
103. Geniaris, N., Concentration of tea. U.S. Pat. 3,598,608, Aug. 10, 1971.
104. Gurkin, M., Sanderson, G. W., and Graham, H. N., Process for making a spray-dried instant tea of desired bulk density. U.S. Pat. 3,666,484, May 30, 1972.
105. Seltzer, E. and Harriman, A. J., Process for preparing a soluble tea product. U.S. Pat. 2,,891,865, June 23, 1959.
106. Fobes, A., Process for preparing a soluble tea product. U.S. Pat. 3,151,985, Oct. 6, 1964.
107. Roberts, E. A. H. and Myers, M. *J. Sci. Food Agric.* 10: 172-176, 1959.
108. Nagalakshmi, S., Jayalaksmi, R., and Seshadri, R. *J. Food Sci. Tech.* 22: 198-201, 1985.
109. Marks, V. and Kelly, J. F., Absorption of caffeine from tea, coffee, and coca cola. *Lancet*, 14:827, 1973. Corrected in Lancet, 9:1313, 1973.
110. Stagg, G. V. and Millin, D. J., The nutritional and therapeutic value of tea — a review. *J. Sci. Food Agri.*, 26:1439, 1975.
111. Czok, G., Schmidt, B., Lang, K., Comparative animal experiments with coffee and tea. *Z. Ernahrung.*, 9:103, 1969.
112. Das, D. N., Ghosh, J. J., and Guha, B. C., Studies on tea. Part I. Nutritional aspects. *Ind. J. Appl. Chem.*, 27:6, 1964.

113. Ho, C. T. *Phenolic Compounds in Food and their Effects on Health I.* Ho, C. T., Lee, C. Y., and Huang, M. T., Eds., American Chemical Society, Washington D.C. 1992. pp. 2-7.
114. Yang, C. S. and Wang, Z.-Y., *J. National Cancer Inst.*, 85: 1038-1049, 1993.
115. Ding, Z.-H., Chen, Y., Zhou, M., and Fang, Y.-Z. *Chinese J. Pharm. Toxicol.* **6**: 263-266, 1992.
116. Kim, Y. H., Shim, J. S., Kang, M. H., Roh, J. K., Roberts, C., and Lee, I. P. *Proc. American Assoc. Cancer Res.* 34: abstract #3309, 1993.
117. Stich, H. F., Rosin, M. P., and Bryson, L., Inhibition of mutagenicity of a model nitrosation reaction by naturally occurring phenolics, coffee, and tea. *Muta. Res.*, 95:119, 1982.
118. Wang, Z.-Y., Hong, J.-Y., Huang, M-T., Reuhl, K. R., Conney, A. H., and Yang, C. S. *Cancer Res.*, 52: 1943-1947, 1992.
119. Glock, C. Y., Fiske, M., and Sills, D. L., They Changed to Tea, A Study in the Dynamics of Consumer Behavior, Columbia University Report, 1954.

Chapter 4

TEA IN CHINA

David Lee Hoffman

Tea is found in every shape and size, grown and processed everywhere across a wide belt throughout China. In the U.S., we are used to only a few types of tea; however, the varieties of *Camellia sinensis* found in China are almost endless. Each of them is given a name that often reflects the romantic and almost metaphysical nature of tea in Chinese culture. Probably nowhere else in the world is tea worshipped as a mystical and ceremonial beverage as in Asian countries, and especially in China, where *C. sinensis* finds its roots.

The flavors of Chinese teas range from extremely mild white teas to astringent green teas to heavy, black, strong-flavored varieties.

Often the leaves of *C. sinensis* are prepared in a very unique manner, such as in Tibet, where, for example, tea leaves are boiled overnight on an open fire, with a pinch of alkaline soda added. After the tea is strained, yak butter and salt are added and the concoction is vigorously pumped in a churn to a frothy brew. The tea is then poured back into the pot, reheated and served.

Table 1 lists Chinese names of teas and, when possible, their English translations, as well as the provinces in China where these teas are grown. Table 2 shows the many varieties of black, green, Oolong, Pu-erh, and white teas.

0-8493-2647-8/98/$0.00+$.50

TABLE 1

List of 85 Rare and Tribute Teas in the 1996 National Tea Competition in China

Province/name of tea	English translation	Farm name
Anhui Province		
Bai Bei Xiang Ya	Fragrant Buds	Jiunanshan Tea Plantation
Ci Shan Cui Kui	Ci Shan Green Shoot	Cishangang Tea Plantation
Ci Shan Jian Ya	Ci Shan Green Bud	Cishangang Tea Plantation
Ding Gu Da Fang		Wuhu Tea Corporation
Gan Lu Qing Feng	Sweet Dew Green Peak	Dongzhi Tea Plantation
Huang Hua Yun Jian		Lingou Tea Factory
Huang Shan Mao Feng		Wuhu Tea Corporation
Jing Shang Tian Hua	Add Flowers to the Brocade	Shexian Famous Tea
Jing Ting Lu Xue		Jing Ting Shan Tea
Jing Xian Ti Kui		Wuhu Tea Corporation
Jiu Shan Bi Hao	Jiu Shan White Hair	Jiunanshan Tea Plantation
Jiu Shan Cui Jian	Jiu Shan Green Sword	Jiunanshan Tea Plantation
Jiu Shan Cui Ya	Jiu Shan Green Bud	Jiunanshan Tea Plantation
Jiu Shan Qu She	Jiu Shan Bird Tongue	Jiunanshan Tea Plantation
Leu An Gua Pian		Jinzhai Tea Factory
Lu Mu Dan		Shexian Famous Tea
Rui Cao Kui		Shizipu Tea Plantation
Shen Quan Zhen Zhu Lu	Spring Green Pearl of the Gods	Dongzhi Tea Plantation
Tai Ping Hou Kui		Taiping Tea Corporation
Tan Kou Que She	Tang Kou Bird Tongue	Tangkou Tea Plantation
Wan Xi Zao Hua		Shuchen Tea Plantation
Xiang Shan Yun Jian		Dongzhi Tea Plantation
Ye Que She	Wild Bird Tongue	Tongnin Wushong Tea
Yong Xi Huo Qing		Wuhu Tea Plantation
Yong Xi Huo Qing		Yongxi Tea Factory
Yue Xi Cui Lan	Yue Xi Green Orchid	Yue Xi Tea Corporation
Fujian Province		
Bai Long Zhu		Yongan Tea Factory
Ge Heng Fu Xin Cha	Rich in Zinc Content Tea	Hanjiang Tea Plantation
Li Zhi Cha	Litchi Tea	Dengyun Tea Plantation
Guangxi Province		
Cha Lei	Flower Stamen	Baise Tea Factory
Cui Ye Cha	Green Leaves Tea	Jiangfunfeng Tea Factory
Nin Xiang Cei Min	Good Flavored Green Tea	Zhaopin Tea Factory
Guizhau Province		
Fan Jing You Lu	Best Green Tea in Fan Jing	Fan Jing Shan Tea
Fan Jing Cui Feng	Fan Jing Green Peak	Yin Jiang Tea Plantation
Fan Jing Xue Feng	Fan Jing Snow Peak	Fan Jing Shan Tea

TABLE 1 (continued)

List of 85 Rare and Tribute Teas in the 1996 National Tea Competition in China

Province/name of tea	English translation	Farm name
Henan Province		
Xing Yang Chun Hao	Xingyang Spring White Hair	Xingyang Famous Tea
Xing Yang Mao Jian		Xingyang Famous Tea
Xing Yang Xue Pian	Xing Yang Snowflake	Xingyang Famous Tea
Hubai Province		
Bao Quan Cha		Xianfeng Tea Factory
Jin Shui Cui Feng	Jin Shui Green Peak	Hubai Tea Research
Qing Long Que She	Like a Tongue of a Bird	Xianfeng Tea Factory
Song Feng Cha	Song Peak Tea	Yangloudong Tea
Song Feng Yun Wu	Song Feng Clouds & Mist	Yangloudong Tea
Jiangsu Province		
Bi Luo Chun	Green Snail in Spring	Dongnin Tea Plantation
Bi Luo Chun	Green Snail in Spring	Nanquan Tea Plantation
Dong Lin Mao Jian	Dong Lin Spear-Shape Tea	Donglin Tea Plantation
Er Qian Yin Hao	Er Qian Silver Hair Tea	Dafulin Tea Plantation
Er Qian Yin Hao	Er Qian White Hair Tea	Dafulin Tea Plantation
Tai Hu Cui Zhu		Xuelang Tea Plantation
Tai Hu Cui Zhu	Green Bamboo in Tai Hu Lake	Bashi Tea Plantation
Wu Xi Hao Cha	Wu Xi White Hair Tea	Jiangsu Bashi Tea
Xi Mei Hao Cha	Xi Mei White Hair Tea	Meiyuan Tea Factory
Xue Lang You Lu	Best Green Tea in Xue Lang	Xuelang Tea Plantation
Yin Hu Hao Cha	Yin Lake White Hair Tea	Yaojin Tea Factory
Yixing Chun Yue	Yixing Spring Moon	Shanjuan Tea Factory
Jiangxi Province		
Xiao Bu Yan Cha		Xiaobu Tea Farm
Sichuan Province		
Fu Xi Hua Cha	Rich in Selenium Flower Tea	Tianxiang Tea Factory
Tian Gong Cui Lu		Huangshan Tea Plantation
Yunnan Province		
Zu He Tuo Cha	Combined Tuo Cha	Kunming Lubao Tea
Zhejiang Province		
Bai Mu Dan	White Peony	Jinghua Tea Factory
Chen Tian Zue Long	Chen Tian Snow Dragon	Xuelong Tea Plantation
Da Fo Long Jing		Xingchang Famous Tea

TABLE 1 (continued)

List of 85 Rare and Tribute Teas in the 1996 National Tea Competition in China

Province/name of tea	English translation	Farm name
Dao Ren Feng Cha	Taoist Peak Tea	Dao Ren Feng Tea
Dong Keng Cha		Linmu Tea Factory
Fun Yun Qu Hoa	Curly White Hair	Lishui Famous Tea Factory
Hu Yuan Yun Lu		Xinghe Tea Factory
Jing Jiang Hui Ming		Yuhang Famous Tea
Kai Hua Long Ding		Kaihua Tea Experiment
Lin An Cui Lan		Linan Tea Factory
Lin Hai Pan Hao		Linhai Pan Hao Tea
Lu Mu Dan	Green Peony	Jiangshan Tea Plantation
Ping Yang Lu Yun	Ping Yang Green Cloud	Pingyang Tea Plantation
Qian Yu Gao Lu	Qian Yu High Grade Green Tea	Yuhang Tea Factory
San Bei Xiang		Taishueng Farm
Song Yang Yin Hou	Silver Monkey	Songyang Tea Factory
Sui Chang Gao Liu	Sui Chang High Grade	Sui Chang Tea Corporation
Tai Shun Cui Long	Tai Shun Green Dragon	Taishun Tea Plantation
Tian Mu Shan Qing Ding	Tian Mu Shan Green Peak	Linan Tea Factory
Wu Lin Cha	Wu Peak Tea	Xiongfeng Tea Factory
Xi Hu Long Jing	West Lake Yellow Dragon	Tea Research Institute
Xian Yu Cui Ya	Xian Yu Green Bud	Xianyu Tea Plantation
Xue Shui Lu Ya	Snow Water Green Bud	Tonglu Tea Factory
Xue Shui Yun Lu		Xinhe Tea Factory
Ying Guo Cha	Silver Hook	Jinyun Tea Plantation
Yun He Lu Shuang		Yunhe Tea Plantation

Reproduced with permission of Silk Road Teas.

TABLE 2

Examples of Varieties of Black, Green, Oolong, Pu-erh, and White Chinese Teas

Name of Tea	Province
Black Tea	
Golden Monkey	Fujian
Golden Needle	Fujian
Guangdong Black	Guangdong
Hunan Brick Tea	Hunan
Jiantsu Mountain Red	Jiangsu
Leubao Black	Guangxi
Zhejiang Black	Zhejiang
Green Tea	
Anhui Green	Southern Anhui
Bi Luo Chun	Fujian
Bi Luo Chun	Zhejiang
Bi Luo Chun "Snow"	Northern Fujian
Dragon Peak Rare Green Tea	Zhejiang
Dragon Pearls	Fujian
Dragon Tooth	Fujian
Dragon Well	Zhejiang
Farmer Yang's Green	Zhejiang
Fujian Mao Feng	Fujian
Golden Dragon	Zhejiang
Green Pearls	Fujian
Green Sea Anemone	Anhui
Huangshan Mao Feng	Anhui
Huangshan Maojian	Southern Anhui
Jade Spring	Zejiang
Kiahua Long Ding	Zhejiang
Litchi Nut	Fujian
Rare Anhui Green	Southern Anhui
Rare Fujian Green	Fujian
Snow Dragon	Zhejiang
Spring Blossom Pekoe	Fujian
Spring Bud Rosette	Zhejiang
Spring Bud Rosette	Fujian
Spring Bud Wafer	Zhejiang
Taiping Hou Kui	Anhui
Tongyu Mountain Green	Fujian
Yang Xian	Jiangsu
Yellow Mountain Green	Southern Anhui
Yellow Mountain Green	Southern Fujian
Zhejiang Mao Feng	Zhejiang
Oolong Tea	
Anxi Oolong	Fujian
Ben Shan	Fujian
Dai Bamboo	Yunnan
Dragon Balls	Fujian

TABLE 2 (continued)

Examples of Varieties of Black, Green, Oolong, Pu-erh, and White Chinese Teas

Name of Tea	Province
Dragon Beard	Fujian
Golden Water Turtle	Fujian
Hairy Crab	Fujian
Huangshan Mao Feng	Anhui
Jade Oolong	Fujian
Phoenix Select	Fujian
Ti Kwan Yin	Fujian
Ti Kwan Yin	Southern Fujian
Pu-Erh Tea	
Beencha Pu-erh	Yunnan
Pu-erh	Yunnan
Pu-erh Beencha '88	Yunnan
Pu-erh Tuocha "Camel"	Yunnan
Tibetan Mushroom Pu-erh	Yunnan
White Tea	
Baihao Cha	Fujian
Drum Mountain White Cloud	Fujian
Fujian White Tea	Northern Fujian
Gold Tip Silver Needle	Northern Fujian
Green Leaf Silver Needle	Zhejiang
Silver Needle	Fujian
White Peony	Fujian

Reproduced with permission of Silk Road Teas.

Chapter 5

The Coffee Plant and Its Processing

Monica Alton Spiller

CONTENTS

0-8493-2647-8/98/$0.00+$.50

I. INTRODUCTION

Outlines of coffee cultivation and the production of coffee ready for use as a beverage are presented in this chapter.[1-7] It is hoped that the information given, in conjunction with Chapter 6, will serve as a background for those studying the physiological effects of coffee. Coffee is such a variable and complex beverage that it seems imperative that the coffee used in a biological study should be defined. In particular, is the coffee Arabica or Robusta? Was the coffee wet- or dry-processed? What are the extent and conditions of the roasting? Decaffeinated and instant coffees need separate consideration and description.

An attempt has been made to bring out any variations there may be in processing methodology that would produce a different chemical pattern in the final beverage.

II. COFFEE: BOTANY, CULTIVATION, AND DISTRIBUTION

The two main species of commercial interest in the genus *Coffea* are *Coffea arabica* and *Coffea canephora* var. *robusta*. They are conveniently referred to as Arabica and Robusta, respectively. Each genus covers a number of varietals; there are at least 13 varieties of Arabica coffees, for example. The genus is in the botanical family of *Rubiaceae*.

A. *Coffea arabica*

Coffea arabica is a glossy-leaved shrub or small tree with fragrant white flowers and red berry fruit. It was introduced into Arabia, in Yemen, in the fifteenth century where it soon became used as the preferred beverage. *C. arabica* is actually indigenous to Ethiopia, Arabia's neighbor across the Red Sea. The Dutch, French, and English introduced *C. arabica* into their tropical colonies from the late seventeenth century onwards. By 1723, Brazil had obtained seed and to this day Brazil is one of the world's major suppliers of coffee.

The growth of *C. arabica* is best between the two tropics, but at an elevation such that the temperature does not rise much above 72°F or below 64°F and where the rainfall is fairly evenly spread throughout the year and is 40 to 60 in. The usual elevation is 4,000 to 5,000 ft. It can tolerate cooler temperatures but is killed by frost. Shading of the plants does not seem essential, although some shading prevents overbearing and weakening of the trees. Mulching is advantageous so that the roots are kept cool. For the most part, when *C. arabica is* grown in these conditions it is relatively disease-resistant, but where it has been planted at a warmer and wetter elevation the plants have been lost to fungal disease. In particular, the leaf spot disease *Hemileia vastatrix* has caused great losses. Plantations that thrived initially in Sri Lanka have been essentially destroyed by this disease. In Brazil during the mid-1970s vast plantations were lost to frost damage.

B. *Coffea canephora* var. *robusta*

Coffea canephora var. *robusta* was not recognized until 1895, when it was seen as the indigenous *Coffea* species in the African Congo. C. *canephora* var. *robusta* thrives at elevations between the tropics, where the rainfall is about 75 in. and the temperature is 60 to 80°F. Optimal rainfall and temperature conditions favored by the two species are very similar; the distinction comes in the tolerance of more extreme conditions. C. *canephora* var. *robusta* can tolerate more humid conditions without being attacked by *Hemileia vastatrix,* for example.

C. World Distribution of Plantations and Markets

Coffee is grown in countries situated between the Tropics of Capricorn and Cancer. C. *arabica* is the most widely grown, but regions where temperature and humidity are rather high have been replanted with C. *canephora* var. *robusta.* Robusta coffees are thus the major species grown in the less mountainous regions closest to the equator.

Production of coffee in Brazil was 42% of the world crop in 1960. However, by 1980, although the actual amount was still high, Brazil's proportional contribution to world exports was halved. African Robusta coffees instead now represent over 25% of all coffee used in the U.S. and Europe.

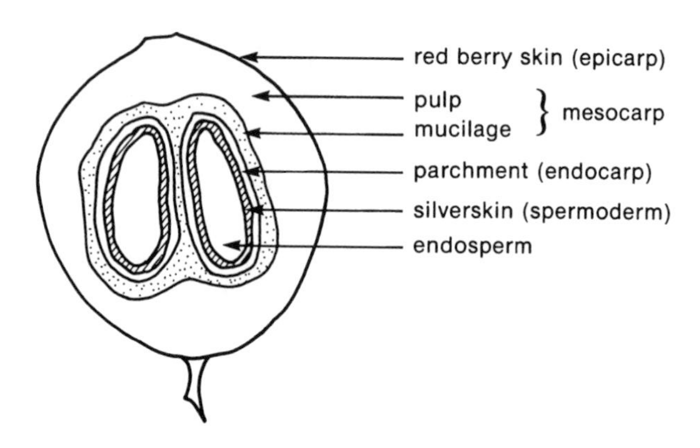

FIGURE 1
The coffee berry in a cross-sectional diagram.

Per capita consumption of coffee has been steadily decreasing in the U.S. and Sweden, despite an overall increase in coffee production. This increase is taken up by the increase in population and the increased popularity of coffee in Japan, the Soviet Union, and the U.K.

III. COFFEE PROCESSING

A. Green Coffee Bean Processing

The production of green coffee beans involves successive removal of the outermost red skin and the pulp of the coffee berry, followed by removal of the mucilage, parchment covering, and, finally, the silverskin surrounding the green coffee bean (endosperm) (Figure 1).

There are two methods currently used to produce green coffee beans; they will be described here as the "wet" and the "dry" methods. However, an alternative nomenclature is often used: "washed" and "natural processing", respectively, and to avoid a misunderstanding it is often necessary to obtain a definition of the processing used on a given batch of coffee beans.

1. Green Coffee Bean Processing by the Wet Method

This is relatively intricate and is best carried out with uniformly ripe coffee berries that are still firm. To achieve this uniformity the coffee berries are selectively handpicked. As soon as possible they are sorted further in a water-flotation system and sent directly to a pulping machine. Here the berries have the outermost skin and pulp removed and the mucilage layer is exposed.

Removal of the mucilage is brought about in concrete fermentation tanks, where the beans are slurried with water. A fermentation occurs that is mainly due to lactobacilli and yeasts. Enzymes are produced that dissolve away the mucilage. The beans are washed free from the mucilage and the parchment layer is exposed. Now the beans are dried in the sun or more usually in mechanical driers. Hulling completes the process. The parchment layer and most of the silverskin are removed in a hulling machine. Green coffee beans produced in this way are now ready for storage and shipping.

2. *Green Coffee Bean Processing by the Dry Method*

Ideally in this process the coffee berries should be uniformly ripened, but often in practice they are harvested by stripping all the berries at once from the trees and collecting them on the ground beneath. The berries are gathered from the ground and spread out in the sun where they are raked so that they are evenly exposed. Initially the microorganisms and the enzymes inherent in the coffee berry alter the pulp and mucilage. Then the red skin, pulp, mucilage, and parchment fuse to produce a thick hull as they dry out. The coffee is called "pergamino" at this stage. This hull is removed in a hulling machine that simultaneously polishes off most of the silverskin layer. Both Arabica and Robusta coffees can be processed in this way, but an additional step is necessary for the Robusta beans, which have a particularly tough silverskin. Before the tough silverskin can be removed, the beans must be soaked in water. The moistened silverskin can then be removed mechanically and the beans are dried again before storage and shipping.

The dry method produces green coffee beans much less expensively than the wet method. A high proportion of Brazilian Arabica coffee is processed in this way, and almost all Robusta coffees are treated in this way. The final beverage produced from dry-processed coffee has a full flavor that is often described as hard and sometimes is characteristic of a region, for example Rio coffees.

The dry method is generally the less controlled of the two main methods. The stages where extra care could be introduced after harvesting are where the coffee berries may be washed and sorted by flotation before being dried and during the drying itself. The risk of fungal damage to the berries and consequently to the beans is very high if the berries are too heaped. They need to be spread out very thinly, to be frequently raked, and not resoaked by rainfall.

B. Storage and Shipment of Green Coffee Beans

Ideally, coffee is bagged with a standard moisture content of 12%, in the country of origin, and it is kept below 70°F until close to the time when it can be placed on a ship. Some coffee is also stored in silos, but this is usually just for a few days. The coffee beans need to be stored at low temperatures once on-board ship, and away from any strong-smelling cargo. Ideally, the journey would be as short as possible and any subsequent movement of the beans would be at 70°F and low humidity. This is quite difficult to achieve in practice and the risk of developing molds is high. Another risk is that compounds will be leached or volatilized from the green coffee beans so that they will not yield a pleasing beverage. Green coffee beans are reasonably stable for one year at 70°F and 40 to 60% relative humidity.

C. Decaffeination

Decaffeination of green coffee beans is most usually carried out with a water/solvent partition system. The green coffee beans are first steamed until they are hot, wet, and swollen, to make the caffeine available. Solvent is then used to extract the caffeine out of the aqueous phase of the beans. Finally, the beans are steamed to drive off residual solvent. The coffee beans lose their wax surface covering in the process, as well as some flavor components. For this reason, the Robusta and Brazilian Arabica coffees that are dry-processed and have the most powerful flavors are usually the types that are decaffeinated. They become milder in the process. Mechanical polishing is used to improve the appearance of decaffeinated green coffee beans if they are not to be roasted immediately. Extra care is required, however, to store these decaffeinated beans since the loss of wax covering as well as caffeine renders them much more susceptible to fungal attack.

Methylene chloride is probably the most generally used solvent for decaffeination processes, but others, some of which are already found in small amounts in coffee beans, are coming into use. For example, ethyl acetate,[8] formaldehyde-dimethylacetal, ethanol, methanol, acetone,[9] propane,[10] benzyl alcohol,[11] carbon dioxide,[12] and supercritical carbon dioxide with an acid[13] are used. Generally the pressure and temperature of the system are adjusted to keep the solvent in the liquid state. Coffee oil itself is even described for this use in one patent.[14]

A great deal of effort has been put into methods for removing only the caffeine from the extracting solvent, and somehow returning all of the other components to the coffee beans for reabsorption. The principle of the method most generally seen involves exposure of the extract-laden solvent to a caffeine-specific adsorbent. Once the solvent has been treated in this way, it is returned to remove more caffeine. However, the solvent is already saturated with the other solvent-soluble components and does not extract them from the second and subsequent batches of steamed green coffee beans. Adsorbants used for this purpose include activated char-

TABLE 1

Coffee Roasting Styles Correlated with Approximate Value for Green Coffee Bean Weight Loss, Color, and Temperature

Roast style	Green bean weight loss (%)	Final color	Final temperature (°F)
Light city	14	Cinnamon	390
City	15	Brown	410
Full city	15.5	Deep brown	
Brazilian	16		
Viennese	17	Dark brown	
French	18	Very dark brown with oil on surface	440
Ice	19		
Italian	20	Extremely dark brown to black, shiny oil on surface	465

coal,[15-17] resins,[18-20] clay,[21] and treated carob pods.[22] In yet another scheme, sucrose solution, instead of water, is partitioned with the chosen solvent. Caffeine is still extracted, but the taste of the final beverage is improved.[16,23] The subtleties of the individual methods are guarded by numerous patents. Microbiological and electrochemical methods to remove caffeine specifically have also been developed.[24,25]

D. Roasting, Grinding, and Storage of Roasted Coffee

1. Roasting

Green coffee contains about 12% water and most of this is lost in the early stages of roasting, followed by a loss of up to 8% of the dry bean material. The total loss in roasting is therefore 14 to 20%. In general, bean color indicates the extent of this loss, and bean temperatures can be correlated with these color changes. While water is still present the bean remains light in color, but by the time the bean temperature has risen to 465°F, the bean is extremely dark brown and has decreased in weight by about 20%. These correlations and some of the names given to roasting extents are given in Table 1. Eight color grades are distinguishable.

Roast style is a matter of personal taste, but for the most part the mildest Arabica coffees are the lightest roasted. Some Arabica coffees even become bitter if they are roasted to too high a temperature. Dry-processed Robustas and Brazilian Arabicas, on the other hand, benefit from deeper roasting.

The present largest Jabez Burns coffee roasters in the U.S. were brought into use around 1950. They are continuous in operation. Hot gases at

500°F, produced by natural gas combustion in air, are used to heat the beans in a perforated steel rotating drum. Relatively small quantities at a time are heated for a total of only 5 min. When the beans have reached the selected internal temperature and corresponding color, they have already been moved through the oven to a heat lock. At this point they are released and rapidly cooled, with a fine water spray or air draft, so that further pyrolytic changes in the bean are prevented.

The economy of this method is enhanced by the recycling of the hot gases that have passed over and from the beans. However, it is known that this practice causes changes in the compounds lost from the coffee, and a lot of soot and tar are produced. If some of this soot and tar coats the coffee beans, there will be a significant increase in their aromatic and polycyclic content. The beverage produced will no longer have a clean taste. Darker roasts, which produce more oil and combustible volatiles, need extra supervision, so that only the lighter roasts are most usually prepared in this system.

Another economy sometimes practiced in this process is that of spraying enough water to cool the beans, as well as to compensate for some of the weight loss that occurs during roasting.

The chaff, which is the bean silverskin caught in the fold of the bean, flies off the bean during roasting and can be collected, pelletized, and mixed with roasted beans which are to be ground, even though it may impart a bitter flavor to the final beverage.

One of the major advantages seen in this method is the relatively low temperature, 500°F, to which the coffee is exposed. An earlier version of these roasters brought out in 1935 subjects the beans to a temperature of 850°F.

A high proportion of coffee in the U.S. is produced in this way. However, some roasters have been designed to have a once-through hot gas flow. One example is that designed by Sivetz.

German coffee-roasting equipment (Probat or Gothot) is quite different from that made in the U.S. The rotating steel drum holding the coffee beans is solid and has a double wall so that heat can be supplied by passing hot gases between the cylinder walls. Hot gases can also be passed into the cylinder from one end. No recycling of coffee effluent or hot gases occurs. At the end of the roast, the beans are discharged into a cooling cart. Roasting time is 10 min at the most.

It is evident that different roasting practices will produce a variety of chemical effects in the bean. Recycling of hot effluent gases, perforation of the rotating drum, and use of radiant heat will each give different chemical character to the final roasted coffee bean.

Yet another consideration is the fact that the sugar content of the beans causes roast variation. For example, high-grown Arabica coffees have the highest relative sucrose content and these will achieve the darkest roast under a set of specified conditions.

2. Grinding and Storage of Roasted Coffee

The most generally used industrial grinders are roll and breaker bar systems. The roasted beans are rolled past toothed rollers, where they are cut. A series of these rollers gives a successively finer grind. Any chaff that separates is reground and mixed in with the ground coffee beans. Inclusion of the chaff tends to impart a bitter flavor to the coffee and the mixing process contributes to oil release from the ground bean particles and early staling. Other systems used on a large scale are hammer mills with cutting blades.

The roasted beans need to be cool, hard, and brittle. Light-roast beans are relatively pliable and tend to be flattened rather than ground. Dark-roasted beans grind the most readily. Large amounts of carbon dioxide are released from roasted coffee, along with other volatile compounds, during the grinding process. These afford temporary protection to the freshly ground coffee from the oxygen and moisture in the air. Ground coffee is usually extracted or packed within 8 h of grinding. It is best stored in an evacuated and sealed container; roasted and ground coffee stored in this way best resists staling if it is kept at -10°F (-20°C). When roasted and ground coffee is stored in an evacuated and sealed container, its shelf life is of the order of weeks at room temperatures. Whole roasted coffee beans, however, have a shelf life of the order of months with respect to staling.[26]

E. Instant Coffee Production

In outline, a percolation process is used to produce an aqueous coffee extract, which in turn is dehydrated to yield water-soluble solids. Instant and soluble coffees are synonymous for these water-soluble coffee extract solids. Usually some of the volatile aroma and flavor compounds, which are lost during the processing, are added back immediately before packaging.

1. Percolation

Roasted and ground coffee is packed into columns and percolated by the passage of hot water under pressure at about 340°F. The use of pressurized boiling water not only brings about the dissolution of the most readily water-soluble coffee extractables, it also causes the solubilization and possibly the hydrolysis of complex carbohydrates. Water-soluble compounds of a smaller molecular weight are produced. The extent of possible hydrolysis is enhanced by the inherent acidity of the coffee extract as it passes through the column. The pH in the spent grounds can be as low as 3.4. The presence of these hydrolyzed carbohydrates gives a total yield of 36% or more water-soluble extract from the original roasted and ground coffee, compared with 21% using boiling water under normal atmospheric pressures. These hydrolyzed carbohydrates are used as the bulk on which the more flavorful part of the extract can be adsorbed and they are the body of the final free-flowing powder. Occasionally the coffee is defatted prior to this type of percolation, with a resultant 30% increase in extractable solubles. The final product is bulkier, but this is not necessarily an advantage.

Optimization of this percolation process involves using a roast, usually somewhat lighter than a French roast. This is ground to a particle size that gives suitable flow characteristics for the extracting water as it passes through the columns. Ideally the finest particles act as a filter for unwanted tars and remain evenly distributed throughout the columns without causing compacting. Contact time with the coffee is 20 to 30 min in each of a series of six columns, so that each batch of coffee extract is produced in about 3 h. The solution issuing from the columns is cooled to 40°F to reduce the loss of volatile flavor compounds and to prevent microbial growth.

Dehydration is effected as soon as possible after the extract leaves the percolation columns, but still after the elapse of enough time for some sedimentation to occur. The sediment is discarded.

2. Spray Drying

One of the most widely used spray-drying techniques for coffee extract involves spraying percolated coffee extract at 40°F into the top of a baffled tower of hot air at 480°F initially. The cooler wet air is removed toward the bottom of the tower and finally a powder of the coffee extract solids leaves the tower at about 90°F. These solids are in the form of hollow beads and contain 3% moisture.

Variations in equipment and techniques can be used to retain the aroma and flavor volatiles. In one scheme, the coffee extract is fractionated. The first fraction obtained from the percolation columns is rich in the most volatile components. The second fraction contains the simple sugars and the final fraction contains larger molecular weight compounds resulting from carbohydrate hydrolysis, as well as polymerized sugars and proteins. By spray drying the second and third fractions initially and then combining these with the first fraction, the volatile aroma and flavor compounds are more likely to be retained, by adsorption onto the carbohydrates. The hollow of the spray-dried beads is also important as a haven for the flavor and aroma compounds. The trapping of these compounds in this way can be optimized by bead size selection and the prevention of agglomeration. In general, however, aroma and flavor volatiles are lost and a mild-tasting product leaves the spray-drying equipment.

The dry-processed coffees, especially Robustas, are often selected for the production of instant coffees since they have less-popular powerful flavors that are rendered mild in the production of an instant coffee. There is also economy in the use of Robusta coffees in this way, since they are produced much less expensively than wet-processed Arabicas. Before the instant coffee is marketed, it can be flavored with the coffee oil obtained from a wet-processed Arabica coffee to improve the acceptability of the product.

3. Freeze Drying

As a coffee extract freezes, the soluble coffee solids separate out. During freeze drying the water separates as ice, and it can be removed by sublimation under vacuum. Various systems are available to do this. In general, the coffee solids are produced as flakes or as a slab, which is then broken up and granulated so that it has the appearance of roasted and ground coffee beans. Freeze drying is a more expensive process than spray drying, but offers the advantages of very quickly producing soluble flakes, even in cold water, as well as retained "brew colloids". These contribute to a smoother-tasting, richer, and slightly opaque-looking final beverage. However, volatile aroma and flavor compounds are lost from the coffee during freeze drying just as they are during spray-drying processes. Therefore, the less expensive dry-processed Robusta and Brazilian Arabica coffees are most generally used. The loss of some harsher and less-acceptable flavor and aroma compounds is an advantage. The product is relatively mild and can still have flavor compounds added.

Freeze-drying conditions can be optimized, however, and where there is a demand, the very best coffees can be used to yield a final beverage that is very close in quality to freshly brewed roast and ground coffee prepared from the same beans.

4. Flavor and Aroma Addition

Spray- and freeze-dried coffee extracts have generally lost their original volatile flavor and aroma compounds. Several techniques for collecting the flavor and aroma components that are given off during roasting, grinding, and percolation have been developed so that the "flavor and aroma" can be added back to the soluble coffee before it is packaged. These aroma and flavor compounds must be protected from moisture and oxygen during short storage times and they must be added back as late as possible before packaging the soluble coffee in evacuated or inert gas-filled containers.

Solvent-extracted coffee oil contains about half the lipids present in freshly roasted and ground coffee; this coffee oil carries with it a high proportion of the flavor and aroma compounds. The most volatile solvents are preferred over halogenated hydrocarbons, which may be incompletely stripped from the coffee oil at a later stage. Thus, preferred solvents for the extraction of coffee oil include carbon dioxide, methane, ethane, and methylamine, often in mixtures to span the polarity range of the compounds to be extracted. The dangers of using nitrous oxide as a supercritical fluid for extracting materials such as coffee, became obvious when an explosion occurred during an attempted extraction.[27] Alcohols and aldehydes are also used in mixed solvent systems, to specifically extract the flavor and aroma compounds. Once the solvents have been stripped away, usually to be recycled, a coffee oil remains that is quite reasonably stable, since it is dry. This oil can be stored under refrigeration without undue loss or degeneration of flavor and aroma compounds.

Expelled coffee oil differs from solvent-extracted coffee oil in that it can only be produced from roasted coffee that has been softened by steam treatment. The oil is expelled at temperatures close to 180°F. Expelled coffee oil quickly stales unless the densest fraction is centrifuged away.

Both solvent-extracted and expelled coffee oils can be sprayed directly onto soluble coffee solids. The oil is adsorbed without degradation, provided moisture and oxygen are absent. However, the most volatile compounds do tend to leave the coffee powder and fill the head space of the container.

Methods of "fixing" the volatile aroma and flavor compounds separately from the instant coffee powder have been developed. The volatile mixture can be mixed with aqueous gelatin or gum arabic and spray dried. The oily droplets of the flavor and aroma compounds are coated with gelatin or gum arabic in a dry lattice. This powder can be mixed in with instant coffee powder and is relatively stable in the presence of air. Emulsification with sugar is also a highly effective way of trapping and preserving coffee volatiles, but is of limited use for instant coffees.

IV. COFFEE BEVERAGES

A. Coffee Beverage Preparation Methods

1. Ideal Preparation Methods

The coffee beans with the most desirable flavor to many tastes are the highest grown Arabicas prepared by the wet method. Coffee beverages need to be prepared within 8 h of grinding the freshly roasted coffee beans if the volatile flavor and aroma compounds are to be retained. Brew preparation is best when the ground coffee is thoroughly wet by 200°F water, but then drained from the water within 3 min. The amount of coffee used should correspond to 40 to 50 cups of beverage per pound of roast and ground coffee. A standard brew uses 5 g/100 ml of water. Examples of methods for producing coffee beverage under these conditions are the steeping and draining through a flannel or muslin bag (quador) as used in Brazil, and the espresso methods of Italy, provided only stainless steel or ceramic surfaces are exposed to the coffee.

In the early 1980s the observation was made that Norwegian boiled coffee tended to raise serum cholesterol, whereas filtered coffee did not. From this it was discovered that it is the coffee oils that contain the cholesterol raising factors, cafestol and kahweol. So, coffee making methods that remove these oils from the brew are desirable. These oils are successfully removed from the coffee brew by paper and, presumably, cloth filters. The cake of spent coffee grounds resulting from espresso coffee preparation also holds back at least some of these damaging coffee oils, from the final cup of coffee beverage. Turkish and Greek style coffee beverages contain all of the oils extracted during the brewing.[28-30]

2. *Water for Coffee Beverage Preparation*

The quality of an ideally prepared coffee beverage can still be reduced or even spoiled if the water quality affects the coffee. Hardness is one of the main problems in the U.S. because it is usually associated with alkalinity. The acidity, which is a substantial part of the flavor character of coffee, is partly neutralized by hard water. Ion-exchange softened water is even worse, since the excess sodium ions present form soaps with the fatty acids in the roasted coffee. Demineralization of the water is the most effective way to obtain water for the preparation of a clean-flavored cup of coffee in hard-water areas. Oxygen in the water is easily removed by boiling. Chlorine in the water can spoil the flavor of a good coffee, as can organic matter and metal ions, such as iron and copper.

3. *Other Preparation Equipment*

The use of copper and iron for coffee brewing equipment produces a dark color and an off flavor, presumably as a result of their interaction with coffee phenols. Aluminum is frequently used for brewing equipment but it has the disadvantage of being dissolved into the brew.[31,32] American home percolators made from aluminum do corrode.

Filter papers offer advantages in clean up and preparation of a clear beverage. Ideally the filter papers should be made from carefully chosen paper, that is, for example, dioxin-free.[33] They should be stored so that they cannot pick up foreign odors that might be transferred from the filter to the coffee brew.

4. *Coffee Blends*

The coffees commanding the highest prices are also those with the most desirable taste quality. An order of decreasing value for some coffees follows: wet-processed high-grown and then low-grown Arabicas, followed by dry-processed Arabicas and Robustas. Blends are made, in general, to reduce the cost.

B. Comparison of Beverages from Arabica and Robusta Coffees

In the U.S. the per capita consumption of coffee has declined by one-third since 1960. Parallel with this has been a change in the proportion of Robusta coffees imported into the U.S. In 1950 only 6% of the imported coffees were Robustas whereas by 1975, 35% were Robustas. In the 1950s, Robustas were mainly used for instant coffee; now they also constitute a significant part of the roast and ground coffee blends. These Robustas are used to the highest extent in vending machines, restaurants, decaffeinated blends, and instant coffees.

One of the most significant differences between Arabica and Robusta coffees is in the caffeine content. Robusta coffees contain almost twice the caffeine found in Arabica coffees. There are some other differences recognized thus far: Robustas contain almost no sucrose and only very small amounts of the kaurane and furokaurane-type diterpenes; they contain higher proportions of phenols, complex carbohydrates (both soluble and hydrolyzable), volatile fatty acids on roasting, and sulfur compounds, all in comparison with Arabicas. References to these distinctions can be found in Chapter 6 of this book.

C. Instant Coffee Beverages

Instant coffee beverages are markedly different from coffee prepared from roast and ground coffee directly. As has already been described in Section III.E, instant coffees contain extra water-soluble carbohydrates obtained from hydrolyzed complex carbohydrates. The high extraction rate means that about 100 cups of instant coffee can be prepared from 1 lb of coffee, compared with 40 to 50 cups per pound of normally brewed coffee.

Additionally Robusta coffees are frequently used to prepare instant coffees and the result is a distinctly brown beverage; Arabicas give a reddish colored beverage.

If the instant coffee has been spray-dried, then the brew colloids will have been broken down and the beverage will have lost some of its "smoothness". The generally mild taste of instant coffees is usually offset by the addition of flavor and aroma compounds from roasted and ground coffee just before packaging.

D. Decaffeinated Coffee Beverages

Methods for the decaffeination of green coffee beans, mainly with solvents after a steaming, have already been described. Even with the selective adsorption techniques to remove only caffeine, it is unlikely that the full character of the starting beans can be realized in a final decaffeinated beverage; the result is that Robusta coffees are generally used to prepare decaffeinated coffee. The cost is kept down and the treatment, anyway, reduces any harsh or bitter flavor that the Robusta coffee may have had. The resulting beverage will be relatively caffeine-free, but Robusta coffee will contribute more soluble carbohydrates, phenols, and volatile fatty acids, and much less of the diterpenes found in Arabica coffees.

V. CONCLUSIONS

Coffee is a widely variable beverage. The parameters necessary to define a particular beverage include the coffee species, altitude of growth, method for green bean production, manner and style of roasting, and brewing method or soluble coffee technique applied. Further considerations include the uses made of pesticides and the storage conditions of the green and of the roasted coffee.

ACKNOWLEDGMENTS

The author would like to thank Dr. Kenneth Hirsh and Dr. William Ryder for reading an earlier edition of this chapter, written in 1983, and offering many helpful comments.

REFERENCES

1 Sivetz, M. and Desrosier, N. W., *Coffee Technology*, AVI, Westport, 1979.
2 Haarer, A. K., *Modern Coffee Production*, Leonard Hill, London, 1962.
3 Schapira, J., Schapira, D., and Schapira, K., *The Book of Coffee and Tea*, St. Martin's, New York, 1975.

4 Wilbaux, R., *Farm Products Processing, Informal Working Bulletin Number 20, Agricultural Engineering, Coffee Processing*, Rome: Agricultural Engineering Branch, Land and Water Development Division, Food and Agriculture Organization of the United Nations, 1963.
5 Illy, A. and Vianni, R., Eds., *Espresso Coffee: The Chemistry of Quality*, Academic Press, London, 1995.
6 Clarke, R. J. and Macrae, R., Eds., *Coffee Volume 2: Technology, Coffee*, Elsevier Applied Science, London, 1987.
7 Clarke, R. J. and Macrae, R., Eds., *Coffee Volume 4: Agronomy*, Elsevier Applied Science, London, 1987.
8 Anon, Secondary direct food additives permitted in food for human consumption; ethyl acetate. Fed Regist 47(2, BK. 1),145, 1982. (CA96:67362v)
9 Peter, S. and Brunner, G., Decaffeinating coffee with solvents at high pressure, Ger. Offen. 2,737,794, 1979. (CA90:150500k)
10 Coenen, H. and Kriegel, E., Decaffeination of raw coffee, Ger. Offen. 2,846,976, 1980. (CA93:44393e)
11 Strobel, R. G. K., Caffeine free coffee. Ger Offen 2,740,628, 1978. (CA89:4867y)
12 Studiengesellschaft Kohle m.b.h, Decaffeinating coffee. Belg 856,955, 1978. (CA89:4866x)
13 Kazlas, P. T., Novak, R. D., and Robey, R. J., Supercritical carbon dioxide decaffeination of acidified coffee, U. S. 5,288,511, 1994. (CA120:190235x)
14 Fout, G. W., Mishkin, A. R., and Roychoudhury, R. N., Decaffeinization of plant material, Ger Offen, 2,651,128, 1977. (CA87:66878v)
15 Green, D. and Blanc, M., Caffeine adsorption, Eur. Pat. Appl. EP 40,712, 1981. (CA96:84409h)
16 Fischer, A. and Kummer, P., Decaffeinization of raw coffee, Eur. Pat. Appl. 8,398, 1980. (CA93:24812n)
17 Heilmann, W., A modified Secoffex process for green bean decaffeination, *Colloq. Sci. Int. Cafe*, 14th, 349, 1992. (CA117:110460s)
18 Blanc, M. and Margolis, G., Caffeine extraction, Eur. Pat. Appl. EP 49,357, 1982. (CA97:22433y)
19 Kramer, F., Henig, Y. S., Garin, T. A., and Vogel, G. J., Selective adsorption from solutions such as coffee extracts, UK Pat. Appl. 2,027,576, 1980. (CA93:69060g)
20 Thijssen, H. A. C., Selective extraction of a number of soluble components contained in a fine- granular material, Ger. Offen. 2,832,360, 1979. (CA90:170823w)
22 Farr, D. R. and Horman, I., Treatment of an aqueous extract of plant material for reducing the content of caffeine and/or chlorogenic acid, Ger. Offen. 2,826,466, 1979. (CA90:166789x)
22 Sakanaka, S. and Nakamura, I., Removal of caffeine from solutions with clay, Jpn. Kokai Tokkyo Koho JP 06,142,405, 1994. (CA121:156270r)
23 Lando, F. and Teitelbaum, C. L., Decaffeinated coffee of improved flavor, US 4,044,162, 1977. (CA87: 166375x)
24 Farr, D. R., Decaffeination method, Patentschrift (Switzerland) CH 626,791, 1981. (CA96: 121244y)
25 Kummer, P., Caffeine removal, Swiss 623,994, 1981. (CA95:131206f)
26 Clarke, R. J., The shelf life of coffee, *Dev. Food Sci., 33(Shelf Life Studies of Foods and Beverages)*, 801, 1993. (CA121:33355q)
27 Raynie, D. E., Warning concerning the use of nitrous oxide in supercritical fluid extractions, *Anal. Chem.*, 65(21), 3127, 1993. (CA119:187552x)
28 Katan, M. B. and Urgert, R., The cholesterol-elevating factor from coffee beans, *Colloq. Sci. Int. Cafe*, 16th (Vol.1), 49, 1995. (CA124:173701m)
29 Peters, A., Brewing [of coffee] makes the difference, *Colloq. Sci. Int. Cafe*, 14th, 165, 1992. (CA117:47053u)

30 Ratnayake, W. M. N., Hollywood, R., O'Grady, E., and Stavric, B., Lipid content and composition of coffee brews prepared by different methods, *Food Chem. Toxicol.*, 31(4), 263, 1993. (CA119:27040a)
31 Erba, D., Ciappellino, S., Bermano, G., and Testolin, G., Aluminum level and availability in home-made coffee, *Riv. Sci. Aliment.*, 24(2), 203, 1995. (CA123:337992q)
32 Mueller, J. P., Steinegger, A., and Schlatter, C., *Z. Lebens.-Unters. Forsch.*, 197(4), 332, 1993. (CA120:132591z)
33 Hashimoto, S., Ito, H., and Morita, M., Elution of polychlorinated dibenzo-*p*-dioxins and dibenzofurans from coffee filters, *Chemosphere*, 25(3), 297, 1992. (CA118:21237c)

Chapter 6

The Chemical Components of Coffee

Monica Alton Spiller

CONTENTS

0-8493-2647-8/98/$0.00+$.50

I. INTRODUCTION

An understanding of coffee chemistry is made easier by remembering that the coffee bean is the seed of the coffee plant and as such it can be expected to contain the full complement of plant cell material. Roasting the coffee bean will result in thermal transformation of the plant materials.

Plant cell walls are constructed from cellulose, hemicelluloses, and pectins with varying amounts of lignin, tannins, gums, proteins, minerals, pigments, fats, waxes, and oils, all according to the cell's location and function.

Each plant cell contains various organelles arranged within the cytoplasm. They are separated from each other with specialized membranes of phospholipids and sometimes sulfo-lipids and proteins. Among the organelles, there are chloroplasts that contain proteins, lipids, chlorophyll, and carotenoids particularly. There is a nucleus, rich in nucleic acids. Ribosomes are present that generate proteins and there are dictyosomes that generate enzymes. The mitochondria support respiration in the cell with a full complement of coenzymes, including nicotinamide adenine dinucleotide (NAD) and its phosphate (NADP), flavine mononucleotide (FMN), coenzyme A, as well as cytochromes. Plant hormones will also be present to influence the growth pattern of a new plant.[1,2] All of this is stated as an explanation for the tremendous variety and complexity of compounds that have been seen in green and roasted coffee beans.

A list of the main components of roasted coffee, in highly approximated proportions, is given in Table 1.

The two major species of coffee grown commercially are *Coffea arabica* and *Coffea canephora* var. *robusta*. For ease of reference in the following pages they are described as Arabica and Robusta, respectively. They are mentioned separately because they do show differences in their chemical composition. For example, Robusta contains approximately twice as much caffeine as Arabica.

This chapter is essentially a list of the chemical components of coffee beans and beverages.

Compounds are discussed in terms of their structure. For example, fatty acids are discussed as aliphatic compounds, even though their presence is the result of carbohydrate breakdown.

Most of the lists that follow were based on those written by O. G. Vitzthum,[3] with permission of the publisher, Springer-Verlag.

The compounds given off during the roasting of coffee are not necessarily found in the finally roasted bean, and so only a few such compounds are included. In a list of volatile components in foods which is regularly brought up to date[4] more than 800 volatile compounds are listed for coffee when it is roasted, and of these 60 to 80 contribute to coffee aroma.[5] Comparison of the 14 most potent odorants from roasted Arabica and Robusta coffees, revealed significant differences,[6] (see Table 2).

II. ALIPHATIC COMPOUNDS

A. Sources

The principal sources of aliphatic compounds in roasted coffee are fragmented carbohydrates and proteins.

TABLE 1

The Approximate Composition of Roasted Arabica Coffee[3]

Components		Total (%)	Water soluble (%)
Protein	As amino acids	9	1.5
Carbohydrates	Polysaccharides:		
	Water insoluble	24	—
	Water soluble	6	6
	Sucrose	0.2	0.2
	Glucose, fructose, arabinose	0.1	0.1
Lipids	Triglycerides	9.5	—
	Terpenes: free, esters, glycosides	2	Some
Volatile acids	Formic acid	0.1	0.1
	Acetic acid	0.2	0.2
Nonvolatile acids	Lactic, pyruvic, oxalic, tartaric, citric acids	0.4	0.4
	Chlorogenic acids	3.8	3.8
Alkaloids	Caffeine	1.2	1.2
	Trigonelline	0.4	0.4
Ash	Minerals	4	3.5
Water	—	2.5	2.5
Partially known	Volatile aroma compounds	0.1	0.1
	Browning compounds, phenols, etc.	35	7.5
Total		100	27.5

Free aliphatic acids are generated during the thermal transformation of complex carbohydrates. In a model system designed to be comparable with green coffee beans, cellulose and arabinogalactan produced citric, formic, acetic, oxalic, malonic, and succinic acids.[7] In green beans themselves, formic, acetic, and lactic acids have been seen to increase markedly with light roasting and are the cause of a more acidic beverage, pH 5.1, than is obtained from a deeply roasted coffee, which has lost these most volatile acids. The pH of a deeply roasted coffee beverage rises to 5.9.[8,9] These free volatile fatty acids, formed during roasting, are easily lost during the storage of roasted coffee, as is evidenced by a decrease in acid value.[10] The volatile fatty acids are found in a higher proportion in roasted Robusta coffees than in roasted Arabicas.[3] Free fatty acids also apparently form during the storage of green coffee beans under tropical conditions.[11]

The carboxylic acids formed in this way are themselves a source of other aliphatic compounds, so that free carbon acids above C-10 are found only in traces.[3] Citric acid yields itaconic acid and citraconic acid during

TABLE 2

Potent Odorants From Roasted Arabica and Robusta Coffees[6]

Compound	Concentration in Arabica coffee (mg/kg)	Concentration in Robusta coffee (mg/kg)
2-Furfurylthiol	1.08	1.73
Methional	0.24	0.095
3-Mercapto-3-methylbutyl formate	0.13	0.115
2-Ethyl-3,5-dimethylpyrazine	0.33	0.94
2,3-Diethyl-5-methylpyrazine	0.095	0.31
Guaiacol	4.2	28.2
4-Vinylguaiacol	64.8	177.7
4-Ethylguaiacol	1.63	18.1
Vanillin	4.8	16.1
(E)-β-damascenone	0.195	0.205
4-Hydroxy-2,5-dimethyl-3(2H)-furanone	109	57
3-Hydroxy-4,5-dimethyl-2(5H)-furanone	1.47	0.63
5-Ethyl-3-hydroxy-4-methyl-2(5H)-furanone	0.16	0.085
5-Ethyl-4-hydroxy-2-methyl-3(2H)-furanone	17.3	14.3

the roasting (see Figure 1).[3] The decarboxylation of aliphatic acids produces a series of hydrocarbons when coffee is roasted.[3]

Other carbonyl compounds are also formed from carbohydrates.[3] Glyoxal, methyl glyoxal, and diacetyl are among those identifed in ground coffee.[12] Browning reactions involving aldose sugars and amino compounds can account for the production of such compounds as acetol ($CH_3.CO.CH_2OH$) and diacetyl (CH_3-CO-CO-CH_3).[13]

Model systems indicate that aldehydes may also be produced by the action of polyphenoloxidases on amino acids in the presence of catechin, all of which are present in coffee beans at some stage between green and roasted. For example, valine yields isobutanal, leucine yields isopentanal, and isoleucine yields 2-methyl-butanal.[14] Some of these aldehydes probably undergo condensation reactions in the acidic medium of the roasted bean when moisture is present.[15] Some dienals in green coffee beans have recently been identified as (E,E)-2,4- and (E,Z)-2,4-nonadienal and (E,E)-2,4- and (E,Z)-2,4-decadienal.[16]

The aliphatic polyamines, putrescine, spermine, and spermidine, are present in green coffee beans, but they are all decomposed during the roasting process.[17]

Sulfur-containing amino acids, such as methionine and cystine, are probably the precursors of the mercaptans, sulfides, and disulfides.[3] Dimethyl sulfide yields dimethyl sulfoxide and its oxidized product dimethyl

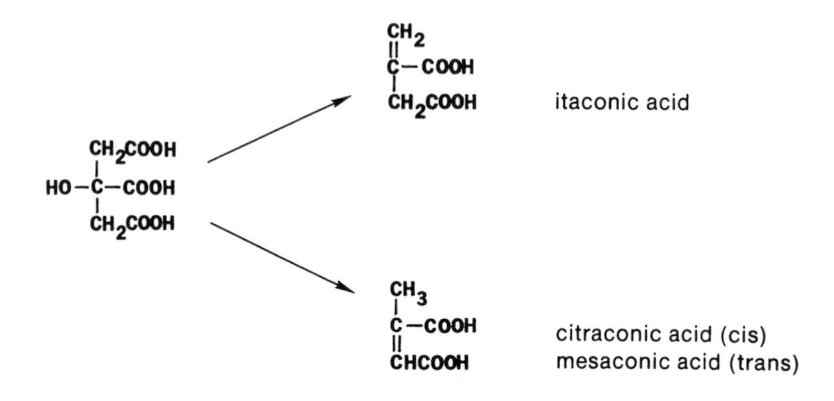

FIGURE 1
Citric acid yields itaconic, citraconic, and mesaconic acids during coffee roasting.[3]

sulfone, both of which are probably present in green and roasted coffee beans.[18] Dimethyltrisulfide has also recently been recognized in coffee beans.[19] Freshly roasted coffee contains only trace amounts of alkyl di- and trisulfides, but these concentrations are increased in processed or stale coffee.[19]

B. Aliphatic Aroma and Flavor Compounds

Several of the lower molecular weight aliphatic compounds, in a mixture, are part of the roasted coffee aroma. A nine-compound mixture with roasted coffee aroma contained isopentane, *n*-hexane, acetaldehyde, dimethyl sulfide, propanal, isobutanal, isopentanal, methanol, and 2-methylfuran.[20] In addition, the freshness of aroma and taste has been correlated with 2-methylpropanal and diacetyl. When the concentration of these falls off, so does the taste.[21] Other aliphatic compounds that are steadily lost from ground roasted coffee, unless it is vacuum packaged, include methyl formate, methyl acetate, methyl thioacetate, and acetone.[22] The concentrations in roast coffee for four compounds whose contribution to the fresh flavor have long been known are dimethyl sulfide (4 ppm), methyl formate (12 ppm), isobutanal (20 ppm), and diacetyl (40 ppm). The taste thresholds are 0.1, 0.5, 0.5, and 1.0 ppm, respectively, in the brew made with 5 g coffee per 100 ml water.[15]

A stale odor, on the other hand, is noticed when moisture and oxygen are present. They probably cause condensation reactions among the aldehydes and the oxidation of dimethyl sulfide.[15]

The most volatile aliphatic compounds are largely lost at some stage of the roasting process. For example, acetaldehyde was among 12 volatile compounds evolved after an 8-min roast of coffee beans at 220°C.[23] Waste gases from a coffee-roasting factory contained methanol, acetone, and acetic acid.[24] Some moderately volatile aliphatic compounds present in instant coffee are at a higher concentration than might have been expected. They are produced during the percolation solubilization of carbohydrates at temperatures around 172°C and are presumably strongly adsorbed in the carbohydrate matrix. Such compounds include acetaldehyde, propanal, acetone, and methylethyl ketone.[15]

There are some other mixtures that are predominantly aliphatic that are associated with "stinker" beans. These contain extraordinarily increased amounts of methanol, ethanol, acetone, acetic acid, 2-butanediol, butanols, 2,3-pentanedione, 3-pentanone, and butane.[25]

A list of aliphatic compounds that have been recognized in green and roasted coffees is given in Table 3.

III. ALICYCLIC COMPOUNDS

Preliminary roasting of coffee produces low molecular weight fragments, which in turn form alicyclic carbonyl compounds via the aldol condensation.[3] The cyclopentadiones probably arise from fructose specifically.[3]

Several alicyclic compounds identifiable in roasted coffee are terpenes and these contribute presumably to the coffee oil. The kaurane and furokaurane type diterpenes are discussed in Section VIII.D.

The characteristic earthy and harsh flavor and aroma of roasted Robusta coffees is largely attributed to 2-methylisoborneol. Amounts found in green Robusta coffee beans were 0.03 to 0.3 ppb, and this could be completely removed by steam heating or roasting.[26] There is approximately ten times as much 2-methylisoborneol in roasted Robusta coffee beans than in similarly treated Arabica coffee.[27]

The phytate content of coffee beans is 1.2 to 5.4 mg/g, and only a portion of this is water extractable.[28,29] Inositol with six phosphate groups (IP6) is decomposed to inositol with fewer phosphate groups, on roasting.[30] A list of alicyclic compounds found in coffee is given in Table 4.

IV. AROMATIC COMPOUNDS

A. Aromatic Hydrocarbons

Although the aromatic polycyclic hydrocarbons are usually associated with tar and soot formation, in a firing or roasting process, compounds such as fluoranthrene and pyrene have also been found in green

TABLE 3

Aliphatic Compounds Found in Green and Roasted Coffee[3]

Compound	Empirical formula	Source[a]
Hydrocarbons		
Methane	CH_4	R
Ethane	C_2H_6	G
n-Butane	C_4H_{10}	R
Isobutane	C_4H_{10}	G R
n-Pentane	C_5H_{12}	G R
Isopentane	C_5H_{12}	G R
Isohexane	C_6H_{14}	G R
Isoheptane	C_7H_{16}	G R
Octane	C_8H_{18}	G R
Isooctane	C_8H_{18}	G R
n-Nonane	C_9H_{20}	G R
Isononane	C_9H_{20}	G R
n-Decane	$C_{10}H_{22}$	R
Isodecane	$C_{10}H_{22}$	G
Isoundecane	$C_{11}H_{24}$	G
n-Tetradecane	$C_{14}H_{30}$	R
n-Pentadecane	$C_{15}H_{32}$	R
n-Heptacosane	$C_{27}H_{56}$	R
Nonacosane	$C_{29}H_{60}$	G
Ethylene	C_2H_4	G R
Butene	C_4H_8	R
Pentene	C_5H_{10}	R
Isopentene	C_5H_{10}	R
Hexene	C_6H_{12}	R
Isohexene	C_6H_{12}	R
Octene	C_8H_{16}	G R
Isooctene	C_8H_{16}	G R
Isononene	C_9H_{18}	G
Isodecene	$C_{10}H_{20}$	G
Penta-1,4-diene	C_5H_8	R
Isoprene	C_5H_8	R
Hexadiene	C_6H_{10}	
Myrcene	$C_{10}H_{16}$	R
Squalene	$C_{30}H_{50}$	G
Octyne	C_8H_{14}	R
Alcohols, ketoalcohols		
Methanol	CH_4O	R
Ethanol	C_2H_6O	R
2-Propanol	C_3H_8O	R
Isobutyl alcohol	$C_4H_{10}O$	R
tert-Butyl alcohol	$C_4H_{10}O$	R
l-Pentanol	$C_5H_{12}O$	R
Isoamyl alcohol (3-methyl-1-butanol)	$C_5H_{12}O$	R
2-Methyl-2-butanol	$C_5H_{12}O$	R

TABLE 3 (continued)

Aliphatic Compounds Found in Green and Roasted Coffee[3]

Compound	Empirical formula	Source[a]
l-Hexanol	$C_6H_{14}O$	R
2-Heptanol	$C_7H_{16}O$	R
3-Octanol	$C_8H_{18}O$	R
3-Methylbut-2-en-1-ol	$C_5H_{10}O$	R
Oct-l-en-3-ol	$C_8H_{16}O$	R
Linalool (3,7-dimethyl-octa-1,6-dien-3-ol)	$C_{10}H_{18}O$	R
Acetol (hydroxyacetone)	$C_3H_6O_2$	R
Acetoin (butan-2-ol-3-one)	$C_4H_8O_2$	R
Butan-1-ol-2-one	$C_4H_8O_2$	R
2-Hydroxy-pentan-3-one	$C_5H_{10}O_2$	R
3-Hydroxy-pentan-2-one	$C_5H_{10}O_2$	R
Aldehydes		
Formaldehyde	CH_2O	R
Acetaldehyde	C_2H_4O	G R
Propanal	C_3H_6O	R
Butanal	C_4H_8O	R
Isobutyl aldehyde	C_4H_8O	G R
Pentanal	$C_5H_{10}O$	G R
Isopently aldehyde	$C_5H_{10}O$	R
2-Methylbutanal	$C_5H_{10}O$	G R
2-Methylpentanal	$C_6H_{12}O$	R
n-Hexanal	$C_6H_{12}O$	R
Acrolein (propenal)	C_3H_4O	R
Butenal	C_4H_6O	R
2-Methylacrolein	C_4H_6O	R
Dimethylacrolein	C_5H_8O	R
2-Methyl-3-ethylacrolein	$C_6H_{10}O$	R
2-Methylbutenal	C_5H_8O	G R
trans-2-Nonenal	$C_9H_{16}O$	R
Glyoxal[12]	$C_2H_2O_2$	R
Methylglyoxal[12]	$C_3H_4O_2$	R
Dimethylacetal	$C_4H_{10}O_2$	R
Ketones, diketones		
Acetone	C_3H_6O	G R
l-Methyl-isobutan-2-one	$C_5H_{10}O$	R
Methylethylketone	C_4H_8O	G R
Pentan-2-one	$C_5H_{10}O$	R
Pentan-3-one	$C_5H_{10}O$	R
Hexan-3-one	$C_6H_{12}O$	R
Heptan-2-one	$C_7H_{14}O$	R
Octan-2-one	$C_8H_{16}O$	R
Octan-3-one	$C_8H_{16}O$	R
Nonan-2-one	$C_9H_{18}0$	R
Decan-2-one	$C_{10}H_{20}O$	R

TABLE 3 (continued)

Aliphatic Compounds Found in Green and Roasted Coffee[3]

Compound	Empirical formula	Source[a]
Undecan-2-one	$C_{11}H_{22}O$	R
Tridecan-2-one	$C_{13}H_{26}O$	R
6,10,14-Trimethyl-pentadecan-2-one	$C_{18}H_{36}O$	R
6,10-Dimethyl-undecan-2-one	$C_{13}H_{26}O$	R
6-Methylhept-5-en-2-one	$C_8H_{14}O$	R
Pent-3-en-2-one	C_5H_8O	R
trans-Pent-2-en-4-one	C_5H_8O	R
Mesityl oxide	$C_6H_{10}O$	R
Methylvinyl ketone	C_4H_6O	R
O-Acetylacetol	$C_5H_8O_3$	R
l-Acetoxybutan-2-one	$C_6H_{10}O_3$	R
l-Acetoxypentan-2-one	$C_7H_{12}O_3$	R
2-Acetoxypentan-3-one	$C_7H_{12}O_3$	R
O-Propionylacetol	$C_6H_{10}O_3$	R
Diacetyl	$C_4H_6O_2$	G R
4-Methylpentan-2,3-dione	$C_6H_{10}O_2$	R
Pentan-2,3-dione	$C_5H_8O_2$	R
Pentan-2,4-dione	$C_5H_8O_2$	R
Hexan-2,3-dione	$C_6H_{10}O_2$	R
Hexan-2,5-dione	$C_6H_{10}O_2$	R
Hexan-3,4-dione	$C_6H_{10}O_2$	R
Heptan-2,5-dione	$C_7H_{12}O_2$	R
Heptan-3,4-dione	$C_7H_{12}O_2$	R
Octan-2,3-dione	$C_8H_{14}O_2$	R
5-Methylhexan-2,3-dione	$C_7H_{12}O_2$	R
5-Methylheptan-3,4-dione	$C_8H_{14}O_2$	R
6-Methylheptan-3,4-dione	$C_8H_{14}O_2$	R
Carboxylic acids		
Formic acid	$C\ H_2O_2$	R
Acetic acid	$C_2H_4O_2$	R
Propionic acid	$C_3H_6O_2$	R
Butyric acid	$C_4H_8O_2$	R
Isobutyric acid	$C_4H_8O_2$	R
Pentanoic acid	$C_5H_{10}O_2$	G R
Isopentanoic acid	$C_5H_{10}O_2$	R
Methylethylacetic acid	$C_5H_{10}O_2$	R
Caproic acid	$C_6H_{12}O_2$	R
Heptanoic acid	$C_7H_{14}O_2$	R
Octanoic acid	$C_8H_{16}O_2$	R
Pelargonic acid	$C_9H_{18}O_2$	R
Decanoic acid	$C_{10}H_{20}O_2$	R
Palmitic acid	$C_{16}H_{32}O_2$	R
C12:0-C2:20[109]		R
α-Methylcrotonic acid	$C_5H_8O_2$	R
Dimethylacrylic acid	$C_5H_8O_2$	R

TABLE 3 (continued)

Aliphatic Compounds Found in Green and Roasted Coffee[3]

Compound	Empirical formula	Source[a]
Oxalic acid	$C_2H_2O_4$	R
Itaconic acid	$C_5H_6O_4$	R
Citraconic acid	$C_5H_6O_4$	R
Mesaconic acid	$C_5H_6O_4$	R
Citric acid	$C_6H_8O_7$	R
Malonic acid	$C_3H_4O_4$	R
Pyruvic acid	$C_3H_4O_3$	R
Lactic acid	$C_3H_6O_3$	R
Succinic acid	$C_4H_6O_4$	R
Glutaric acid	$C_5H_8O_4$	R
Tartaric acid	$C_4H_6O_6$	R
Malic acid	$C_4H_6O_5$	R
Fumaric acid	$C_4H_4O_4$	R
Maleic acid	$C_4H_4O_4$	R
trans-Crotonic acid	$C_4H_6O_2$	R
cis-Crotonic acid	$C_4H_6O_2$	R
Methacrylic	$C_4H_6O_2$	R
Tiglic acid	$C_5H_8O_2$	R
Glycolic acid	$C_2H_4O_3$	R
Levulinic acid	$C_5H_8O_3$	R
Esters, ethers		
Methyl formate	$C_2H_4O_2$	G R
Ethylformate	$C_3H_6O_2$	R
Isopropyl formate	$C_4H_8O_2$	R
Methyl acetate	$C_3H_6O_2$	G R
Ethyl acetate	$C_4H_8O_2$	G R
n-Butyl acetate	$C_6H_{12}O_2$	G R
Isoamyl acetate	$C_7H_{14}O_2$	R
Isopentenyl acetate	$C_7H_{12}O_2$	R
Hexyl acetate	$C_8H_6O_2$	G
Propionyl acetate	$C_4H_4O_2$	G R
Propyl propionate	$C_6H_{12}O_2$	G
Methyl butyrate	$C_5H_{10}O_2$	G R
Ethyl butyrate	$C_6H_{12}O_2$	G
Methyl isopentanoate	$C_6H_{12}O_2$	R
Ethyl pentanoate	$C_7H_{14}O_2$	G
Methyl caproate	$C_7H_{14}O_2$	G R
Methyl palmitate	$C_{17}H_{34}O_2$	R
Nitrogen compounds		
Methylamine	$C\ H_5N$	R
Trimethylamine	C_3H_9N	R
Acrylonitrile	C_3H_3N	R
3-Butenenitrile	C_4H_5N	R
n-Butyraldoxime	C_4H_9NO	R
Putrescine[17]	$C_4H_{12}N_2$	G

TABLE 3 (continued)

Aliphatic Compounds Found in Green and Roasted Coffee[3]

Compound	Empirical formula	Source[a]
Spermine[17]	$C_{10}H_{26}N_4$	G
Spermidine[17]	$C_7H_{19}N_3$	G
Sulfur compounds		
Methyl mercaptan	$C H_4S$	R
Ethyl merceptan (tentative)	C_2H_6S	R
Propyl mercaptan	C_3H_8S	R
Carbon disulfide	CS_2	G R
Dimethylsulfide	C_2H_6S	G R
Methylethyl sulfide	C_3H_8S	R
Dimethyl disulfide	$C_2H_6S_2$	R
Methylethyl disulfide	$C_3H_8S_2$	R
Diethyl disulfide	$C_4H_{10}S_2$	R
Dimethyl trisulfide[19]	$C_2H_6S_3$	R
Methylethyl trisulfide[19]	$C_3H_8S_3$	R
Dimethyl sulfoxide, tentative[18]	C_2H_6OS	R
Dimethyl sulfone, tentative[18]	$C_2H_6O_2S$	R
1-Methylthiobutan-2-one	$C_5H_{10}O S$	R

[a]G, in green coffee; R, in roasted coffee.

TABLE 4

Alicyclic Compounds Found in Green and Roasted Coffee[3]

Compound	Empirical formula	Source[a]
1,2-Dihydrotoluene	C_7H_{10}	R
Limonene	$C_{10}H_{16}$	R
3-Isopropenyl-1-methylcyclohexene	$C_{10}H_{16}$	R
α-Terpineol	$C_{10}H_{18}O$	R
Cyclopentanone	C_5H_8O	R
3-Methylcyclopentanone[76]	$C_6H_{10}O$	R
2-Cyclopenten-1-one	C_5H_6O	R
2-Methyl-2-cyclopenten-1-one	C_6H_8O	R
2,3-Dimethyl-2-cyclopenten-1-one	$C_7H_{10}O$	R
2-Ethyl-2-cyclopenten-1-one	$C_7H_{10}O$	R
2,3,5-Trimethyl-2-cyclopenten-1-one	$C_8H_{12}O$	R
2-Hydroxy-3-methyl-2-cyclopenten-1-one	$C_6H_8O_2$	R
Cyclohexylmethylketone[76]	$C_8H_{14}O$	R
2-Cyclohexen-1-one	C_6H_8O	R
2-Methyl-2-cyclohexen-1-one	$C_7H_{10}O$	R
Cyclopentan-1,2-dione	$C_5H_6O_2$	R
3,4-Dimethylcyclopentan-1,2-dione	$C_7H_{10}O_2$	R
3,5-Dimethylcyclopentan-1,2-dione	$C_7H_{10}O_2$	R
3-Methylcyclopentan-1,2-dione	$C_6H_80_2$	R
3-Ethylcyclopentan-1,2-dione	$C_7H_{10}O_2$	R
3-Methylcyclohexan-1,2-dione	$C_7H_{10}O_2$	R

[a]G, in green coffee; R, in roasted coffee.

coffee.[3] Amounts present in coffees will be highly dependent on roasting conditions (see Chapter 5). Some quantities given in the literature follow. Benzo-(a)-pyrene has been seen at the 1-4 μg/Kg level in roasted ground coffee, and below 1 μg/Kg in soluble coffee.[31] When Arabica coffee is carefully kept free from soot and silverskin, and the hot gases are released from the roasting system, the benzo-(a)-pyrene levels are 1 μg/Kg. If the hot gases are recycled, the value rises to about 3 μg/Kg, but if the soot and silverskin have accumulated with the coffee, the value rises sharply to 350 μg/Kg for benzo-(a)-pyrene.[32] However, in an Italian study, benzo(a)-pyrene that was present in green coffee was not seen after roasting.[33] But then, the darkest roasts such as Italian are not usually carried out in a system where hot gases are recycled.[15]

The most abundant polycyclic hydrocarbon, 2,3-benzofluorene was seen at the 22 μg/Kg level in green coffee and was decreased to 12 μg/Kg in an Italian roasting process.[33]

Coffee beans have been found to contain small amounts of styrene (1.57 to 7.85 ng/g), which could not be attributed to contact with plastic.[34]

B. Phenols

A high proportion of the aromatic compounds in coffee beans are phenolic and presumably they are derived from the lignin and tannin of the cell structure.[2] Hydroquinone is present in coffee beverages, 0.3 ppm, either in the free form or as its β-D-glucopyranoside, arbutin.[35]

The extraction of the flavanols (catechol and 4-ethylcatechol), from steam-treated green coffee beans[36] (Figure 2), can be correlated with the presence of the so-called condensed tannins.[37]

Trihydroxybenzene carboxylic acid esters with a sugar are characteristic of "hydrolyzable tannins".[37] These, too, may be present in coffee

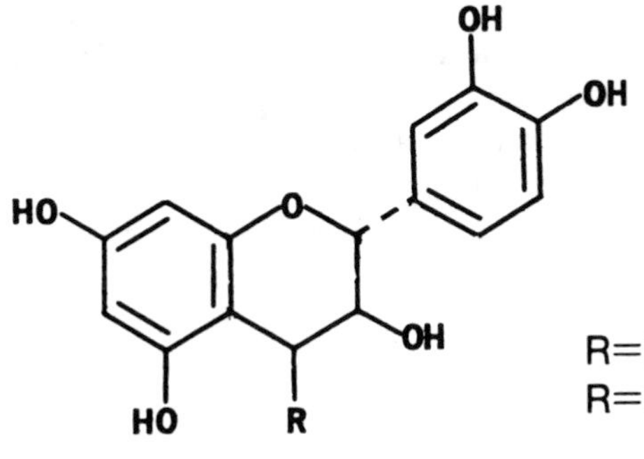

OH
OH
HO
O
OH
HO
R

R=H, catechol (flavan-3-ol)
R=C_2H_5, 4-ethylcatechol

FIGURE 2
Some flavanols obtained from steam-treated green coffee beans.[36]

pyrogallol

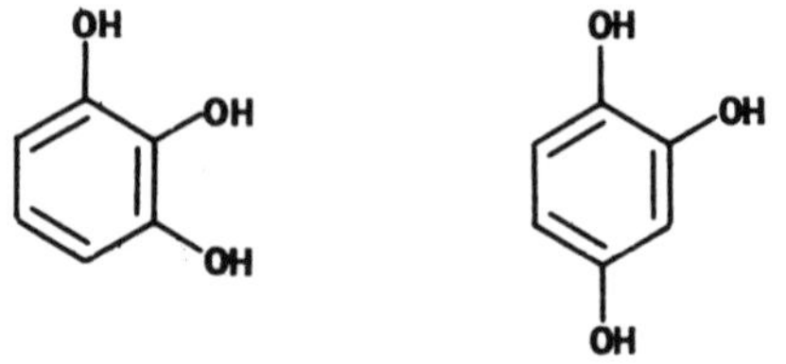

1, 2, 4-trihydroxybenzene

FIGURE 3
Some trihydroxybenzenes obtained from roasted coffee beans.[38]

beans, as evidenced by the presence of pyrogallol[3] and 1,2,4-trihydroxybenzene[38] (Figure 3), in roasted coffee beans.[38] However, the source of trihydroxybenzenes from coffee is much more likely to be quinic acid.[39] For this reason, coffee is not usually described as tannin-containing. Nevertheless, the tannin contents of green and roasted coffee beans, in terms of a protein precipitation method, have been determined: green coffee beans contained 6.6 mg/g and roasted coffee beans contained 18 mg/g tannic acid equivalents.[40]

In coffee there is a series of phenolic compounds that is characteristically present, which are derived from caffeic and ferulic acids. These acids are present as esters of quinic acid, and are known as chlorogenic and feruloylquinic acids, respectively (Figure 4). The pattern of the chlorogenic acids in green and roasted coffees can be used to distinguish between them.[41] The inclusion of immature green coffee berries has a negative effect on flavor in the final beverage. So, it is interesting to recognize that immature green coffee berries of *Caffea arabica cv Catuai vermelho* have a higher ratio of monocaffeoylquinic acid: dicaffeoylquinic acid.[42] Free quinic acid is used as a taste-improving agent in beverages, and it can be obtained in quantity from coffee beans.[43]

Chlorogenic acids are well recognized as antioxidants, which are in some circumstances more powerful than a-tocopherol or ascorbic acid,[44] and have value as free radical scavengers *in vivo*.[45] A water soluble antioxidant mixture containing caffeic and chlorogenic acid has been developed for use as an alternative to synthetic antioxidants.[46] Coffee imported from different countries had superoxide anion scavanging activity values ranging from 470 to 1360 superoxide dismutase units/mL of coffee extract, and is correlated to metal ion content.[47] Instant coffee has been shown to be a pro-oxidant with respect to ascorbic acid, as well as a superoxide radical scavenger.[48] At least part of the antibacterial nature of coffee has been attributed to the 5-caffeoyl quinic acid content of roasted coffee,[49] whereas in coffee residue, 3′,4′-dihydroxy-acetophenone was recognized as an antimicrobial.[50]

Amounts of chlorogenic acids found in roasted coffee are given in Table 5.

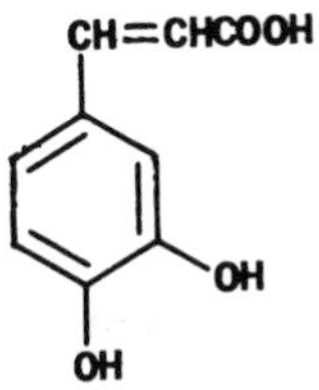

caffeic acid 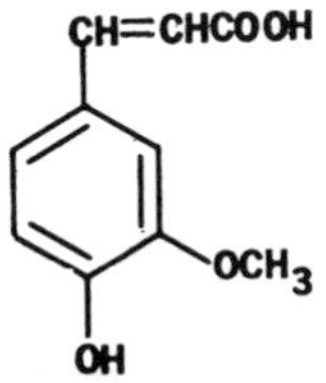 ferulic acid 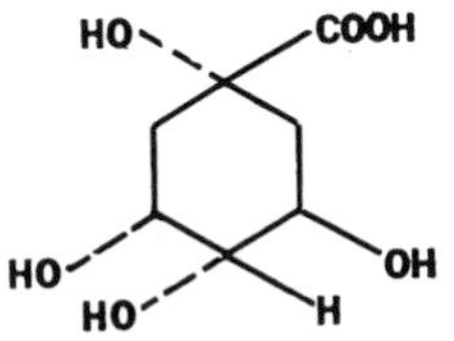 quinic acid

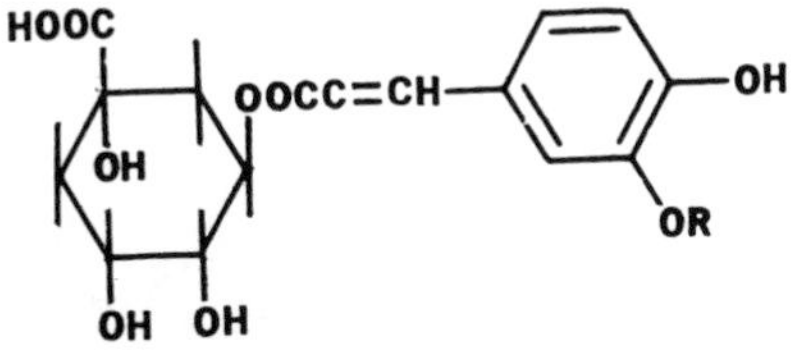

R=H, chlorogenic acid (3′-caffeoylquinic acid)
R=CH_3, feruloylquinic acid

FIGURE 4
Some phenolic compounds found in coffee beans.[3]

TABLE 5
Amounts of Chlorogenic Acids Found in Roasted Coffee[3]

Chlorogenic acids in roasted coffee	Amount (%)
3-caffeoylquinic acid (chlorogenic acid)	2.0
4-caffeoylquinic acid (cryptochlorogenic acid)	0.2
5-caffeoylquinic acid (neochlorogenic acid)	1.0
3,4-dicaffeoylquinic acid (isochlorogenic acid a)	0.01
3,5-dicaffeoylquinic acid (isochlorogenic acid b)	0.09
4,5-dicaffeoylquinic acid (isochlorogenic acid c)	0.01

More recently, a series of 11 chlorogenic acids has been recognized in green Robusta coffee beans.[51]

The treatment and environment of green coffee beans affects the concentrations of both caffeoyl- and feruloyl-quinic acids,[52] and several decomposition products have been recognized. Some of these products, in this case from steam-treated green coffee beans, are given in Figure 5.[53]

Soaking the green coffee beans in water for 48 h results in a 40% loss of chlorogenic acid, even though the beans swell very little. The bean weight gain is only 5.5%.[54] Infestation of coffee beans by the coffee borer can lead to increased concentrations of chlorogenic acid.[55] On the other hand, γ-radiation treatment does not seem to change either the chlorogenic acid or caffeic-acid concentration.[56]

3, 4-dihydroxystyrene

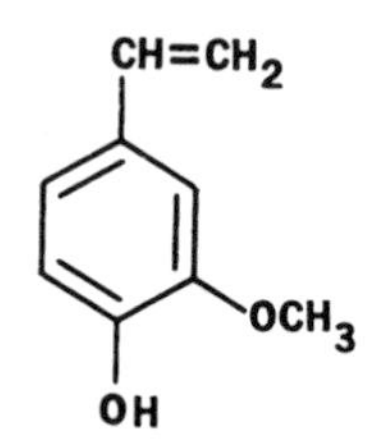

3-methoxy-4-hydroxystyrene

3, 4-dihydroxybenzaldehyde

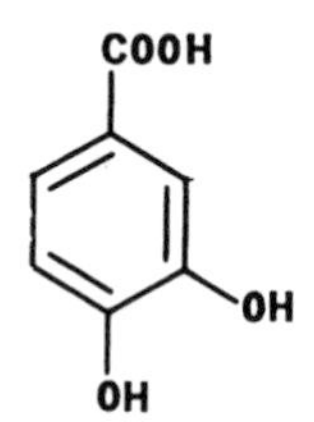

3, 4-dihydroxybenzoic acid

FIGURE 5
Examples of compounds obtained from coffee during steam treatment.

Roasting causes a decrease in chlorogenic acid from 7 to 4.3%.[57] This is accompanied by an initial increase in quinic acid. In deeply roasted coffee the quinic acid is, however, decreased. This suggests that inherent sugars may be reacting with the chlorogenic acid to release quinic acid.[58] The quinic acid content in increasingly roasted coffee beans is given in Table 6.[58]

In addition to the changing amounts of quinic acid present as roasting proceeds, the quinic acid isomer concentrations change and the degree of isomerization can be correlated with roasting degree regardless of the coffee's origin.[59]

Chlorogenic acid loss is also correlated with its incorporation in browning products.[3] During roasting, the diphenols, 4-ethylpyrocatechol and pyrocatechol are formed from the caffeic acid moiety and the quinic acid moiety yields phenol and benzoic acid as well as all the di- and trihydroxybenzenes.[39]

Chlorogenic acid lactones are produced in roasted coffee and range from 1.5 to 3.5 g/kg in commercial roasted coffee samples. Two lactones that have been identified in roasted coffee are 3-caffeoyl- and 4-caffeoylquinic acid-γ-lactone.[60]

Perhaps eugenol (Figure 6), seen in roasted coffee, is from another series similar to tannins.[3]

TABLE 6

The Quinic Acid Content of Increasingly Roasted Coffee Beans[58]

Roast style in order of increasing roast	Quinic acid (%)
Green beans	1.3
Medium roast	1.4
French roast	3.5
Ice roast	2.0
Italian roast	1.7

Polyphenoloxidase activity also determines the distribution of phenolic compounds in coffee beans. "Condensed tannins" are believed to be produced via quinones by free radical mechanisms, in a polyphenoloxidase-catalyzed oxidation of catechol.[61] Certainly quinone production has been correlated with high polyphenoloxidase activity.[62] This polyphenoloxidase activity decreases quickly during coffee bean storage unless they are canned or in a plastic bag.[63] There is an order of magnitude increase in this enzyme when coffee beans germinate.[64] Bean color is associated with enzyme activity in general,[65] although there is not total agreement.[66] It has been found that polyphenoloxidase activity decreased in the same way as a taste classification by experts.[62, 67] A high polyphenoloxidase coffee extract can even be added to a poor-tasting coffee extract to give a total resultant taste improvement.[68]

There is also another group of polyphenolic compounds, thus far only known through their biological activity as thrombogenic haptens.[69]

Opiate receptor binding activity has been recognized in coffee. It is ether extractable and not modifiable by enzymic digestion with papain; it has a molecular weight in the range of 1,000 to 3,500.[70]

Robusta coffee has a somewhat higher phenolic content than Arabica (see Table 7). The feruloylquinic and dicaffeoylquinic acid content in Robusta is higher than in Arabica coffee beans.[71, 72]

Bearing in mind that most Robusta coffees are prepared by the dry method and most Arabicas by the wet method, it is interesting to read the following: Tannin formation in coffee bean pulp begins soon after pulp removal from the beans. When this pulp is sun-dried, glycosides are hydrolyzed with the liberation of phenolic groups otherwise bound in esters and ethers.[73] It can be speculated that at least part of the high phenolic concentration in Robusta beans might come from the pulp as the beans dry out, and recent studies have shown this to be the case.[74]

Crossing the boundaries of phenolic compounds and amino acids in coffee, caffeoyl tryptophan, and *p*-coumaryl-(L)-tryptophan have both been identified recently in green Robusta coffee beans.[51] A

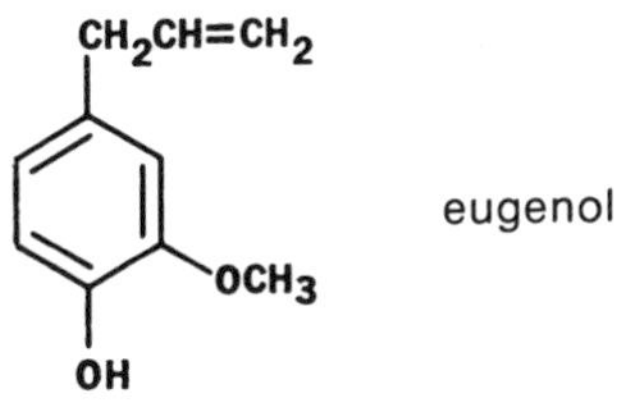

FIGURE 6
Eugenol.

TABLE 7

The Concentration of Some Phenolic Components in Roasted Coffee[39]

Compound	Arabica (ppm)	Robusta (ppm)
Pyrocatechol	80	120
4-Methylpyrocatechol	16	13
Hydroquinone	40	30
4-Ethylpyrocatechol	37	80
4-Vinylpyrocatechol	25	25
Vanillin	3	3
Pyrogallol	45	55
3,4-Dihydroxybenzaldehyde	20	9
1,2,4-Trihydroxybenzene	20	13
3,4-Dihydroxycinnamaldehyde	10	12

similar type of compound caffeoyl-tyrosine seems to be unique to Robusta coffees produced in Angola.[75]

A list of aromatic compounds that have been found in coffee is given in Table 8.

V. HETEROCYCLIC COMPOUNDS

Almost all the heterocyclic compounds listed are volatile and have been recognized as present in roasted coffee or its aroma, suggesting that almost all are thermal transformation products rather than compounds present in the green coffee bean.

A. Oxygen Heterocyclics

The furans are mostly 2- and 2,5-substituted and are formed from the sugars that are largely destroyed during roasting.[3] Glucose heated alone yields over 20 furans, of which at least 9 have been seen in roasted coffee.[3] The vinylmethylfurans and alkenylfurans included in Table 11, have been reported in heat-processed foods.[76] Possible sources of furans specific to coffee are kahweol, a furokaurene, and similar compounds that contain the furan moeity.[3] The fresh taste quality of roasted coffee can be estimated from the concentration of 2-methylfuran.[21] Furfural, with its haylike odor, is characteristic of instant coffees and is probably formed along with furan when carbohydrates are subjected to 172°C water to produce the coffee extract.[15] In roasted coffee, arabinogalactan has been recognized as the precursor of furfural.[77] On the other hand, a furfuryl alcohol-containing fraction obtained from roasted coffee has been regarded as an unde-

TABLE 8

Aromatic Compounds Found in Green and Roasted Coffee[3]

Compound	Empirical formula	Source[a]
Hydrocarbons, polycyclic hydrocarbons		
Benzene	C_6H_6	G R
Toluene	C_7H_8	G R
Ethylbenzene	C_8H_{10}	G R
Xylene	C_8H_{10}	G R
1,2,4-Trimethylbenzene	C_9H_{12}	R
p-Cymene	$C_{10}H_{14}$	R
1,2,4,5-Tetramethylbenzene	$C_{10}H_{14}$	R
Styrene	C_8H_8	R
p-Isopropenyltoluene	$C_{10}H_{12}$	R
Naphthalene	$C_{10}H_8$	R
l-Methylnaphthalene	$C_{11}H_{10}$	R
2-Methylnaphthalene	$C_{11}H_{10}$	R
Dimethylnaphthalene	$C_{12}H_{12}$	R
2-Ethylnaphthalene	$C_{12}H_{12}$	R
Trimethylnaphthalene	$C_{13}H_{14}$	R
Tetramethylnaphthalene	$C_{14}H_{16}$	R
Diphenyl	$C_{12}H_{10}$	R
3-Methyldiphenyl	$C_{13}H_{12}$	R
Indene	C_9H_8	R
Fluorene	$C_{13}H_{10}$	R
Anthanthracene	$C_{22}H_{12}$	R
Benzanthracene	$C_{18}H_{12}$	R
3,4-Benzfluoranthene	$C_{20}H_{12}$	R
11,12-Benzfluoranthene	$C_{20}H_{12}$	R
1,12-Benzperylene	$C_{22}H_{12}$	G R
Benzo-(a)-pyrene	$C_{20}H_{12}$	G R
Benzo-(e)-pyrene	$C_{20}H_{12}$	R
Coronene	$C_{24}H_{12}$	R
Chrysene	$C_{18}H_{12}$	R
1,2,5,6-Dibenzanthracene	$C_{22}H_{14}$	R
Fluoranthene	$C_{16}H_{10}$	G R
Indenopyrene	$C_{25}H_{14}$	R
Perylene	$C_{20}H_{12}$	R
Phenanthrene[33]	$C_{14}H_{10}$	G R
Pyrene	$C_{16}H_{10}$	G R
2,3-benzofluorene[33]	$C_{17}H_{12}$	G R
Phenols		
Phenol	C_6H_6O	G R
m-Cresol	C_7H_8O	R
o-Cresol	C_7H_8O	R
p-Cresol	C_7H_8O	R
2,3-Dimethylphenol	$C_8H_{10}O$	R
2, 5-Dimethylphenol	$C_8H_{10}O$	R
2, 6-Dimethylphenol	$C_8H_{10}O$	R

TABLE 8 (continued)

Aromatic Compounds Found in Green and Roasted Coffee[3]

Compound	Empirical formula	Source[a]
3,4-Dimethylphenol	C_8H_6O	R
2-Ethylphenol	$C_8H_{10}O$	R
4-Ethylphenol	$C_8H_{10}O$	R
2,3,5-Trimethylphenol	$C_9H_{12}O$	R
4-Vinylphenol	C_8H_8O	G
Catechin[36]	$C_{15}H_{14}O_6$	G
4-Ethylcatechin[36]	$C_{17}H_{18}O_6$	G
l-Ethyl-3,4-dihydroxybenzene[38]	$C_8H_{10}O_2$	R
2,3-Dihydroxytoluene[38]	$C_7H_8O_2$	R
1,2,4-Trihydroxybenzene[38, 39]	$C_6H_6O_3$	R
Pyrocatechol	$C_6H_6O_2$	R
4-Methylpyrocatechol[39]	$C_7H_8O_2$	R
3-Methylpyrocatechol[39]	$C_7H_8O_2$	R
4-Ethylpyrocatechol[39]	$C_8H_{10}O_2$	R
4-Vinylpyrocatechol	$C_8H_8O_2$	R
Resorcinol	$C_6H_6O_2$	R
Hydroquinone	$C_6H_6O_2$	R
Pyrogallol	$C_6H_6O_3$	R
2,3-Dihydroxyacetophenone	$C_8H_8O_3$	R
3,4-Dihydroxystyrene[36]	$C_8H_8O_2$	G
Alcohols, aldehydes, ketones		
Benzyl alcohol	C_7H_8O	G
β-Phenylethyl alcohol	$C_8H_{10}O$	G R
Benzaldehyde	C_7H_6O	G R
3,4-Dimethoxybenzaldehyde	$C_9H_{10}O_3$	G
o-Toluylaldehyde	C_8H_8O	R
m-Toluylaldehyde (tentative)	C_8H_8O	R
Phenylacetaldehyde	C_8H_8O	G R
Salicylaldehyde	$C_7H_6O_2$	R
3,4-Dihydroxybenzaldehyde[24, 39]	$C_7H_6O_3$	G
o-Hydroxyacetophenone	$C_8H_8O_2$	R
1 -Phenylpropan- 1,2-dione	$C_9H_8O_2$	R
Propiophenone	$C_9H_{10}O$	R
5-Methyl-2-hydroxy-acetophenone	$C_9H_{10}O_2$	R
4-Hydroxy-2-methoxy-acetophenone	$C_9H_{10}O_3$	R
3,4-Dihydroxycinnamaldehyde[39]	$C_9H_8O_3$	R
Phenol-carboxylic acids		
3, 4-Dihydroxybenzoic acid[24]	$C_7H_6O_4$	G
2, 4-Dihydroxybenzoic acid[24]	$C_7H_6O_4$	G
Caffeic acid	$C_9H_8O_4$	G R
Chlorogenic acid	$C_{16}H_{18}O_4$	G R

TABLE 8 (continued)

Aromatic Compounds Found in Green and Roasted Coffee[3]

Compound	Empirical formula	Source[a]
Ferulic acid	$C_{10}H_{10}O_4$	G R
3-Feruloylquinic acid	$C_{17}H_{20}O_9$	G R
4-Feruloylquinic acid	$C_{17}H_{20}O_9$	G R
5-Feruloylquinic acid	$C_{17}H_{20}O_9$	G R
Cryptochlorogenic acid	$C_{16}H_{18}O_9$	G R
Isochlorogenic acid a	$C_{25}H_{24}O_{12}$	G R
Isochlorogenic acid b	$C_{25}H_{24}O_{12}$	G R
Isochlorogenic acid c	$C_{25}H_{24}O_{12}$	G R
Neochlorogenic acid	$C_{16}H_{18}O_9$	G R
p-Coumaric acid	$C_9H_8O_3$	G R
3-*p*-Coumarylquinic acid	$C_{16}H_{18}O_8$	G R
4-*p*-Coumarylquinic acid	$C_{16}H_{18}O_8$	G R
5-*p*-Coumarylquinic acid	$C_{16}H_{18}O_8$	G R
3,4-Dimethoxycinnamic acid	$C_{11}H_{12}O_4$	G
Esters, ethers		
Guaiacol	$C_7H_8O_2$	R
2(4)-Methylphenetol	$C_9H_{12}O$	R
4-Ethylguaiacol	$C_9H_{12}O_2$	R
4-Vinylguaiacol	$C_9H_{10}O_2$	G R
Eugenol	$C_{10}H_{12}O_2$	R
Isoeugenol	$C_{10}H_{12}O_2$	G
3,4-Dimethoxystyrene	$C_{10}H_{12}O_2$	R
Vanillin	$C_8H_8O_3$	G
Benzyl formate	$C_8H_8O_2$	R
Benzyl acetate	$C_9H_{10}O_2$	R
2-Ethylphenyl formate	$C_9H_{10}O_2$	R
Methyl benzoate	$C_8H_8O_2$	R
Methyl salicylate	$C_8H_8O_3$	G
4-Hydroxy-3-methoxystyrene[24]	$C_9H_{10}O_2$	G
Nitrogen compounds		
Aniline	C_6H_7N	G
N-methylaniline	C_7H_9N	G
N-ethylaniline	$C_8H_{11}N$	G
o-Toluidine	C_7H_9N	G
o-Anisidine	C_7H_9NO	G
m-Aminoacetophenone	C_8H_9NO	G
Methylanthranilate	$C_8H_9NO_2$	G
Sulfur Compounds		
Thioanisole	C_7H_8S	R
o-Hydroxythioanisole	C_7H_8OS	R

[a]G, in green coffee; R, in roasted coffee.

sirable flavor component.[78] Furfuryl alcohol itself can, however, be significantly decreased in concentration during the steam treatment of green coffee.[36]

The distribution of oxygen heterocyclic compounds differs in Robusta and Arabica roasted coffees; some concentration values are given in Table 9.[39] Roasted Robusta contains relatively high proportions of furfuryl alcohol and the caramel flavored maltol (Figure 7) in comparison with roasted Arabica.[39]

TABLE 9

The Concentration of Some Furan and Pyrone Components in Roasted Coffee[39]

Compound	Arabica (ppm)	Robusta (ppm)
Furfuryl alcohol	300	520
Furan carboxylic acid	80	55
5-(Hydroxymethyl)-2-furaldehyde	35	10
Furaneol	50	25
Ethylfuraneol	8	2
Isomaltol	8	1.5
Maltol	39	45
5-Hydroxymaltol	15	6
5-Hydroxy-5,6-dihydromaltol	13	10

Lactones and acid anhydrides are also seen in roasted coffee, presumably secondarily to the production of the corresponding acid, which finds enhanced stability as an anhydride or a lactone.

Scopoletin and dihydroactinidiolide (Figure 8) are found in green coffee.[3]

B. Nitrogen and Sulfur Heterocyclics

Nitrogen and sulfur heterocyclics are formed during roasting when sugars and furans react with amino acids (Figure 9). For example, model systems containing sucrose in the presence of serine and heated to 225°C yield mostly pyrazines, pyridines, quinoxalines, as well as furans. Alkyl and alkenyl pyrazines and pyrroles are obtained when the serine is replaced by threonine.[79] Similarly, model systems of L-proline and L-hydroxyproline with sucrose gave a series of N-furyl pyrroles that have been identified as a main constituent of coffee aroma.[80] Some aroma contributing S-components in roasted coffee are formed from furfural, 5-methylfurfural, cysteine, and methionine.[80] Various schemes have been described for the reactions between sugars and amino acids. Among the best known is that due to Hodges, with an Amadori reaction as the first reaction be-

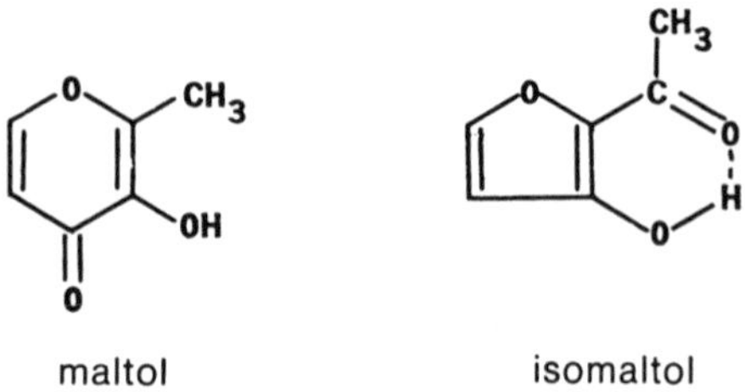

FIGURE 7
Maltol and isomaltol.

maltol

isomaltol

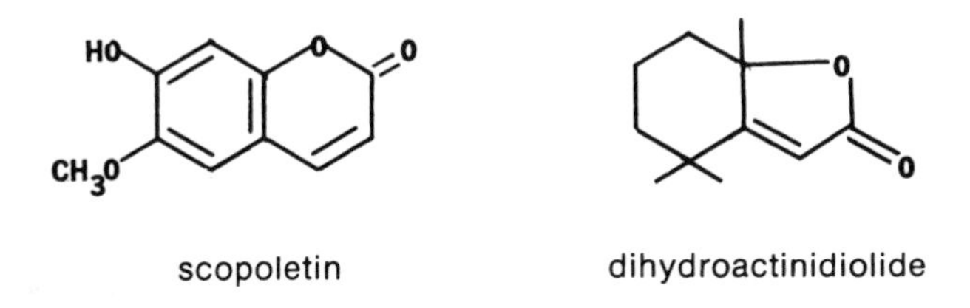

FIGURE 8
Scopoletin and dihydroactinidiolide.

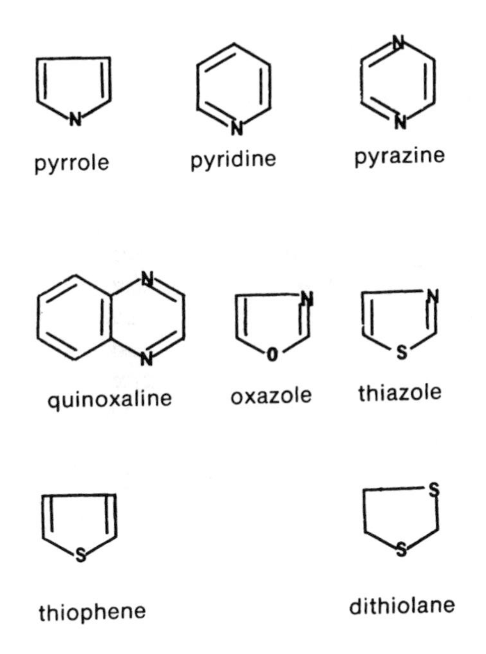

FIGURE 9
Some nitrogen and sulfur heterocyclic systems produced in roasted coffee.

tween an aldose sugar and an amino compound.[3, 14] Pyrazine formation can be accounted for by the scheme given in Figure 10,[3] where a diketone reacts initially with an amino compound. A scheme for oxazole formation is given in Figure 11.[3]

Another source of pyrroles is probably the chlorophyll present in the coffee beans.[15]

Some of the more volatile heterocyclic compounds in ground roasted coffee are substantially lost after 2 weeks; for example, thiophene-3-aldehyde is 80 to 90% lost in this time.[21]

Kahweofuran is an unusual heterocyclic found particularly in coffee (see Figure 12).[3]

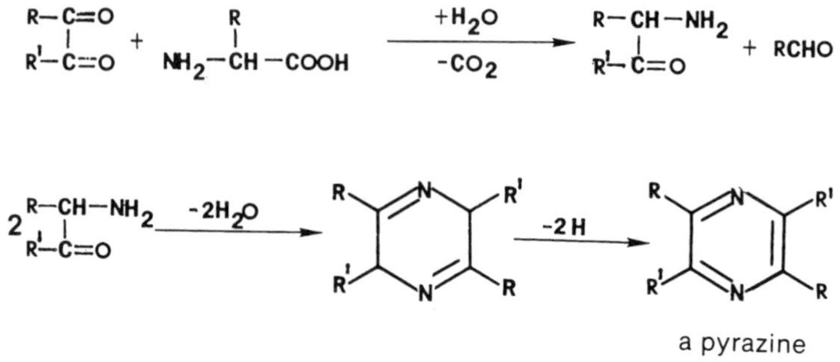

FIGURE 10.
A suggested scheme for pyrazine formation in roasted coffee.[3]

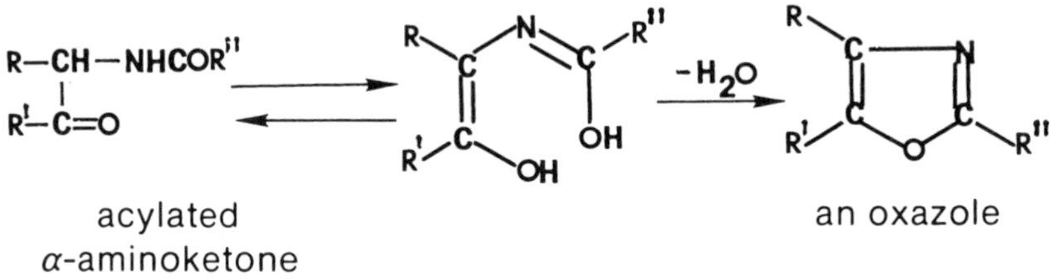

FIGURE 11
A suggested scheme for the formation of oxazoles from a-aminoketones.[3]

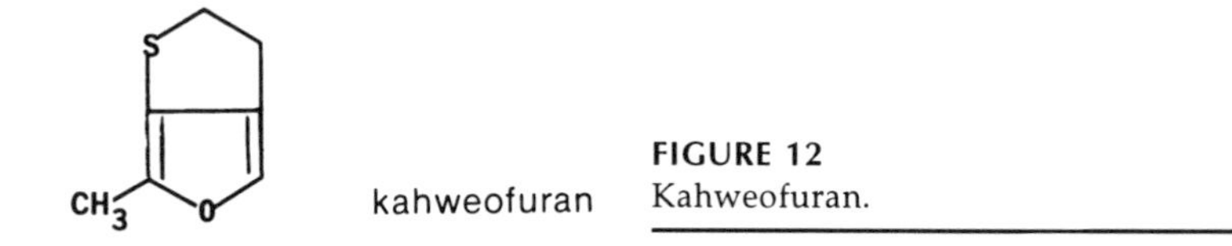

FIGURE 12
Kahweofuran.

Pyrrolidin-2-one is commonly found in coffee products in amounts in the mg/kg range.[81] This has importance if coffee products come into contact with nitrites, because N-nitrosopyrrolidin-2-one is then produced, which can explain observed methylating activity.[82]

Sulfur-containing compounds are significantly more concentrated in Robusta coffees than in Arabicas. This difference can be used to recognize Robusta in coffee blends with Arabica.[83]

C. Aroma and Flavor Heterocyclics

Various heterocyclic compounds contribute particular flavor and aroma notes; some examples follow: Furfural is haylike,[15] N-furyl pyrroles pos-

TABLE10

Sulfur-Containing Furans in Arabica, Robusta, and Instant Coffees, 10 Days After Roasting[19]

Compound	Arabica (ppb)	Robusta (ppb)	Instant (ppb)
Furfurylmercaptan	1100	2000	3900
Furfurylmethyl sulfide	1100	2200	2800
Furfurylmethyl disulfide	120	650	600
(5-Methylfurfuryl)mercaptan	190	110	10
(5-Methylfurfuryl)methyl sulfide	90	60	40
(5-Methylfurfuryl)methyl disulfide	30	20	15
Furfurylethyl sulfide	+	10	–
Difurfuryl sulfide	60	130	–
2-Methyl-3-(methylthio)furan	+	25	–
2-Methyl-3-(methyldithio)furan	+	10	–
Kahweofuran	1160	850	600

sess green notes,[80] the odor of pyrazines is that of roasted nuts and that of pyridines is burnt or tarry.[3] The concentrations of several heterocyclic compounds with sulfur group substituents, 10 d after roasting, are given in Table 10.[19]

Sulfur compounds such as furfuryl mercaptans have a rotten odor but in small amounts are coffee-like.[15] Furfuryl mercaptan itself has an odor threshold of 0.005 ppb in water but at 10 ppb in water it imparts a distinctly stale odor.[19] The particular precursors of furfuryl mercaptan seem to be the coffee cell wall material which contains both arabinogalactan as a pentose sugar source and protein such as glutathione.[84] Other sulfur compounds such as kahweofuran and methyldithiofurans impart a meaty odor if their concentrations are high enough.[19]

Pyridine is formed from trigonelline during roasting.[3] It is presumed to contribute to the flavor, especially in the darker coffee roasts.[15]

A list of heterocyclic compounds found in coffee is given in Table 11.

VI. PROTEINS, AMINO ACIDS AND NUCLEIC ACIDS

The protein content of green and roasted coffee beans as a percentage of the whole bean, in each case, is of the same order of magnitude. However, a roasted coffee will have sustained a 14 to 20% weight loss.[15] Roasted coffee contains about 10% protein when estimated in terms of the amino acids released on hydrolysis.[3] Protein nitrogen is lost and redistributed during roasting, when the proteins react with the carbohydrates in browning reactions, and heterocyclic compounds are produced.

The proportions of the amino acids obtained by hydrolysis in green and roasted coffee beans differs (see Table 12).[3] Arginine, cystine, histi-

TABLE 11

Heterocyclic Compounds Found in Green and Roasted Coffee[3]

Compound	Empirical formula	Source[a]
Oxygen compounds		
Furan	C_4H_4O	G R
2-Methylfuran	C_5H_6O	G R
3-Methylfuran	C_5H_6O	R
2,5-Dimethylfuran	C_6H_8O	R
2,3,5-Trimethylfuran[76]	$C_7H_{10}O$	R
2-Ethylfuran	C_6H_8O	R
2-Methyl-5-isopropylfuran[76]	$C_8H_{12}O$	R
2-Propylfuran	$C_7H_{10}O$	R
2-Isopropylfuran[76]	$C_7H_{10}O$	R
2-Butylfuran	$C_8H_{12}O$	R
2-Amylfuran	$C_9H_{14}O$	G R
2-Vinylfuran[76]	C_6H_6O	R
2-Vinyl-3-methylfuran[76]	C_7H_8O	R
2-Vinyl-4-methylfuran[76]	C_7H_8O	R
2-Vinyl-5-methylfuran[76]	C_7H_8O	R
2-Propenylfuran[76]	C_7H_8O	R
2-Vinyl-3,5-dimethylfuran[76]	$C_8H_{10}O$	R
2-Vinyl-4,5-dimethylfuran[76]	$C_8H_{10}O$	R
2-Methyl-5-*n*-propenylfuran[76]	$C_8H_{10}O$	R
2-Isobutenylfuran[76]	$C_8H_{10}O$	R
2-Acetylfuran	$C_6H_6O_2$	G R
2-Propionylfuran	$C_7H_8O_2$	R
2-Furancarboxylic acid	$C_5H_4O_3$	R
5-Methylfurfural	$C_6H_6O_2$	G R
5-Methyl-2-acetylfuran	$C_7H_8O_2$	R
5-Methyl-2-propionylfuran	$C_8H_{10}O_2$	R
2-Butyrylfuran	$C_8H_{10}O_2$	R
1-(2'-Furyl)-propan-2-one	$C_7H_8O_2$	R
1-(2'-Furyl)-butan-2-one	$C_8H_{10}O_2$	R
1-(2'-Furyl)-butan-3-one	$C_8H_{10}O_2$	R
Benzofuran (cumaron)	C_8H_6O	R
2-Methylbenzofuran	C_9H_8O	R
3-Phenylfuran	$C_{10}H_8O$	R
Furfuryl alcohol	$C_5H_6O_2$	G R
5-Methylfurfurylalcohol[76]	$C_6H_8O_2$	R
5-Methyl-2-methylfuryl sulfide	C_6H_8OS	R
Furfurylmethylether	$C_6H_8O_2$	R
Furfuryl formate	$C_6H_6O_3$	R
Furfurylacetate	$C_7H_8O_3$	G R
Furfuryl propionate	$C_8H_{10}O_3$	R
Furfuryl butyrate	$C_9H_{12}O_3$	R
Furfuryl isobutyrate	$C_9H_{12}O_3$	R
Furfuryl isovalerate	$C_{10}H_{14}O_3$	R
Furfuryl 2-methylbutyrate	$C_{10}H_{14}O_3$	R
Furfurylcrotonate	$C_9H_{10}O_3$	R
Furfuryl β,β'-dimethylacrylate	$C_{10}H_{12}O_3$	R

TABLE 11 (continued)

Heterocyclic Compounds Found in Green and Roasted Coffee[3]

Compound	Empirical formula	Source[a]
Difurfurylether	$C_{10}H_{10}O_3$	R
5-Methyldifurfurylether	$C_{11}H_{12}O_3$	R
Furfurylmercaptan	$C_5H_6O\ S$	R
Furfurylmethyl sulfide	$C_6H_8O_2S$	R
Furfurylthioacetate	C_7H_8OS	R
Difurfuryl sulfide	$C_{10}H_{10}O_2S$	R
Furfural	$C_5H_4O_2$	G R
1-(5'-Methyl-2'-furyl)-propan-2-one	$C_8H_{10}O_2$	R
1-(5'-Methyl-2'-furyl)-butan-2-one	$C_9H_{12}O_2$	R
1-(5'-Methyl-2'-furyl)-butan-3-one	$C_9H_{12}O_2$	R
3-(2'-Furyl)-propenal	$C_7H_6O_2$	R
1 -(2'-Furyl)-propan-1,2-dione	$C_7H_6O_3$	R
1-(2'-Furyl)-butan-1,2-dione	$C_8H_8O_3$	R
1-(5'-Methyl-2'-furyl)-propan-1,2-dione	$C_8H_8O_3$	R
1-(5'-Methyl-2'-furyl)-butan-1,2-dione	$C_9H_{10}O_3$	R
Methyl furoate[76]	$C_6H_6O_3$	R
Ethyl furoate[76]	$C_7H_8O_3$	R
Methyl thiofuroate	$C_6H_6O_2S$	R
5-Methyl-2-furonitrile	C_6H_5NO	R
2,2'-Difuryl	$C_8H_6O_2$	R
2,2'-Difurylmethane	$C_9H_8O_2$	R
5-Methyl-2,2'-difurylmethane	$C_{10}H_{10}O_2$	R
bis-(5-Methyl-2-furyl)-methane	$C_{11}H_{12}O_2$	R
4-(2'-Furyl)-but-2-en-2-one	$C_8H_8O_2$	R
2-Furfuryloxyacetone	$C_7H_8O_3$	R
2-Isobutyrylfuran	$C_8H_{10}O_2$	R
3-(2'-Furyl)-propanal (tentative)	$C_7H_8O_2$	R
Hydroxymethylfurfural	$C_6H_6O_3$	R
Tetrahydrofuran	C_4H_8O	R
2-Methyltetrahydrofuran	$C_5H_{10}O$	R
2-Acetyltetrahydrofuran	$C_6H_{10}O_2$	R
2-Isopropenyl-5-vinyl-5-methyl-tetrahydrofuran	$C_{10}H_{16}O$	R
2-(2'-Hydroxy-2'-propyl)-5-vinyl-5-methyl-tetrahydrofuran (*cis*-linalool oxide)	$C_{10}H_{18}O_2$	R
trans-Linalool oxide	$C_{10}H_{18}O_2$	R
2,3-Dihydrobenzofuran	C_8H_8O	R
2-Methyltetrahydrofuran-3-one	$C_5H_8O_2$	R
2,4,5-Trimethyl-2H-furan-3-one	$C_7H_{10}O_2$	R
2,5-Dimethyl-2H-furan-3-one	$C_6H_8O_2$	R
Furaneol (2,5-dimethyl-4-hydroxy-3(2H)-furanone)[39]	$C_6H_8O_3$	R
Ethylfuraneol[39]	$C_6H_8O_3$	R
γ-Butyrolactone	$C_4H_6O_2$	

TABLE 11 (continued)

Heterocyclic Compounds Found in Green and Roasted Coffee[3]

Compound	Empirical formula	Source[a]
γ-Valerolactone	$C_5H_8O_2$	R
α-Methyl-g-butyrolactone	$C_5H_8O_2$	R
Crotonolactone	$C_4H_4O_2$	R
2,3-Dimethylbut-2-en-1,4-lactone	$C_6H_8O_2$	R
3,4-Dimethylbut-2-en-1,4-lactone	$C_6H_8O_2$	R
2,3,4-Trimethylbut-2-en-1 ,4-lactone	$C_7H_{10}O_2$	R
6-Methoxy-7-hydroxycoumarin (scopoletin)	$C_{10}H_8O_4$	G
Dihydroactinidiolide	$C_{11}H_{16}O_2$	G
5-Methyl-2-furfurylmethyl sulfide	$C_7H_{10}OS$	R
Methylmaleic anhydride	$C_5H_4O_3$	R
Dimethylmaleic anhydride	$C_6H_6O_3$	R
2-Ethyl-3-methylmaleic anhydride	$C_7H_8O_3$	R
Maltol (2-methyl-3-hydroxy-γ-pyrone)	$C_6H_6O_3$	R
Isomaltol[39]	$C_6H_6O_3$	R
5-Hydroxymaltol[39]	$C_6H_6O_4$	R
5-Hydroxy-5,6-dihydromaltol[39]	$C_6H_8O_4$	R
Nitrogen compounds		
Pyrrole	C_4H_5N	R
N-methylpyrrole	C_5H_7N	G R
2-Methylpyrrole	C_5H_7N	R
N,2-dimethylpyrrole	C_6H_9N	R
2,4-Dimethylpyrrole	C_6H_9N	R
2-Ethylpyrrole[76]	C_6H_9N	R
N-ethylpyrrole	C_6H_9N	R
N-*n*-butylpyrrole	$C_8H_{13}N$	R
2-Isobutylpyrrole	$C_8H_{13}N$	R
2,4-Dimethyl-3-ethylpyrrole	$C_8H_{13}N$	R
N-*n*-pentylpyrrole	$C_9H_{15}N$	R
N-isopentylpyrrole	$C_9H_{15}N$	R
2-*n*-Pentylpyrrole	$C_9H_{15}N$	R
N-(2-methylbutyl)-pyrrole	$C_9H_{15}N$	R
N-acetylpyrrole[76]	C_6H_7NO	R
2-Acetylpyrrole	C_6H_7NO	G R
2-Propionylpyrrole[76]	C_7H_9NO	R
2-Pyrrole aldehyde	C_5H_5NO	R
N-methylpyrrole-2-al	C_6H_7NO	R
5-Methylpyrrole-2-al	C_6H_7NO	R
N-methyl-2-acetylpyrrole	C_7H_9NO	R
N-ethyl-2-acetylpyrrole	$C_8H_{11}NO$	R
N-ethylpyrrole-2-al	C_7H_9NO	R
N,5-dimethylpyrrole-2-al	C_7H_9NO	R
N-isopentylpyrrole-2-al	$C_{10}H_{15}NO$	R
N-(2-methylbutyl)-pyrrole-2-al	$C_{10}H_{15}NO$	R
1-(2'-Pyrryl)-butan-1,2-dione	$C_8H_9NO_2$	R

TABLE 11 (continued)

Heterocyclic Compounds Found in Green and Roasted Coffee[3]

Compound	Empirical formula	Source[a]
N-methyl-(2'-pyrryl)-butan-1,2-dione	$C_8H_9NO_2$	R
N-furfurylpyrrole	C_9H_9NO	R
N-furfuryl-2-methylpyrrole[76]	$C_{10}H_{11}NO$	R
N-propionylpyrrole	C_7H_9NO	R
N-acetyl-2-methylpyrrole[76]	C_7H_9NO	R
2-Acetyl-5-methylpyrrole[76]	C_7H_9NO	R
N-furfurylpyrrole-2-al	$C_{10}H_9NO_2$	R
N-furfuryl-2-acetylpyrrole	$C_{11}H_{11}NO_2$	R
N-(5'-methylfuryl)-pyrrole	$C_{10}H_{11}NO$	R
Indole	C_8H_7N	R
2-Methylindole	C_9H_9N	R
3 Oxindole	C_8H_7NO	R
2-Methylindoline (tentative)	$C_9H_{11}N$	G
Pyridine	C_5H_5N	G R
2-Methylpyridine (α-picoline)	C_6H_7N	G R
3-Methylpyridine (β-picoline)	C_6H_7N	R
3-Ethylpyridine	C_7H_9N	G R
2-Acetylpyridine	C_7H_7NO	G R
3-Acetylpyridine	C_7H_7NO	G R
2-Acetyl-methylpyridine	C_8H_9NO	R
3-Phenylpyridine	$C_{11}H_9N$	R
Methylnicotinamide	$C_7H_7NO_2$	R
2,6-Dimethylpyridine	C_7H_9N	G
2-Ethylpyridine	C_7H_9N	G
4-Vinylpyridine	C_7H_7N	G
Quinoline	C_9H_7N	G
3(4)-Methylquinoline	$C_{10}H_9N$	G R
3-Methylcarbostyril (2-hydroxy-3-methylquinoline)	$C_{10}H_9NO$	R
Pyrazine	$C_4H_4N_2$	R
2-Methylpyrazine	$C_5H_6N_2$	G R
2-Ethylpyrazine	$C_6H_8N_2$	G R
2-Propylpyrazine	$C_7H_{10}N_2$	R
2,3-Dimethylpyrazine	$C_6H_8N_2$	G R
2,5-Dimethylpyrazine	$C_6H_8N_2$	G R
2,6-Dimethylpyrazine	$C_6H_8N_2$	G R
2-Ethyl-3-methylpyrazine	$C_7H_{10}N_2$	R
2-Ethyl-5-methylpyrazine	$C_7H_{10}N_2$	G R
2-Ethyl-6-methylpyrazine	$C_7H_{10}N_2$	G R
2,5-Diethylpyrazine	$C_8H_{12}N_2$	R
2,6-Diethylpyrazine	$C_8H_{12}N_2$	R
2-Methyl-6-*n*-propylpyrazine	$C_8H_{12}N_2$	R
2-Methyl-5-*n*-propylpyrazine	$C_8H_{12}N_2$	R
2-Methyl-5-isopropylpyrazine	$C_8H_{12}N_2$	R
2-Isobutyl-3-methylpyrazine	$C_9H_{14}N_2$	R
2,3,5-Trimethylpyrazine	$C_7H_{10}N_2$	G R

TABLE 11 (continued)

Heterocyclic Compounds Found in Green and Roasted Coffee[3]

Compound	Empirical formula	Source[a]
2,3-Dimethyl-5-ethylpyrazine	$C_8H_{12}N_2$	R
2,6-Dimethyl-3-ethylpyrazine	$C_8H_{12}N_2$	R
2-Ethyl-3,5-dimethylpyrazine	$C_8H_{12}N_2$	G R
3-Ethyl-2,5-dimethylpyrazine	$C_8H_{12}N_2$	G R
2,3-Diethyl-5-methylpyrazine	$C_9H_{14}N_2$	R
2,5-Diethyl-3-methylpyrazine	$C_9H_{14}N_2$	R
2,6-Diethyl-3-methylpyrazine	$C_9H_{14}N_2$	R
2,5-Dimethyl-3-isobutylpyrazine	$C_{10}H_{16}N_2$	R
Tetramethylpyrazine	$C_8H_{12}N_2$	R
2-Ethyl-3,5,6-trimethylpyrazine	$C_9H_{14}N_2$	R
Diethyl-dimethylpyrazine	$C_{10}H_{16}N_2$	R
2-Vinylpyrazine	$C_6H_6N_2$	R
2-Methyl-5-vinylpyrazine	$C_7H_8N_2$	R
2-Methyl-6-vinylpyrazine	$C_7H_8N_2$	R
2-(*trans*-1-Propenyl)-pyrazine	$C_7H_8N_2$	R
2-Methyl-6-(*trans*-1-propenyl)-pyrazine	$C_8H_{10}N_2$	R
2-Methyl-5-(*trans*-1-propenyl)-pyrazine	$C_8H_{10}N_2$	R
2-Ethyl-6-*n*-propylpyrazidine	$C_9H_{14}N_2$	R
2-Methoxy-3-methylpyrazine	$C_6H_8N_2O$	G
2-Methoxy-3-ethylpyrazine	$C_7H_{10}N_2O$	G
2-Methoxy-3-isopropylpyrazine	$C_8H_{12}N_2O$	G
2-Methoxy-3-isobutylpyrazine	$C_9H_{14}N_2O$	G R
2-Acetylpyrazine	$C_6H_6N_2O$	R
2-Acetyl-3-methylpyrazine	$C_7H_8N_2O$	R
2-Acetyl-5-methylpyrazine	$C_7H_8N_2O$	R
2-Acetyl-6-methylpyrazine	$C_7H_8N_2O$	R
2-Acetyl-3,5-dimethylpyrazine	$C_8H_{10}N_2O$	R
2-Acetyl-3,6-dimethylpyrazine	$C_8H_{10}N_2O$	R
2-Acetyl-5,6-dimethylpyrazine	$C_8H_{10}N_2O$	R
2-(2'-Furyl)-pyrazine	$C_8H_6N_2O$	R
2-(2'-Furyl)-3-methylpyrazine	$C_9H_8N_2O$	R
2-(2'-Furyl)-5-methylpyrazine	$C_9H_8N_2O$	R
2-(2'-Furyl)-6-methylpyrazine	$C_9H_8N_2O$	R
2-(2'-Furyl)-3,5-dimethylpyrazine	$C_{10}H_{10}N_2O$	R
2-(2'-Furyl)-3,6-dimethylpyrazine	$C_{10}H_{10}N_2O$	R
2-(2'-Furyl)-5,6-dimethylpyrazine	$C_{10}H_{10}N_2O$	R
2-(2'-5'-Methylfuryl)-3-methylpyrazine	$C_{10}H_{10}N_2O$	R
2-(2'-5'-Methylfuryl)-6-methylpyrazine	$C_{10}H_{10}N_2O$	R
2-(2'-4'-Methylfuryl)-3-methylpyrazine	$C_{10}H_{10}N_2O$	R
2-(2'-4'-Methylfuryl)-5-methylpyrazine	$C_{10}H_{10}N_2O$	R
2-(2'-4'-Methylfuryl)-6-methylpyrazine	$C_{10}H_{10}N_2O$	R

TABLE 11 (continued)

Heterocyclic Compounds Found in Green and Roasted Coffee[3]

Compound	Empirical formula	Source[a]
2-(2'-4',5'-Dimethylfuryl)-5(6)-methylpyrazine	$C_{11}H_{12}N_2O$	R
6,7-Dihydro-5H-cyclopentapyrazine	$C_7H_8N_2$	R
5-Methyl-6,7-dihydro-5H-cyclopenta-pyrazine	$C_8H_{10}N_2$	R
2(3),5-Dimethyl-6,7-dihydro-5H-cyclopentapyrazine	$C_9H_{12}N_2$	R
3(2),5-Dimethyl-6,7-dihydro-5H-cyclopentapyrazine	$C_9H_{12}N_2$	R
5,7-Dimethyl-6,7-dihydro-5H-cyclo-pentapyrazine	$C_9H_{12}N_2$	R
2,3-Dimethyl-6,7-dihydro-5H-cyclo-pentapyrazine	$C_9H_{12}N_2$	R
2,5,7-Trimethyl-6,7-dihydro-5H-cyclo-pentapyrazine	$C_{10}H_{14}N_2$	R
2,3,5-Trimethyl-6,7-dihydro-5H-cyclo-pentapyrazine	$C_{10}H_{14}N_2$	R
2-Ethyl-6,7-dihydro-5H-cyclopenta-pyrazine	$C_9H_{12}N_2$	R
5-Ethyl-6,7-dihydro-5H-cyclopenta-pyrazine	$C_9H_{12}N_2$	R
2-Methyl-3-ethyl-6,7-dihydro-5H-cyclopentapyrazine	$C_{10}H_{14}N_2$	R
2-Methyl-6,7-dihydro-5H-cyclopenta-pyrazine	$C_8H_{10}N_2$	R
Quinoxaline	$C_8H_6N_2$	R
5-Methylquinoxaline	$C_9H_8N_2$	R
Methylquinoxaline	$C_9H_8N_2$	R
Dimethylquinoxaline	$C_{10}H_{10}N_2$	R
2,3-Dimethylquinoxaline	$C_{10}H_{10}N_2$	R
5,6,7,8-Tetrahydroquinoxaline	$C_8H_{10}N_2$	R
2-Methyl-5,6,7,8-tetrahydroquinoxaline	$C_9H_{12}N_2$	R
5-Methyl-5,6,7,8-tetrahydroquinoxaline	$C_9H_{12}N_2$	R
2,3-Dimethyl-5,6,7,8-tetrahydro-quinoxaline	$C_{10}H_{14}N_2$	R
2-Ethyl-5,6,7,8-tetrahydroquinoxaline	$C_{10}H_{14}N_2$	R
Sulfur compounds		
Thiophene	C_4H_4S	R
2-Methylthiophene	C_5H_6S	R
2-Methyl-4-ethylthiophene	$C_7H_{10}S$	R
2-*n*-Propylthiophene[76]	$C_7H_{10}S$	
2-*n*-Butylthiophene[76]	$C_8H_{12}S$	R

TABLE 11 (continued)

Heterocyclic Compounds Found in Green and Roasted Coffee[3]

Compound	Empirical formula	Source[a]
3-Vinylthiophene	C_6H_6S	R
Thenyl alcohol (2-hydroxymethylthiophene)	C_5H_6OS	R
2-Acetylthiophene	$C_6H_6O\ S$	R
3-Acetylthiophene	$C_6H_6O\ S$	R
2-Thiophene aldehyde	$C_5H_4O\ S$	R
5-Methylthiophene-2-al	$C_6H_6O\ S$	R
3-Methylthiophene-2-al[76]	$C_6H_6O\ S$	R
2-Propionylthiophene	$C_7H_8O\ S$	R
3-Methyl-2-acetylthiophene	$C_7H_8O\ S$	R
4-Methyl-2-acetylthiophene	$C_7H_8O\ S$	R
5-Methyl-2-acetylthiophene	$C_7H_8O\ S$	R
1-(2'-Thienyl)-propan-1,2-dione	$C_7H_6O_2S$	R
1-(2'-Thienyl-4(5)-methyl)-propan-1,2-dione	$C_8H_8O_2S$	R
1-(3'-Thienyl)-propan-1,2-dione	$C_7H_6O_2S$	R
Methyl thenoate	$C_6H_6O_2S$	R
Thenyl acetate	$C_7H_8O_2S$	R
Thenyl formate	$C_6H_6O_2S$	R
Benzothiophene	C_8H_6S	R
Thienothiophene	$C_6H_4S_2$	R
Kahweofuran	$C_7H_8O\ S$	R
Tetrahydrothiophene-2-one	$C_4H_6O\ S$	R
Tetrahydrothiophene-3-one	$C_4H_6O\ S$	R
2-Methyltetrahydrothiophene-3-one	$C_5H_8O\ S$	R
2-Methyl-3-(methylthio)furan[19]	C_6H_8OS	R
2-Methyl-3-(methyldithio)furan[19]	$C_6H_8OS_2$	R
2,5-Dimethyl-3-(methylthio)furan[19]	$C_7H_{10}OS$	R
2,5-Dimethyl-3-(methyldithio) furan[19]	$C_7H_{10}OS_2$	R
3,3'-Dimethyl-1,2-dithiolane[19]	$C_5H_{10}S_2$	R
3,3'-Dimethyl-4-oxo-1,2-dithiolane[19]	$C_5H_8O\ S_2$	R
Homokahweofuran (2,4-dimethyl-3-oxa-8-thiobicyclo[3.3.0]-1,4-octadiene), tentative[19]	$C_8H_{10}OS$	R
Furfurylmethyl trisulfide, tentative[19]	$C_6H_8O\ S_3$	R
Furfurylethyl sulfide[19]	$C_7H_{10}OS$	R
Difurfuryl disulfide[19]	$C_{10}H_{10}O_2S_2$	R
(5-Methylfurfuryl)mercaptan[19]	$C_6H_8O\ S$	R
5-Methylfurfuryl methyl disulfide[19]	$C_7H_{10}O\ S_2$	R
Di-(5-methylfurfuryl)disulfide[19]	$C_{12}H_{14}O_2S_2$	R
Nitrogen-sulfur compounds		
Thiazole	$C_3H_3N\ S$	R
2-Methylthiazole	$C_4H_5N\ S$	R

TABLE 11 (continued)

Heterocyclic Compounds Found in Green and Roasted Coffee[3]

Compound	Empirical formula	Source[a]
4-Methylthiazole	C_4H_5NS	R
5-Methylthiazole	C_4H_5NS	R
2-Ethylthiazole (tentative)	C_5H_7NS	R
4-Ethylthiazole	C_5H_7NS	R
5-Ethylthiazole	C_5H_7NS	R
2-*n*-Propylthiazole	C_6H_9NS	R
4-*n*-Butylthiazole	$C_7H_{11}NS$	R
2,4-Dimethylthiazole	C_5H_7NS	R
2,5-Dimethylthiazole	C_5H_7NS	R
4,5-Dimethylthiazole	C_5H_7NS	R
2-Methyl-4-ethylthiazole	C_6H_9NS	R
2-Methyl-5-ethylthiazole	C_6H_9NS	R
4-Methyl-5-ethylthiazole	C_6H_9NS	R
2-Ethyl-4-methylthiazole	C_6H_9NS	R
4-Ethyl-5-methylthiazole	C_6H_9NS	R
2,4-Diethylthiazole	$C_7H_{11}NS$	R
2,5-Diethylthiazole	$C_7H_{11}NS$	R
2-*n*-Propyl-5-ethylthiazole	$C_8H_{13}NS$	R
2,4,5-Trimethylthiazole	C_6H_9NS	R
2,4-Dimethyl-5-ethylthiazole	$C_7H_{11}NS$	R
2,5-Dimethyl-4-ethylthiazole	$C_7H_{11}NS$	R
4,5-Dimethyl-2-ethylthiazole	$C_7H_{11}NS$	R
Benzothiazole	C_7H_5NS	R
2-Acetylthiazole	C_6H_5NOS	R
2-Acetyl-4-methylthiazole	C_6H_7NOS	R
2-Propionyl-4-methylthiazole	C_7H_9NOS	R
Nitrogen-oxygen compounds		
2-Ethyloxazole (tentative)	C_5H_7NO	R
4-Ethyloxazole (tentative)	C_5H_7NO	R
5-Ethyloxazole (tentative)	C_5H_7NO	R
2(4)-*n*-Butyloxazole	$C_7H_{11}NO$	R
2,4-Dimethyloxazole	C_5H_7NO	R
2,5-Dimethyloxazole	C_5H_7NO	R
4,5-Dimethyloxazole	C_5H_7NO	R
2-Ethyl-5-methyloxazole	C_6H_9NO	R
2-Methyl-4-ethyloxazole	C_6H_9NO	R
4-Methyl-5-ethyloxazole	C_6H_9NO	R
2-Ethyl-4-methyloxazole	C_6H_9NO	R
4-Ethyl-5-methyloxazole	C_6H_9NO	R
2-Methyl-5-ethyloxazole	C_6H_9NO	R
2-*n*-Propyl-5-methyloxazole	$C_7H_{11}NO$	R
2,4,5-Trimethyloxazole	C_6H_9NO	R
2,5-Dimethyl-4-ethyloxazole	$C_7H_{11}NO$	R
2,4-Dimethyl-5-ethyloxazole	$C_7H_{11}NO$	R
4,5-Dimethyl-2-ethyloxazole	$C_7H_{11}NO$	R
2-*n*-Propyl-4,5-dimethyloxazole	$C_8H_{13}NO$	R

TABLE 11 (continued)

Heterocyclic Compounds Found in Green and Roasted Coffee[3]

Compound	Empirical formula	Source[a]
4-*n*-Butyl-2,5-dimethyloxazole	$C_9H_{15}N\ O$	R
2-Phenyloxazole	$C_9H_7N\ O$	R
5-Acetyl-2-methyloxazole	$C_6H_7N\ O_2$	R
5-Acetyl-2,4-dimethyloxazole	$C_7H_9N\ O_2$	R
2-Methylbenzoxazole	$C_8H_7N\ O$	R
4-Methylbenzoxazole (tentative)	$C_8H_7N\ O$	R
2,5-Dimethylbenzoxazole	$C_9H_9N\ O$	R
2,4-Dimethylbenzoxazole (tentative)	$C_9H_9N\ O$	R
2,6-Dimethylbenzoxazole (tentative)	$C_9H_9N\ O$	R
N,a-Dimethylsuccinimide	$C_6H_9N\ O_2$	R

[a]G, in green coffee; R, in roasted coffee.

TABLE 12

Amino Acids Obtained From Green and Roasted Coffee, by Acidic Hydrolysis, as Percentages of the Total Amino Acid Content[3]

Amino acid	Green coffee (%)	Roasted coffee (%) (17.6% roast)
Alanine	4.75	5.52
Arginine	3.61	0
Aspartic acid	10.63	7.13
Cystine	2.89	0.69
Glutamic acid	19.80	23.22
Glycine	6.40	6.78
Histidine	2.79	1.61
Isoleucine	4.64	4.60
Leucine	8.77	10.34
Lysine	6.81	2.76
Methionine	1.44	1.26
Phenylalanine	5.78	6.32
Proline	6.60	7.01
Serine	5.88	0.80
Threonine	3.82	1.38
Tyrosine	3.61	4.35
Valine	8.05	8.05

dine, lysine, serine, and threonine are the most significantly reduced in proportion after roasting. Glutamic acid and leucine are particularly increased in proportion after roasting.

Aspartic acid has been identified as an iron-binding material in instant coffee, and was found to be approximately 0.4% of the instant coffee by dry weight.[85]

Free amino acids are also present in green coffee. Eighteen amino acids and pipecolic acid have been found, free or as part of the protein.[86] More recently, ornithine, β-alanine, and pipecolic acid have been measured in Arabica and Robusta coffees, and hydroxyproline has been measured in Arabica.[87] Steam pretreatment of coffee reduces the free amino acid content considerably, and roasting can result in no free amino acids remaining.[88] Indeed, a method has been developed for determining the degree of roast in coffee, by determining the relative amounts of both enantiomers of alanine, leucine, phenylalanine, and glutamic acid.[89] Seratonin (5-hydroxy-tryptamine) is found in recoverable amounts in coffee wax, following decaffeination of coffee beans.[90]

Investigation of the nucleopurine content of coffee showed that there was little difference in their nature between Arabica and Robusta coffee. On average the nucleopurine content in coffee is 120mg/kg dry matter. However, the amount in Robusta coffees was higher and this was correlated with the higher caffeine biosynthesis. Roasting coffee reduces the amount of the nucleopurines, and in coffee beverages the amount is less than 1 mg per cup (150 ml).[91]

Some particular proteins, recognizable thus far by little more than their biological effect, have been documented. An allergen in the green coffee bean of between 18,000 and 40,000 da is probably a heterogeneous glycoprotein; it can be precipitated out at pH 4.0 to 4.5.[92, 93]

An acid phosphatase and a trypsin inhibitor[94] also are presumed to form part of the protein complement in green coffee.

A list of protein amino acids and enzyme systems found in coffee is given in Table 13.[3]

VII. CARBOHYDRATES

Green coffee beans, as expected, contain storage polysaccharides such as starch, and structural support compounds such as cellulose and lignin. Mono- and di-saccharides are represented, as well as the related compounds quinic acid and myo-inositol.

A. Polysaccharides

The bulk of the heteropolysaccharides in the green coffee bean are formed from mannan, galactan, and araban.[95, 96] Three fractions can be

TABLE 13

Protein Amino Acids and Enzymes Found in Green and Roasted Coffee[3]

Compound	Empirical formula	Source[a]
Alanine	$C_3H_7NO_2$	G R
γ-Aminobutyric acid	$C_4H_9NO_2$	G
Arginine	$C_6H_{14}N_4O_2$	G R
Aspartine	$C_4H_8N_2O_3$	G
Aspartic acid	$C_4H_7NO_4$	G R
Cysteine	$C_3H_7NO_2S$	G
Cystine	$C_6H_{12}N_2O_4S_2$	G R
Glutamic acid	$C_5H_9NO_4$	G R
Glycine	$C_2H_5NO_2$	G R
Histidine	$C_6H_9N_3O_2$	G R
Hydroxyproline	$C_5H_9NO_3$	G R
Isoleucine	$C_6H_{13}NO_2$	R
Leucine	$C_6H_{13}NO_2$	G R
Lysine	$C_6H_{14}N_2O_2$	G R
Methionine	$C_5H_{11}NO_2S$	G R
Phenylalanine	$C_9H_{11}NO_2$	G R
Pipecolic acid	$C_6H_{11}NO_2$	G
Proline	$C_5H_9NO_2$	G R
Ribonucleic acid		G R
Serine	$C_3H_7NO_3$	G R
Threonine	$C_4H_9NO_3$	G R
Tryptophane (tentative)	$C_{11}H_{12}N_2O_2$	G R
Tyrosine	$C_9H_{11}NO_3$	G R
Valine	$C_5H_{11}NO_2$	G R
Amylase		G
β-Fructofuranosidase		G
2α-D-Galactosidase		G
Catalase		G
Peroxidase		G
Polyphenoloxidase		G
Protease		G
Oxidase		G
Acid phosphatase[94]		G
Trypsin inhibitor[94]		G

[a]G, in green coffee; R, in roasted coffee.

recognized: hollocellulose remains after treatment with a reagent such as "chlorine dioxide", which can dissolve glycoproteins as well as the simple water-soluble carbobydrates. Thus, the glycoproteins, the water-soluble carbohydrates, and the hollocellulose constitute three fractions of heteropolysaccharides in green coffee.

The hollocellulose contains mannan:galactan:cellulose, 2:1:1, and little else.[95]

The glycoproteins and water-soluble polysaccharides contain mainly galactan with some araban.[95]

The elucidation of the molecular characteristics of the arabinogalactans and the galactomannans, present in coffee, continues.[97]

Roasting appears to produce another group of water-soluble polysaccharides containing mannan and galactan, from the hollocellulose; they form 1.8 to 4.4% of the roasted coffee.[98] These galacto-mannans formed on roasting are produced in greater amounts from Robusta coffees than from Arabicas.[99] Galacto-mannans are effective complexing agents and their increased presence in roasted Robusta coffee beverage may account for the higher quantities of water extractables seen from Robustas.[96] It is interesting to note here that Robusta coffee beverage foams in the cup far more than Arabica correspondingly prepared. This is attributable to the larger amount of extractable carbohydrate.[15]

The chemical origin of free radicals in coffee is attributed to the sugars or carbohydrates, rather than phenolic constituents[100].

B. Disaccharides

Green Arabica coffee beans contain 7% sucrose, but this is steadily lost during the roasting process; only 0.05% remains in Italian roasted beans.[101] Green Robusta coffees predominantly contain reducing sugars rather than sucrose.[102] During roasting, an exothermic reaction occurs around 200°C. This seems greatest for those coffees with the highest sucrose content, such as high-grown Arabicas.[15] Carbohydrates in general are lost during the roasting process partly as a result of their interaction with amino acids from protein.

C. Monosaccharides

Monosaccharides, present only in trace amounts in green coffee, increase to 2.6% in roasted coffee due in part to the production of galactose, mannose,[103] arabinose, and ribose,[104] as the heteropolysaccharides are broken down.

D. Melanoidins

Monosaccharides are probably involved in the browning reactions that occur during the roasting of coffee. Caramelization involving the sugars alone, and Maillard reactions, between sugars and free amino acids, produce polymeric yellow to dark brown substances, known as melanoidins. These melanoidins can be extracted into hot water, separated and characterized.[105]

A list of carbohydrates found in coffee is given in Table 14.

TABLE 14

Carbohydrates Found in Green and Roasted Coffee[3]

Compound	Empirical formula	Source[a]
Araban		G R
Arabinogalactan		G
L-Arabinose	$C_5H_{10}O_5$	G R
Cellobiose	$C_{12}H_{22}O_{11}$	G R
Cellulose	$(C_6H_{10}O_5)n$	G
Fructose	$C_6H_{12}O_6$	R
Galactan		G R
D-Galactose	$C_6H_{12}O_6$	G R
D-Galacturonic acid	$C_6H_{10}O_7$	G
Glucan		R
Glucogalactomannan		G
D-Glucose	$C_6H_{12}O_6$	G R
Glucuronic acid	$C_6H_{10}O_7$	G R
Maltose	$C_{12}H_{22}O_{11}$	G R
D-Mannan	$(C_6H_{10}O_5)n$	G R
D-Mannose	$C_6H_{12}O_6$	G R
Melibiose	$C_{12}H_{22}O_{11}$	G
Raffinose	$C_{18}H_{32}O_{16}$	G R
Rhamnose	$C_6H_{12}O_5$	G R
Sucrose	$C_{12}H_{22}O_{11}$	G R
Stachyose	$C_{24}H_{42}O_{21}$	G R
Starch	$(C_6H_{10}O_5)n$	G
Xylose	$C_5H_{10}O_5$	G R
Lignin		G
Myo-inositol	$C_6H_{12}O_6$	
Quinic acid	$C_7H_{12}O_6$	G R
Ribose [65]		R
Pectin [58]		G

VIII. LIPIDS

Coffee bean lipids include triglycerides, sterols, tocopherols, and diterpenes, all of which are mainly found in the coffee oils. The Nβ-alkanoyl-5-hydroxytryptamides are concentrated in the outer coating of coffee bean wax.

A. Coffee Oil

Coffee oil is generally described as the petroleum ether-soluble fraction from green coffee beans. Arabica coffees contain 11.1 to 13.6% oil, whereas Robusta coffees contain only 4.4 to 4.8% oil.[106] Triglycerides constitute 79% of this oil, terpene esters 17%, and the remaining 4% is contributed by sterols, free terpenes, tocopherols, and as yet unknown substances.[3] Palmitic, stearic, oleic, and linoleic are the most frequently seen ester-forming acids. In the triglycerides, the unsaturated acids tend to be in the C-2 position as in most vegetable oils. The unsaturated acids tend to be associated with the triglycerides rather than with the terpenes.[107] Linoleic acid comprises 40% and palmitic acid 30% of the fatty acids in both green and roasted coffee beans,[108] but in coffee grounds palmitic acid predominates over the linoleic acid.[109] Whereas coffee brews filtered through filter paper contained <7 mg lipids per cup, those prepared by boiling without filtering, and espresso coffee, reached 60 to 160 mg lipids per cup. Coffee brew filtered through a metal screen contained 50 mg lipids per cup. Triglycerides and diterpene alcohol esters were the major lipid classes involved.[110]

B. Sterols

Sterols constitute about 5.4% of the total lipids in Arabica coffee. Sitosterol (53%), stigmasterol (21%), campesterol (11%), and cycloartenol (8%) predominate; the remaining sterols are each 5% or less of the total sterol fraction.[111] The C-4 methylated steroids, 24-methylenelophenol and citrostadienol, are found in many plant tissues, as are the C-14 methylated compounds cycloeucalenol and obtusifoliol, and they could have been expected to be present in coffee.[111] Two dehydroavenasterols and 7-dehydrostigmasterol have been recognized in green Arabica coffee more recently.[112] Oxysterols are present only at low levels, if at all, in commercial samples of regular and and decaffeinated coffees. The 7-keto-β-sitosterol was <0.04 mg/kg.[113]

Some sterols found in coffee beans are drawn in Figure 13.

C. Tocopherols

The presence of tocopherols,[114] as well as caffeic acid,[108] accounts for the remarkable stability of green coffee bean oils toward oxidation. In coffee beans from different origins, α-tocopherol concentrations are in the range 89 to 188 μg/kg and (β + γ)-tocopherol concentrations are in the range 252 to 530 μg/kg.[114] Since β- and γ-tocopherols have better antioxidant properties than α-tocopherol,[114] it is not surprising to see coffee oil patented as an antioxidant material.[115-117]

D. Diterpenes

Several diterpenes, free, as their esters or as their glycosides, have been recognized in green coffee beans. Cafestol (a furokaur*ane*) and kahweol (a furokaur*ene*) are the predominant diterpenes. They have been recog-

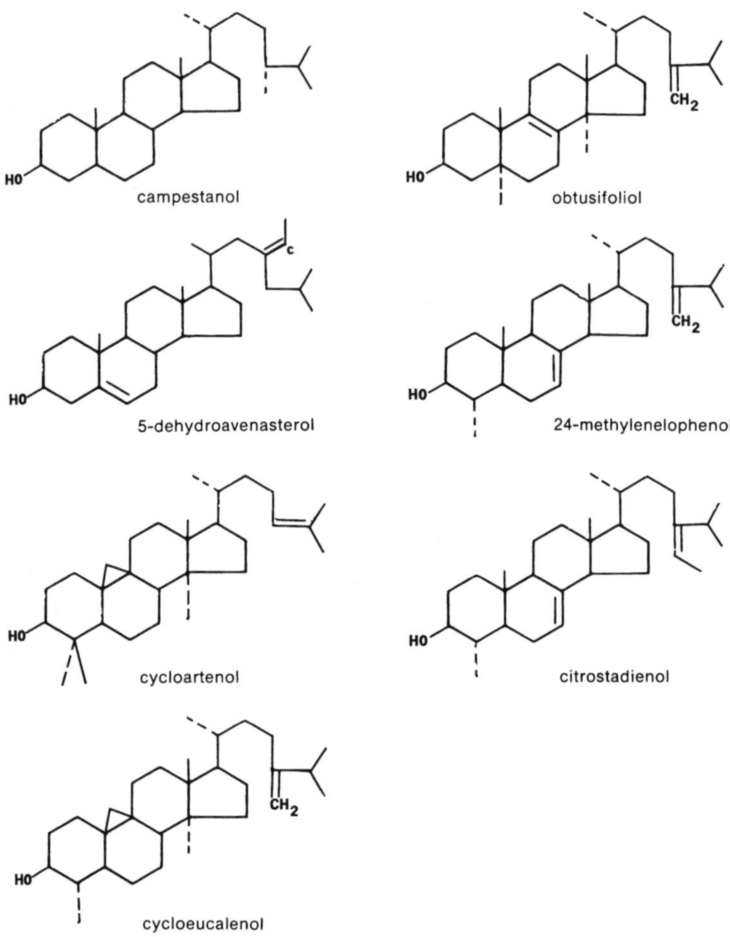

HO campestanol

HO obtusifoliol CH_2

HO 5-dehydroavenasterol

HO 24-methylenelophenol CH_2

HO cycloartenol

HO citrostadienol

HO cycloeucalenol CH_2

FIGURE 13
Some sterols found in green coffee beans.[111, 112]

nized free and as their palmitates in green coffee beans.[118] Cafestol is little affected by various treatments of coffee beans and is one of the components of coffee that remains in spent coffee grounds (1.2%).[119] Kahweol concentrations are various.[106] The kahweol content is reduced during roasting,[3] and is presumably a source of some furan compounds found in roasted coffee. The kahweol content is also used as an indicator for the extent of steam treatments for green coffee beans.[120] In the early 1980s it was discovered in Norway that unfiltered coffee raised cholesterol levels, and that the effect disappeared when the coffee was filtered. The substances responsible for this effect have been identified as cafestol and kahweol. They are present in small amounts in the fat of the coffee beans, and they are not removed by decaffeination.[121, 122] Each 10 mg of cafestol consumed per day elevates cholesterol by 5 mg/dl (0.13 mmol/l). Thus since Scandinavian boiled, French press, and Turkish or Greek style coffees all contain more than 3 mg cafestol per cup, any of these types of coffee brew could apparantly elevate serum cholesterol levels by 8 to 10 mg/dl, if more than five cups were consumed each day. Italian espresso was shown to contain less than 2 mg cafestol per cup, so it would have a reduced effect, raising serum cholesterol levels by 4 mg per day if five cups per day were consumed. Diterpenes in instant, drip filtered, and percolated brews were found to be negligible.[123]

Cafestol from robusta coffee as well as kahweol from arabica coffee were both recognized as capable of elevating serum cholesterol levels.[124]

Dehydrocafestol and dehydrokahweol have been found in roasted coffee, but were not present in the corresponding green coffee.[125]

Large amounts of diterpene mono- and di-alcohols have been found in both Arabic and Robusta coffees, including cafestol, kahweol, and 16-O-methylcafestol.[126] The characteristic differences can be used to quantify the Robusta content of commercial blends with Arabica.[127]

Roasted Robusta coffee contains 16-O-methylcafestol, mostly in its esterified form;[128] and it has been recognized as useful for detecting the addition of Robusta to Arabica coffee because of its stability during roasting.[129]

A furokauranone glycoside has also been recognized in green coffee oil (Figure 14).[130]

Atractyligenin as well as some of its derivatives have also been found, particularly in Arabica coffees[131-134] (Figure 15). These are diterpenes of the kaurane and kaurene type. They are mostly present in coffee beans as glycosides. Green Arabica coffee contains 0 to 0.01 g/kg free atractyligenin and 0.4 to 0.7 g/kg conjugated atractyligenin,[135] which is probably glycoside. The atractyligenin total content decreases by about 35% on roasting.[136] There is a five- to tenfold rise in free atractyligenin on roasting;[135] this is still a small amount compared with the atractyligenin derivatives present. These atractyligenin glycosides (atractylosides) are water soluble and are present in a coffee beverage. For example, when roasted coffee is extracted industrially, atractylosides appear to the greatest extent in the early fractions. About 70% of the total atractyligenin in roast coffee is extracted into a home brew of coffee and about 85% into an industrial extract to be used for soluble coffee preparation.[136] It is interesting to notice that Robusta coffees have been found to contain only one tenth or less of atractyligenin and its derivatives than Arabica coffees.[136]

Some glycosides of atractyligenin from the rhizome *Atractylis gummifera L.* are already known to cause changes in carbohydrate metabolism. Similarly, two coffee atractylosides were also found to cause changes in carbohydrate metabolism; they were 2-O-(2-O-isovaleryl-β-D-glucopyranosyl) atractyligenin and 2-O-β-D-glucopyranosyl atractyligenin.[138]

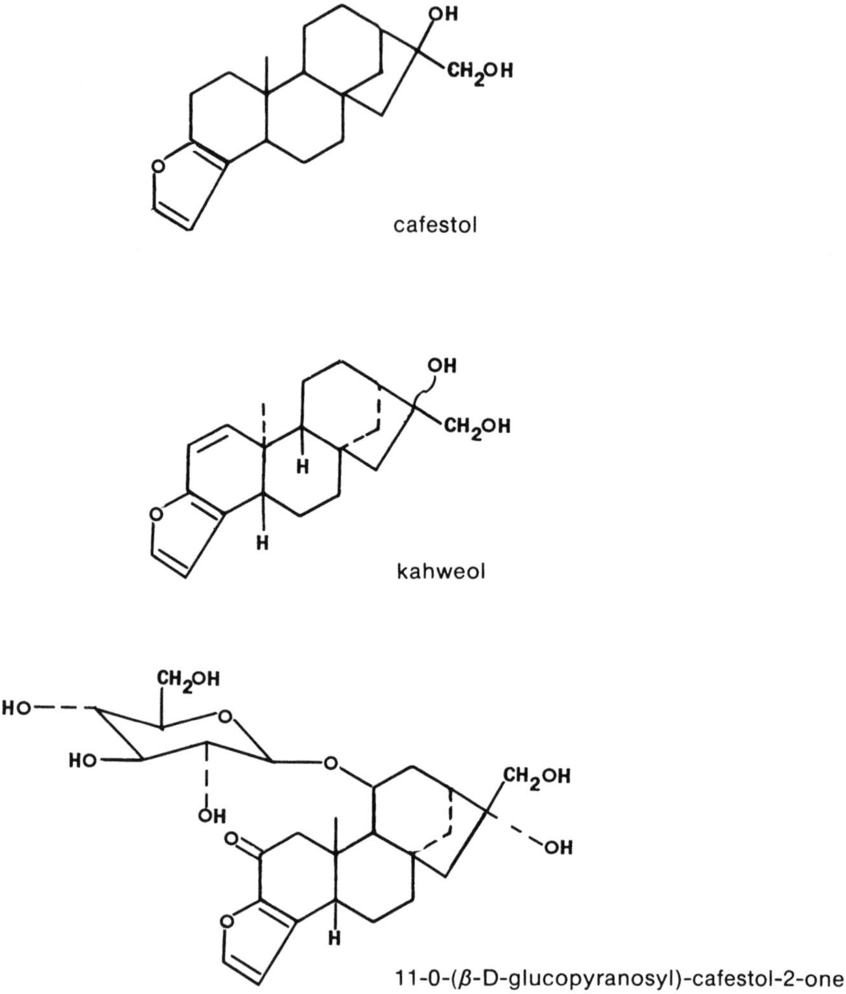

cafestol

kahweol

11-0-(β-D-glucopyranosyl)-cafestol-2-one

FIGURE 14
Some furokauranes and furokaurenes found in coffee beans.[3, 130]

E. Nβ-Alkanoyl-5-Hydroxytryptamides

The most frequently described components of coffee wax are the Nβ-alkanoyl-5-hydroxytryptamides (Figure 16). The range of concentration found on sampling 14 varieties was 401 to 1,099 ppm of the total coffee bean.[139] The relative concentrations of three of the four major 5-hydroxytryptamides are 22.5 to 39.9% with arachic, 49 to 68.9% with behenic, and 7.7 to 12% with lignoceric acids.[139] The fourth major acid involved is stearic.[137] The predominance of Nβ-behenoyl-5-

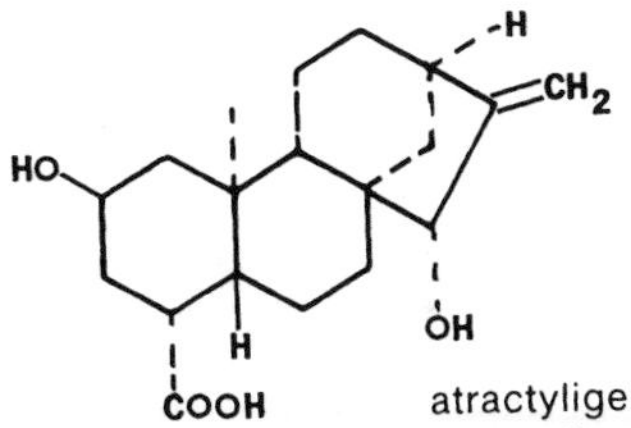

atractyligenin
(2,15-dihydroxy-19-norkaur-16-en-18-oic acid)

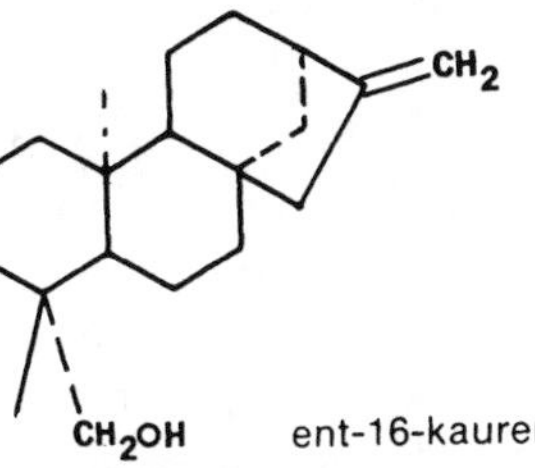

ent-16-kauren-19-ol

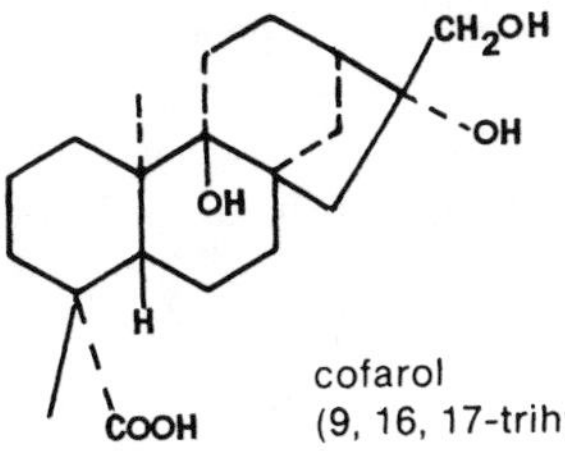

cofarol
(9, 16, 17-trihydroxykauran-18-oic acid)

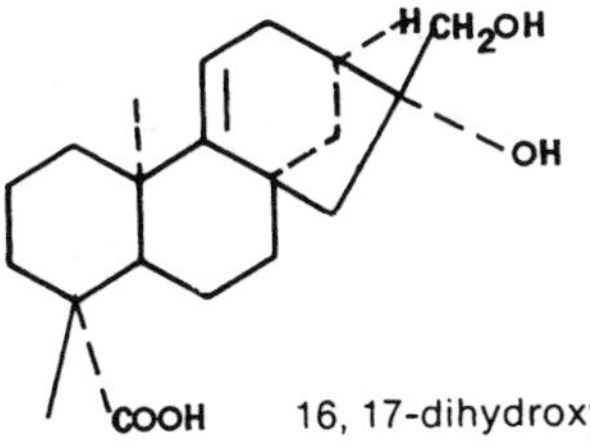

16, 17-dihydroxykaur-9 (11)-en-18-oic acid

FIGURE 15
Some kaurane and kaurene compounds found in green coffee beans; their glycosides are listed in Table 15.

hydroxytryptamide can be used as an indicator for the amount of wax present in green coffee beans.[140] Patents have been taken out for the production of serotonin (5-hydroxytryptamine) from coffee wax.[141-143] Dewaxing of coffee beans is commercially important as a coffee improvement. A solvent is used to remove the wax and removal of the solvent itself

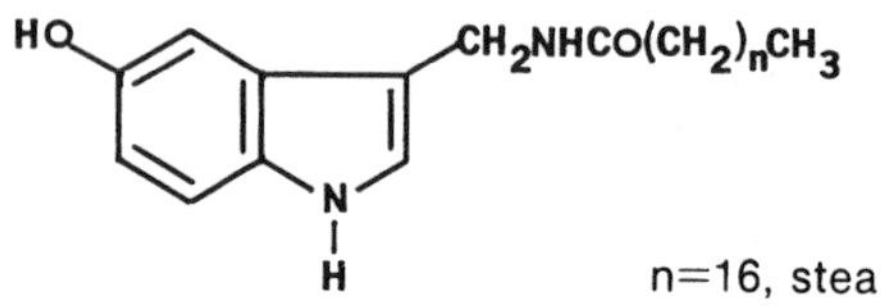

HO — $CH_2NHCO(CH_2)_nCH_3$ — N — H

n=16, stearoyl
n=18, arachidoyl
n=20, behenoyl
n=22, lignoceryl

FIGURE 16
The Nβ-alkanoyl-5-hydroxytryptamides found in coffee bean wax.[137]

is completed during a steam treatment.[144,145] The use of hydrogen peroxide spray to decrease the 5-hydroxytryptamide concentration in coffee wax has been patented.[146] Carbon dioxide under suitable pressure and temperature conditions and in the presence of caffeine is used as one method to extract lipid solubles. Under such conditions the coffee retains most of the original caffeine, but the 5-hydroxytryptamides fall in concentration from 580 to 160 ppm.[147]

However, 5-hydroxytryptamides themselves do not seem to ever become significant in the coffee beverage because they are partly decomposed during roasting and the rest remains in the spent grounds.[148] Any small amount present in a brew is emulsified and could be retained by a filter paper in a drip brew of coffee.[148]

F. Phospholipids

Phospholipids such as lecithin are presumably present in the coffee bean.

A list of those lipids found in green and roasted coffees is given in Table 15.

IX. ALKALOIDS

A. Caffeine

Caffeine is the alkaloid that made coffee fruit and seed so much desired. Caffeine is probably also part of the defense system of the coffee seed, since caffeine has been recognized as an antifungal,[149] a selective phytotoxin,[150] and a chemosterilant toward certain insects.[151]

The caffeine content of coffee is given in Table 16.[15,152,153] Recently determined values for the caffeine content of Brazilian coffees, 0.2 to 109 mg/150 ml (cup),[154] were somewhat lower than those reported in Table 16.

TABLE 15

Lipids Found in Green and Roasted Coffee[3]

Compound	Empirical formula	Source[a]
Choline[b]	$C_5H_{15}NO_2$	G R
Glycerine[b]	$C_3H_8O_3$	G R
Myristic acid[b]	$C_{14}H_{28}O_2$	G R
Palmitic acid[b]	$C_{16}H_{32}O_2$	G R
Palmitoleic acid[b]	$C_{16}H_{30}O_2$	G R
Margaric acid[b]	$C_{17}H_{34}O_2$	G R
Stearic acid[b]	$C_{18}H_{36}O_2$	G R
Oleic acid[b]	$C_{18}H_{34}O_2$	G R
Linoleic acid[b]	$C_{18}H_{32}O_2$	G R
Linolenic[b]	$C_{18}H_{30}O_2$	G R
Arachidic acid[b]	$C_{20}H_{40}O_2$	G R
Arachidonic acid[b]	$C_{20}H_{32}O_2$	G
9,10-Eicosenoic acid[b]	$C_{20}H_{38}O_2$	G R
Behenic acid[b]	$C_{22}H_{44}O_2$	G R
Lignoceric acid[b]	$C_{24}H_{48}O_2$	G R
Montanic acid[b]	$C_{28}H_{56}O_2$	G R
Lignoceroyl-5-hydroxytryptamide	$C_{34}H_{59}N_2O_2$	G R
Arachidoyl-5-hydroxytryptamide	$C_{30}H_{51}N_2O_2$	G R
Behenoyl-5-hydroxytryptamide	$C_{32}H_{55}N_2O_2$	G R
Stearoyl-5-hydroxytryptamide	$C_{28}H_{47}N_2O_2$	G
Sitosterol[111]	$C_{29}H_{50}O$	G
Stigmasterol[111]	$C_{29}H_{48}O$	G
Cycloartenol[111]	$C_{30}H_{50}O$	G
24-Methylenecycloartenol[111]	$C_{31}H_{52}O$	G
Cycloeucalenol[111]	$C_{30}H_{50}O$	G
Cholesterol[111]	$C_{27}H_{46}O$	G
24-Methylenelophenol[111]	$C_{29}H_{48}O$	G
Obtusifoliol[111]	$C_{30}H_{50}O$	G
Cholestanol[111]	$C_{27}H_{48}O$	G
Citrostadienol[111]	$C_{30}H_{50}O$	G
4α-24R-Dimethyl-5α-cholest-7-en-3b-ol[111]	$C_{29}H_{50}O$	G
4α-Methyl-5α-stigmast-7-en-3β-ol[111]	$C_{30}H_{52}O$	G
Campesterol[111]	$C_{28}H_{48}O$	G R
Stigmastanol[111]	$C_{29}H_{52}O$	G R
Campestanol[111]	$C_{28}H_{50}O$	G R
Cycloartanol	$C_{30}H_{52}O$	G R
5-Dehydroavenasterol[112]	$C_{29}H_{48}O$	G
7-Dehydroavenasterol[112]	$C_{29}H_{48}O$	G
7-Dehydrostigmasterol[112]	$C_{29}H_{48}O$	G
Furokauranes, furokaurenes		
Cafestol	$C_{20}H_{28}O_3$	G R
Cafestol palmitate[118]	$C_{36}H_{58}O_4$	G
Kahweol	$C_{20}H_{26}O_3$	G R
Kahweol palmitate[118]	$C_{36}H_{56}O_4$	G

TABLE 15 (continued)

Lipids Found in Green and Roasted Coffee[3]

Compound	Empirical formula	Source[a]
11-O-(β-D-Glucopyranosyl)-cafestol-2-one	$C_{26}H_{38}O_9$	G
Kauranes, kaurenes		
Atractyligenin[131]	$C_{19}H_{28}O_4$	G R
2-O-(2-O-Isovaleryl-β-D-glucopyranosyl)-atractyligenin[134]	$C_{30}H_{46}O_{10}$	G
3'-O-(β-D-Glucopyranosyl)-2'-(O-isovaleryl)-2β-(2-deoxy-atractyligenin)-β-D-glucopyranoside[136]	$C_{36}H_{56}O_{14}$	G R
2-O-(β-D-Glucopyranosyl)-atractyligenin[136]	$C_{25}H_{38}O_9$	G R
ent-16-Kauren-19-ol[132]	$C_{20}H_{32}O$	G
Cofaryloside (β-D-glucopyranosyl-9β,16α,17-trihydroxykauran-18-ate)[133]	$C_{26}H_{42}O_{10}$	G
16,17-Dihydroxy-9(11)-kauren-18-oic acid[131]	$C_{20}H_{30}O_4$	G R
α-Tocopherol	$C_{29}H_{50}O_2$	G
β-Tocopherol	$C_{28}H_{48}O_2$	G
γ-Tocopherol	$C_{28}H_{48}O_2$	G

[a]G, in green coffee; R, in roasted coffee.

[b]These compounds are bound, usually as esters. Free fatty acids are listed in Table 3.

TABLE 16

The Caffeine Content of Coffee

Coffee	Arabica	Robusta
Dry green beans[152]	0.58-1.7% (average 1.16)	1.16-3.27% (average 2.15)
Roasted beans[15]	1%	2%
Beverage[153]	29-176 mg/cup (median 74)	

Some caffeine is evidently lost from the beans during the roasting process by sublimation; indeed in 1977, caffeine was recognized in the air of New York City mainly due to emissions from coffee roasting plants.[155] About 90% of the caffeine is extracted in the first minute of brewing for a coffee beverage.[156] In coffee beverage, the caffeine is mostly associated with chlorogenic acid in a 1:1, π-complex.[3]

Evidence for the pathway for caffeine formation during the ripening of the coffee fruit is seen in the methyltransferase and 7-methyl-N^9-nucleoside hydrolase activities. The path for caffeine formation in Arabica coffees is thought to be from 7-methylxanthosine, to 7-methylxanthine, to theobromine, to caffeine, all occurring in the unripened fruit.[157] Recent investigations have sought to verify this.[158, 159]

Evidence that caffeine contributes antioxidative activity has been shown by the detection of the oxidized caffeine product, 8-oxocaffeine (1,3,7-trimethyluric acid) in roasted, ground and instant coffees, in the range 4 to 35 ppm.[160]

B. Theobromine and Theophylline

Theobromine and theophylline concentrations are relatively low in coffee; the values in green coffee beans are, respectively, 20 and 5 mg/kg.[3]

C. Other Xanthines

Other xanthines present in trace amounts in green coffee are xanthine, hypoxanthine, adenine, and guanine; these are all absent from roasted coffee.[3]

D. Trigonelline

Trigonelline is present in green coffee (1 %),[15] but it is rapidly decomposed on roasting so that only about 0.1% trigonelline is present in a deeply roasted coffee.[161] The products of trigonelline breakdown are evident in roasted coffee and include nicotinic acid and its methylester, pyridine, and β-picoline (Figure 17).[3]

Alkaloids that have been recognized in coffee are listed in Table 17.[3]

X. VITAMINS

Several vitamins have been recognized in green coffee beans, as might be expected in a plant seed. A relatively high ascorbic acid content is associated with fine-grade coffee beans to be used as seeds.[162] Vitamin E has already been mentioned as a component of coffee oil.[114]

Determinations of nicotinamide in green and roasted Robusta coffee are indicative of its much increased content in coffee roasted at or below 240°C. The values are 3 and 46 mg/100 g for green and roasted coffee, respectively.[163] At least part of this increase is from trigonelline as it decomposes on roasting.

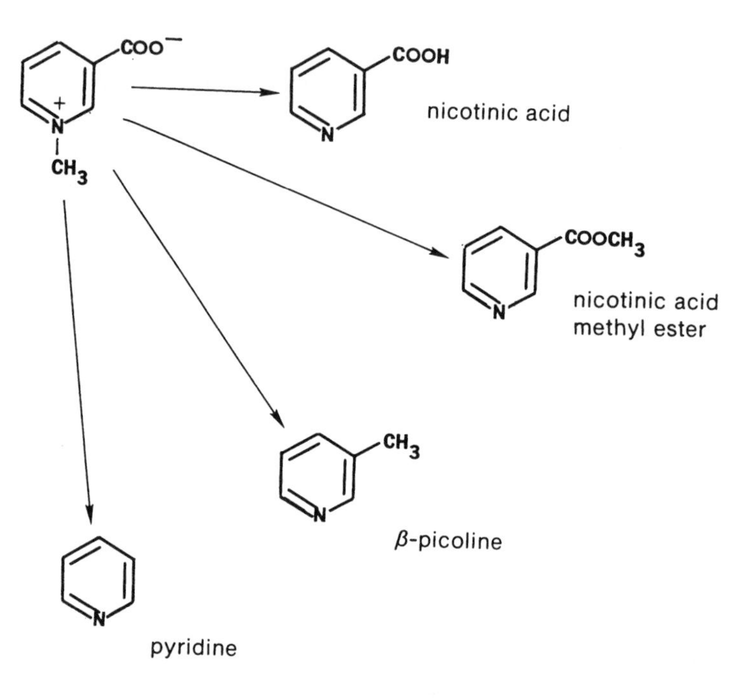

FIGURE 17
The products from trigonelline seen in roasted coffee.[3]

TABLE 17

Alkaloids Found in Green and Roasted Coffee[3]

Compound	Empirical formula	Source[a]
Caffeine	$C_8H_{10}N_4O_2$	G R
Theobromine	$C_7H_8N_4O_2$	G R
Theophylline	$C_7H_8N_4O_2$	G R
Trigonelline	$C_7H_7N\ O_2$	G R
Adenine	$C_5H_5N_5$	G
Guanine	$C_5H_5N_5O$	G
Hypoxanthine	$C_5H_4N_4O$	G
Xanthine	$C_5H_4N_4O_2$	G

[a]G, in green coffee; R, in roasted coffee.

Vitamin B6 (pyridoxine), free and combined, has a total concentration of 2.2 μg/g in green coffee.[164]

Vitamins that have been found in coffee are listed in Table 18.

XI. INORGANIC COMPOUNDS

Some inorganic compounds that have been found in green and roasted coffee are listed in Table 19.[3]

The nitrate and nitrite content of coffees has been determined. Green coffee beans contain between 1 to 109 mg/kg nitrate, and 2.18 to 5.66 mg/kg nitrite. In roasted coffee, the values for nitrate increased to 8.8 to 129 mg/kg, and the values for nitrite decreased to 0.16 to 3.33 mg/kg. One cup of coffee infusion contained up to 1.57 mg nitrates and up to 0.05 mg nitrites.[165]

Hydrogen peroxide levels have been determined. When roasted coffee beans were stored at 30°C for 100 d under sunlight, the beans contained

TABLE 18

Vitamins Found in Green and Roasted Coffee[3]

Compound	Empirical formula	Source[a]
Vitamin B-1 (thiamine)	$C_{12}H_{18}N_4O_2$	G
Vitamin B-2 (riboflavin)	$C_{17}H_{20}N_4O_6$	G R
Nicotinic acid	$C_6H_5N\ O_2$	G R
Nicotinamide	$C_6H_6N_2O$	G R
Pantothenic acid	$C_9H_{17}N\ O_5$	G R
Vitamin B-6 (pyridoxine)	$C_8H_{11}N\ O_3$	G R
Vitamin B-12 (cyanocobalamin)	$C_{63}H_{88}CoN_{14}O_{14}P$	G R
Citrovorum factor	$C_{20}H_{23}N_7O_7$	R
Folic acid	$C_{19}H_{19}N_7O_6$	G R
Vitamin C (ascorbic acid)[162]	$C_6H_8O_6$	G

[a]G, in green coffee; R, in roasted coffee.

TABLE 19

Inorganic Substances Found in Green and Roasted Coffee[3]

Substance	Empirical formula	Source[a]
Ammonia	NH_3	R
Oxygen	O_2	R
Carbon monoxide	CO	R
Carbon dioxide	CO_2	R
Nitrogen	N_2	R
Sulfur dioxide	SO_2	G R
Hydrogen sulfide	H_2S	R
Borate	BO_3^{3-}	G R
Phosphate	PO_4^{3-}	G R
Silica	SiO_2	G R
Sulfite	SO_3^{2-}	G R

[a]G, in green coffee; R, in roasted coffee.

300 μg hydrogen peroxide per gram. Thermal decomposition products from caffeic acid were presumed to contribute largely to the formation of hydrogen peroxide.[166]

XII. ELEMENTAL COMPOSITION

After the elements carbon, hydrogen, and oxygen, the next two major elements in coffee beans are nitrogen (2.6%),[167] and potassium (1.6 to 2.0%).[168] Calcium (0.2%), magnesium (0.2%), phosphorus (0.2%), and sulfur (0.1%) follow. The remaining elements are below 0.1% and are regarded as trace elements. It is likely that the levels of some elements are indicative of the growing plants' microenvironment and can therefore provide a means of differentiating coffees from different geographical regions.[169]

Two of these trace elements, copper and fluorine, have been given particular attention recently. Copper compounds are widely used as fungicides, so copper levels are possibly higher in treated coffee plants. Ground roasted coffee had an average copper content of 17.3 mg/kg.[170] It is interesting to note that copper is 32 mg/kg in a Robusta coffee, which is known to be naturally relatively resistant to fungal attack.[171] Fluorine levels in decaffeinated coffee beans were 6.4 ppm on a dry basis,[172] and in coffee beverages they have been determined to be 28 to 72 mg/kg.[173] Cadmium does not present a problem in coffee; for example, in 20 samples of Arabica and Robusta coffees originating from Central and South America as well as from Africa, only very low cadmium values were observed, 0.02 mg/kg.[174] Example values for some trace heavy metals in coffee beans are: 0.55 ppm nickel, 67 ppm iron, 13.3 ppm copper, 0.1 to 0.3 ppm lead, and no detection of arsenic.[175]

Table 20 lists some elements found in green coffee beans.[3, 171]

XIII. INTRODUCED COMPOUNDS

Coffee beans are cultivated, separated from the whole fruit, dried, stored, shipped, possibly decaffeinated or otherwise "improved", roasted, ground, and packaged all before reaching the consumer. At each of these stages compounds may be deliberately or accidentally introduced. It seems important to appreciate this, especially when coffee is being investigated for its physiological effects. In the following paragraphs a selection from the literature gives examples of additives and contaminants that can be found in some coffee samples.

A. Pesticides

Pesticides of all kinds have potential use during the cultivation and storage of coffee. Jute storage bags impregnated with malathion or Volaton have been used to protect coffee against beetle infestation.[176] Methyl bromide has been successfully used as an insecticide for stored coffee beans. The residues were determined to be less than those legally allowed.[177] In the late 1950s, benzene-hexachloride-treated plants were found to produce brick-flavored beans.[178] Assays in the 1970s indicated no residual benzene hexachloride in such beans,[179] but reports of inferior bean flavor persist.[180] A huge number of pesticides has been investigated for efficacy on coffee plants and some of them also for their final residues in coffee

TABLE 20

Some Elements Present in Green and Roasted Coffee Beans[3, 171]

Element	Symbol	*Coffea arabica*[a]	*Coffea canephora* var. *robusta*[a]	*Coffea* species[a]
Aluminum	Al	—	—	+
Antimony	Sb	0.01	—	
Arsenic	As	0.005	0.005	
Barium	Ba	1	10	
Boron	B	—	—	+
Bromine	Br	0.12	0.06	
Cadmium	Cd	0.1	0.1	
Calcium	Ca	820	1400	
Carbon	C	—	—	+
Caesium	Cs	0.05	0.03	
Chlorine	C1	71	142	
Chromium	Cr	0.025	—	
Cobalt	Co	0.145	0.470	
Copper	Cu	1	32.7	
Fluorine[172]	F	—	—	6.4
Gold	Au	0.0042	0.0012	
Hydrogen	H	—	—	+
Iodine	I	—	—	+
Iridium	Ir	0.00008		
Lanthanum	La	0.005		
Lead	Pb	—	—	+
Lithium	Li	—	—	+
Magnesium	Mg	—	—	0.2%
Manganese	Mn	19.3	14.7	
Mercury	Hg	0.01	0.01	
Molybdenum	Mo	—	—	
Nickel	Ni	—	—	+
Nitrogen[167]	N	—	—	2.6%
Oxygen	O	—	—	+
Phosphorus	P	—	—	0.2%
Potassium	K	13,710	15,240	
Rubidium	Ru	57.4	42.7	
Scandium	Sc	0.0002	0.0009	
Selenium	Se	0.017	0.02	
Silicon	Si	—	—	+
Silver	Ag	0.0083	—	
Sodium	Na	14.5	9.4	
Strontium	Sr	2	11	
Sulfur	S	—	—	0.1%
Thorium	Th	—	—	+
Titanium	Ti	—	—	+
Vanadium	V	—	—	+
Zinc	Zn	6.21	7.10	

[a]Concentration values are in ppm, unless otherwise stated.

beans. Among those pesticides that have been analyzed for their residues in coffee beans are Oxamyl,[181] fentin,[182] heptachlor, heptachlorepoxide, dieldrin,[183, 184] lindane,[185, 186] endosulfan,[185] endrin, DDT, DDD,[184] carbofuran,[187, 188] Bayleton,[189] and methylchlorpyrifos.[190]

Tolerance levels in or on coffee beans, established under the Federal Food, Drug, and Cosmetic Acts, include values for glyphosate and its sulfinyl and sulfonyl metabolites,[191] and N,N-dimethyl-2-(1-naphthalenyloxy)propionamide.[192]

The roasting of coffee significantly reduces the levels of most pesticides,[184, 185] as does brewing the coffee.[193]

Little information has been published on pesticide degradation products, produced in coffee, that may have significant physiological effects. Some information has been published, however, for glyphosate,[191] aldicarb,[194] and carbofuran,[187] although there is some controversy surrounding the carbofuran data.[188]

B. Mycotoxins

Fungal attack following coffee borer beetle damage leads to the formation of "viridic acid". The "viridic acid" test (a color reaction) has been used to estimate the extent of preharvest damage, by the coffee borer beetle, to a batch of coffee beans.[55]

Fungal damage to coffee beans can also occur during fermentation processes used to separate the coffee bean from the coffee berry pulp. However, green coffee beans are highly susceptible to fungal attack if they are stored in warm humid conditions. Ochratoxin A (40 ppb) can be produced in green coffee beans stored in warm humid laboratory conditions, from *Aspergillus ochraceous* growth.[195] Two samples of moldy coffee were found to contain ochratoxin A (10 μg/kg) and sterigmatocystin (12 μg/kg);[196] a single sample found to contain sterigmatocystin (12 mg/Kg) was no longer saleable anyway.[197] Improperly stored coffee was found to contain aflatoxin.[198]

It is very interesting to note that decaffeinated green coffee beans are much more susceptible to fungal attack,[199] than untreated green coffee. Caffeine has an antifungal effect at or above 2mg/g.[200] In addition, decaffeinated beans have lost their protective surface wax covering.[15] Roasting does reduce the levels of several mycotoxins if they are present in green coffee beans.[201, 202] For example, ochratoxin A is reduced by 80 to 90% on roasting contaminated coffee beans,[195] although other researchers have found that roasting causes only a small reduction.[203, 204] A maximum tolerance limit of 20 ng/kg for ochratoxin A was established in 1989 for green coffee beans being exported to Greece and Lebanon.[205] A method for determining ochratoxin A, with a detection limit of 0.3 ppb, has recently been described. In commercial samples of coffee, the range seen for ochratoxin A was 1.43 to 7.54 ppb.[206] Roasting of green coffee beans which were contaminated that ochratoxin A resulted in only a small reduction in ochratoxin A levels, in contrast to earlier observations. Ochratoxin A is eluted into coffee brews, and therefore regular coffee consumption may contribute to exposure of humans to ochratoxin A.[203, 204]

No aflatoxin B1 was detected in a large number of green coffee samples. In order to evaluate aflatoxin B1 in coffee, green coffee beans were artificially contaminated. The aflatoxin B1 in these artificially contaminated green coffee beans was mostly decomposed by roasting and was further decomposed during coffee brew preparation.[207]

C. Solvents

Solvent-assisted decaffeination of coffee can result in residues of solvent reaching the consumer.[208] The use of chlorinated hydrocarbon solvents such as chloroform,[209] methylene chloride, trichloroethylene,[208] and difluoromonochloromethane (Freon),[210] will probably be replaced by compounds already found in roasted coffee. The use of an ethyl acetate and 2-butanone mixture leaves a 26-ppm residue in green coffee, but zero residue in roasted coffee.[211] Other solvent compounds used or suggested for coffee improvement or decaffeination include propane, butane,[212] carbon dioxide,[213, 214] acetone,[215] dimethyl succinate,[216] 1,1-dimethoxymethane, and 1,1-dimethoxyethane.[217] Of all these, supercritical carbon dioxide, ethyl acetate, and methylene chloride are the solvents most used currently in decaffeination processes.

D. Miscellaneous Introduced Compounds

Robusta coffee has undesirable flavor agents that can be masked by the addition of L-aspartyl-L-phenylalaninemethyl ester.[218] The methylxanthine stimulant properties of coffee can be antagonized by spraying freshly roasted coffee beans with nicotinamide and nicotinic acid,[219] quinolinic acid, or trigonelline.[220]

Polyphenoloxidase, produced by *Alternaria* or *Cladosporium*, can be used to improve the brown coloration in a coffee extract.[221]

The freshness of roasted coffees can be maintained with packaged oxygen and carbon dioxide absorbents,[222, 223] or by spraying the coffee beans with a sodium sorbate solution.[224]

Instant coffees may have had small amounts of gelatin, gums, or synthetic flavors added.[15]

Ethrel can be sprayed onto coffee berries still on the tree to enhance and unify the ripening of coffee berries.[225]

Chicory is a well-known coffee extender and caramel coloring is also used with coffees.[15]

Finally, just as in all foods, there are those contaminants that occasionally arise through mismanagement: cashew nut shells were recognized in one batch of coffee,[226] and the solvent from storage bag marking ink has been known to contaminate batches of coffee beans.[15] Nicotine from tobacco[227] can be recognized. Petroleum product contamination leads to the presence of polymethylnaphthalene or polymethylphenanthrene.[228] Sisal fibers are treated with batching oil before spinning. Such oils usually consist of mineral oil products and cause considerable contamination of the packed foods (typically 10 to 100 mg/kg).[229]

XIV. CONCLUSIONS

In conclusion, it can be seen that coffee is a highly variable beverage in terms of its chemical composition. It seems to be essential that studies of the physiological effects of coffee should include a description of the coffee used. In particular the species of coffee, the methods of bean separation, and roasting could be described. This would reduce the possibility of conflicting reports on coffee attributes, and it will allow us to discover how coffee can best be enjoyed.

ACKNOWLEDGMENT

The author would like to express special thanks to Dr. Otto Vitzthum, who read the first edition of this chapter in 1984, and made a number of very helpful comments.

REFERENCES

References Cited

1. Lehninger, A. L., *Biochemistry*, Second Edition. Worth, New York, 1975.
2. Trease, G. E., Evans, W. C., *Pharmacognosy*, Eleventh Edition. Baillère Tindall, London, 1978.
3. Vitzthum, O. G., Chemie und Bearbeitung des Kaffees, in *Kaffee und Coffein, Zweite, Vollig neu Bearbeitete Aufluge*, Eichler, O., Ed., Springer-Verlag, Berlin, 1976, 3.
4. Nijssen, L. M., Ed., *Volatile Compounds in Food, Qualitative and Quantitative Data, 7th Edition*, Division for Nutrition and Food Research TNO, Institute CIVO—Analysis TNO, Zeist, The Netherlands, 1996.

5. Holscher, W., Steinhart, H., Formation pathways for primary roasted coffee aroma compounds, in *ACS Symposium Series 543, Thermally Generated Flavors,* 1994, 206. (CA120:105189t)
6. Semmelroch, P., Laskawy, G., Blank, I., Grosch, W., Determination of potent odorants in roasted coffee by stable isotope dilution assays, *Flavour Fragrance J.* 10(1), 1, 1995.
7. Nakabayashi, T., The quality of coffee. VII. Formation of organic acids from sucrose by roasting, *Nippon Shokuhin Kogyo Gakkaishi,* 25, 257, 1978. (CA91:191684n)
8. Nakabayashi, T., Chemical studies of the quality of coffee. VI. Changes in organic acids and pH of roasted coffee, *Nippon Shokubin Kogyo Gakkaishi,* 25, 142, 1978. (CA91 :106795g)
9. Takahashi, K., Kondo, Y., Sawano, T., Mori, M., Changes in pH of coffee extract depending on temperature and its quality, *Nippon Shokuhin Kogyo Gakkaishi,* 26, 360, 1979. (CA91: 191646b)
10. Hara, S., Okamoto, S., Totani, Y., Lipid constituents of coffee beans and their denaturation, *Seikei Daigaku Kogakubu Kogaku Hokoku,* 27, 1895, 1979. (CA91:18551u)
11. Wajda, P., Walczyk, C., Relation between acid value of extracted fatty matter and age of green coffee beans, *J. Sci. Food Agric.,* 29, 377, 1978. (CA89:145281q)
12. Kasai, H., Kumeno, K., Yamaizumi, Z., Nishimura, S., Nagao, M., Fujita, Y., Sugimura, T., Nukaya, H., Kosuge, T., Mutagenicity of methylglyoxal in coffee, *Gann,* 73, 681, 1982. (CA98: 1512d)
13. Meyer, L. H., *Food Chemistry,* Reinhold, New York, 1960.
14. Motoda, S., Formation of aldehydes from amino acids by polyphenol oxidase, *J. Ferment Technol.,* 57, 395, 1979. (CA92:17776e)
15. Sivetz, M., Desrosier, N. W., *Coffee Technology,* AVI, Westport, 1979.
16. Boosfeld, J., Vitzthum, O. G., Unsaturated aldehydes identification from green coffee, *J. Food Sci.* 60(5), 1092, 1995. (CA123:255207y)
17. Amorim, H. V., Basso, L.C., Crocomo, O. J., Teixeira, A. A. Polyamines in green and roasted coffee *J. Agric. Food Chem.,* 25, 957, 1977. (CA87:37570h)
18. Pearson, T. W., Dawson, H. J., Lackey, H. B., Naturally occurring levels of dimethyl sulfoxide in selected fruits, vegetables, grains and beverages, *J. Agric. Food Chem.,* 29, 1089, 1981. (CA95: 113654w)
19. Tressl, R., Silwar, R., Investigation of sulfur-containing components of roasted coffee, *J. Agric. Food Chem.,* 29:1078, 1981. (CA95:113664z)
20. Osajima, Y., Shimoda, M., Iriki, E., Ito, H., Sakane, Y., Aroma of coffee. I. Head space gas chromatographic method using the internal standard for determination of aroma from roast and ground coffee, *Nippon Shokubin Kogyo Gakkaishi,* 26, 105, 1979. (CA91 :89667x)
21. Radtke-Granzer, R., Piringer, O. G., Problems in the quality evaluation of roasted coffee by quantitative trace analysis of volatile flavor components, *Dtsch Lebensm Rundsch,* 77, 203, 1981. (CA95:95570j)
22. Vitzthum, O. G., Werkhoff, P., Measurable changes of roasted coffee aroma in oxygen permeable bag packs, *Chem. Mikrobiol. Technol. Lebensm.,* 6, 25, 1979. (CA91:54812p)
23. Figueiredo, I. B., Iovaldo, B., Quantitative variations of acetaldehyde in ground coffee after different times of roasting at 220° C, *Colet. Inst. Tecnol. Aliment.,* 6, 361, 1975.(Portuguese) (CA85:122040p)
24. Tijmensen, W. G., Odor abatement in coffee roasting factories, *PT Procestech* 33, 575, 1978. (CA90:109040x)
25. Vincent, J. C., Barel, M., Challot, F., Contribution to the study of defective green coffee beans, *Coll. Int. Chim. Cafes,* 7, 133, 1975. (CA86:3698v)

26. Rouge, F., Gretsch, C., Christensen, K., Liardon, R., Thermal stability of 2-methylisoborneol in Robusta coffee. *Colloq. Sci. Int. Cafe,* 15th(Vol.2), 866, 1993. (CA121:33729q)
27. Bade-Wegner, H., Holscher, W., Vitzthum, O. G., Quantification of 2-methylisoborneol in roasted coffee by GC-MS, *Colloq. Sci. Int. Cafe,* 15th (Vol. 2), 537, 1993. (CA121:33420g)
28. Arnaud, M. J., Metabolism of caffeine and other components of coffee, in Caffeine, Coffee and Health, Garattini, S., Ed., Raven Press Ltd., New York, 1993, 81.
29. Harland, B. F., Oberleas, D., Phytate and zinc contents of coffees, cocoas, and teas, *J. Food Sci.,* 50, 832, 1985.
30. Franz, H., Maier, H. G., Inositol phosphates in coffee and related beverages. Part 2. Coffee. *Dtsch. Lebensm.-Rundsch.* 9(5), 345, 1994. (in German) (CA123:31752j)
31. Levi, C. P., Investigations of contaminants in coffee, *Colloq. Sci. Int. Cafe,* 9, 125, 1980. (CA96: 141318d)
32. Guyot, B., Lahmy, S., Vincent, J. C., Determination of 3,4-benzpyrene in roasted coffee and its roasting by-products, *Cafe Cacao Thé,* 26, 199, 1982. (CA98:33161e)
33. Morgante, A., Aromatic polycyclic hydrocarbons in coffee, *Riv. Merceol.,* 19, 215, 1980. (CA94: 173070s)
34. Steele, D. H., Thornburg, M. J., Stanley, J. S., Miller, R. R., Brooke, R., Cushman, J., Cruzan, G., Determination of styrene in selected foods, *J. Agric. Food Chem.,* 42(8), 1661, 1994. (CA121:106788v)
35. Deisinger, P. J., Hill, T. S, English, C. J., Human exposure to naturally occurring hydroquinone, *J. Toxicol. Environ. Health,* 47(1), 31, 1996. (CA124:281730d)
36. Rahn, W., Meyer, H. W., Koenig, W.A., Effect of steam treatment on the composition of phenolic components of green and roasted coffee, *Z. Lebensm.-Unters. Forsch.* 169, 346, 1979. (CA92:40077m)
37. Windholtz, M., et al., Eds., *The Merck Index,* Ninth Edition, Merck, Rahway, 1976.
38. Rahn. W., Koenig, W. A., GC/MS investigation of the constituents in a diethyl ether extract of an acidified roast coffee infusion, *HRC CC J. High Resolut. Chromatogr. Commun.,* 1, 69, 1978. (CA89: 161806v)
39. Tressl, R., Bahri, D., Kooppler, H., Jensen, A., Diphenols and caramel compounds in roasted coffees of different varieties, II, *Z. Lebensm.-Unters. Forsch.,* 167, 111, 1978, (CA89: 195665p)
40. Savolainen, H., Tannin content of tea and coffee, *J. Appl. Toxicol.,* 12(3), 191, 1992. (CA117:25069b)
41. Bicchi, C. P., Binello, A. E., Pelligrino, G. M., Vanni, A. C., Characterization of green and roasted coffees through the chlorogenic acid fraction by HPLC-UV and principal component analysis, *J. Agric. Food Chem.,* 43(6), 1549, 1995. (CA122:313392x)
42. De Menezes, H. C., The relationship between the state of maturity of raw coffee beans and the isomers of caffeoylquinic acid, *Food Chem.* 50(3),293, 1994. (CA121:33749w)
43. Hatsutori, T., Fujimoto, T., Fujimoto, M., Watanabe, Y., Jpn. Kokai Tokkyo Koho JP 07 08,169 [95 08,169] (Cl. A23F5/24), 13 Jan 1995, Appl. 93/178,499, 28 Jun 1993. (CA122:212613q)
44. Morishita, H., Kido, R., Antioxidant activities of chlorogenic acids , *Colloq. Sci. Int. Cafe,* 16th(Vol.1), 119, 1995. (CA124:134740d)
45. Nakayama, T., Protective effects of caffeic acid esters against hydrogen peroxide-induced cell damage, *Colloq. Sci. Int. Cafe,* 16th(Vol.1), 372, 1995. (CA124:134741e)
46. Zeng, H., Li, J., Feng, Y., Gui, Y., Food antioxidant and caffeine extracted from useless coffee beans, *Huanan Ligong Daxue Xuebao Ziran Kexueban,* 21(2), 31, 1993. (Chinese) (CA121:132585w)

47. Tsuji, A., Oka, S., Sano, Y., Matsushita, R., Takada, J., Sakurai, H., Superoxide scavenging activity and metal contents of coffee, *Biomed. Res. Trace Elem.*, 6(2), 101, 1995. (CA124:230604h)
48. Goodman, B. A., Glidewell, S. M., Deighton, N., Morrice, A. E., Free radical reactions involving coffee, *Food Chem.*, 51(4), 399, 1994. (CA122:30216e)
49. Daglia, M., Cuzzoni, M. T., Dacarro, C., Antibacterial activity of coffee: relationship between biological activity and chemical markers, *J. Agric. Food Chem.*, 42(10), 2273, 1994. (CA121:203869e)
50. Nishina, A., Kajishima, F., Matsunaga, M., Tezuka, H., Inatomi, H., Osawa, T., Antimicrobial substance, 3'4'-dihydroxyacetophenone, in coffee residue, *Biosci. Biotechnol. Biochem.*, 58(2), 293, 1994. (CA120:215727z)
51. Murata, M., Okada, H., Homma, S., Hydroxycinnamic acid derivatives and p-coumaryl-(L)-tryptophan, a novel hydroxycinnamic acid derivative from coffee beans, *Biosci. Biotechnol. Biochem.*, 59(10), 1887, 1995. (CA124:54202q)
52. Balyaya, K., J., Clifford, M. N., Chlorogenic acid and caffeine contents of monsooned Indian Arabica and Robusta coffees compared with wet and dry processed coffees from the same geographic area, *Colloq. Sci. Int. Cafe*, 16th (Vol.1), 316, 1995. (CA124:230587e)
53. Koenig, W. A., Rahn, W., Vetter, R., Identify and quantify emetic active constituents in roast coffee, *Coll. Sci. Int. Cafe*, 9, 145, 1980. (CA96:121183c)
54. Vincent, J. C., Guenot, M. C., Perriot, J. J., Gueule, D., Hahn, J., Effect of different technological treatments on the chemical and organoleptic characteristics of Robusta and Arabusta coffees, *Coll. Sci. Int. Cafe*, 8, 271, 1977. (CA92:162335w)
55. Wurziger, J., Observations on pest-damaged raw coffee, *Coll. Sci. Int. Cafe*, 8, 97, 1977. (CA93:6185f)
56. Deshpande, S. N., Aguilar, A. A., Effects of roasting temperatures and gamma-irradiation on the content of chlorogenic acid, caffeic acid and soluble carbohydrates of coffee, *Int. J. Appl. Radiat. Isot.*, 26, 656, 1975. (CA84:57527r)
57. Goldoni, L., Jovic, V., Milostic, I., Some changes during the roasting of coffee. *Prehrambeno-Tehnol. Rev.*, 12, 31, 1974. (CA85:191018z)
58. Nakabayaishi, T., Kojima, Y., Changes in the quinic acid contents of coffee beans during roasting process, *Nippon Shokuhin Kogyo Gakkaishi*, 27, 108, 1980. (CA93:44318j)
59. Scholtz-Boettcher, B. M., Maier, H. G., Isomers of quinic acid and quinides in roasted coffee: indicators for the degree of roast? *Colloq. Sci. Int. Cafe*, 14th, 220, 1991 (publ. 1992). (CA117:89128c)
60. Bennat, C., Engelhardt, U. H., Kiehne, A., Wirries, F. M., Maier, H. G., HPLC analysis of chlorogenic acid lactones in roasted coffee, *Z. Lebensm.-Unters. Forsch.*, 199(1), 17, 1994. (CA121:178291a)
61. Brown, S. A., Lignin and tannin biosynthesis, in *Biochemistry of Phenolic Compounds*, Harborne, J. B., Ed., Academic Press, London, 1964, 387.
62. Melo, M., Amorim, H. V., Chemistry of Brazilian green coffee and the quality of the beverage. VI, The uv and visible spectral analysis and chlorogenic acids content in TCA soluble buffer extracts, *Turrialba*, 25, 243, 1975. (CA84:57533q)
63. Melo, M., Fazooli, L. C., Teixeira, A., Amorim, H. V., Chemical physical and organoleptic alterations on storage of coffee beans, *Cienc. Cult. (Sao Paulo)*, 32, 468, 1980. (CA93:44277v)
64. Oliveira, J. C., Silva, D. M., Amorim, H. V., Enzymatic activity of polyphenoloxidase and catalase in *Coffea arabica* L. seeds and seedlings, *Cientifica*, 4, 68, 1976. (CA85:139854e)
65. Oliveira, J. C., Amorim, H. V., Silva, D. M., Teixeira, A. A., Polyphenoloxidase enzymic activity of four species of coffee beans during storage, *Cientifica*, 4, 114, 1976. (CA86:68577z)

66. Oliveira, J. C., Silva, D. M., Amorim, H. V., Teixeira, A. A., Effects of the origin, pulping types and storage of coffee on the polyphenoloxidase activity and beverage quality, *Cientifica*, 7, 79, 1979. (CA92:127193v)
67. Oliveira, J. C., Silva, D. M., Teixeira, A. A., Amorim, H. V., Enzymatic activity of polyphenoloxidase, peroxidase and catalase in beans of *Coffea arabica* L. related to the beverage quality, *Turrialba* 27, 75, 1977. (CA87:51839j)
68. Oliveira, J. C., Silva, D. M., Amorim, H. V, Teixeira AA: Effect of the combination of crude coffee bean extracts with high and low polyphenoloxidase activity on 3,4-dihydroxyphenylalanine, *Cientifica*, 3, 332, 1975. (CA84:178461y)
69. Becker, C. G., Van Hamont, N., Wagner, M., Tobacco, cocoa, coffee and ragweed: Crossreacting allergens that activate factor-XII-dependent pathways, *Blood*, 58, 861, 1981. (CA96:33194b)
70. Boublik, J. H., Quinn, M. J., Clements, J. A., Herington, A. C., Wynne, K. N., Funder, J. W., Coffee contains potent opiate receptor binding activity, *Nature*, 301, 246, 1983. (CA98:87914w)
71. Rees, D. I., Theaker, P. D., High pressure liquid chromatography of chlorogenic acid isomers in coffee, *Coll. Sci. Int. Cafe*, 8, 79, 1977. (CA92:196458x)
72. Correia, A. M. N. G., Leitao, A. M. C., Phenolic acids in green and roasted coffee, *Bull. Liaison - Groupe polyphenols*, 16(pt 2), 117, 1992. (CA123:197135k)
73. Vaseo, J. Z., Tabacchi, R., Chemical composition of coffee pulp, *Coll. Sci. Int. Cafe*, 9, 335, 1980. (CA96: 148510u)
74. Belyaya, K. J., Clifford, M. N., Individual chlorogenic acids and caffeine contents in commercial grades of wet and dry processed Indian green robusta coffee, *J. Food Sci. Technol.*, 32(2),104, 1995. (CA123:197159w)
75. Correia, A. M. N. G., Leitao, M. C. A., Clifford, M. N., Caffeoyl-tyrosine and Angola II as characteristic markers for Angolan Robusta coffees, *Food Chem.*, 53(3), 309, 1995. (CA123:8347x)
76. Vitzthum, O. G., Werkoff, P., Steam volatile aroma constituents of roasted coffee, *Z. Lebensm.-Unters. Forsch.*, 160, 277, 1976. (CA84:178488n)
77. De Maria, C. A. B., Trugo, L. C., Aquino, N. F. R., Moreira, R. F. A., Arabinogalactan as a potential furfural precursor in roasted coffee, *Int. J. Food Sci. Technol.*, 29(5), 559, 1994. (CA122:185989h)
78. Shibamoto, T., Harada, K., Mihara, S., Nishimura, O., Yamaguchi, K., Aitoku, A., Fukada, T., Applications of HPLC for evaluation of coffee flavor quality, in Charalambous, G., Inglett, G., Eds., *Qual. Foods Beverages: Chem Technol, Proc. Symp. Int. Flavor Conf. 2nd*, Academic, New York, 1981, 311. (CA96:33486y)
79. Herrman, G., Baltes, W., Model studies on aroma formation in coffee, *Coll. Sci. Int. Cafe*, 9, 77, 1980. (CA96:141420f)
80. Tressl, R., Gruenewald. K. G., Kamperschroer, H., Silwar, R., Formation of pyrroles and aroma contributing sulfur components in malt and roasted coffee, *Prog. Food Nutr. Sci.*, 5, 71, 1981.
81. Mende, P., Ziebarth, D., Preussmann, R., Spiegelhalder, B., Occurrence of the nitrosamide precursor pyrrolidin-2-one in food and tobacco, *Carcinogenesis*,15(4) 733, 1994. (CA120:296984f)
82. Mende, P., Preussmann, R., Spiegelhalder, B., Nitrosamide formation from foodstuffs, in *ACS Symp. Ser. 553, Nitrosamines and related N-Nitroso- compounds*, 314, 1994. (CA121:156110p)
83. Nurok, D., Anderson, J. W., Zlatkis, A., Profiles of sulfur containing compounds obtained from Arabica and Robusta coffees by capillary column gas chromatography, *Chromatographia*, 11, 188, 1978. (CA89:22468y)
84. Parliment, T. H., Stahl, H. D., Formation of furfuryl mercaptan in coffee model systems, *Dev. Food Sci.*, 37A, 805, 1995. (CA123:196907b)

85. Sekiguchi, N., Yata, M., Murata, M., Homma, S., Identification of an iron-binding compound in instant coffee, 2, *Nippon Nogei Kagaku Kaish*, 68(4), 821, 1994. (CA120;321801d)
86. Pereira, A., Pereira, M, M., Free amino acids in green coffee from Huambo (Angola). Separation and identification by electrophoresis and thin layer chromatography, *Coll. Sci. Int. Cafe*, 8, 545, 1977. (CA92:196460s)
87. Arnold, U., Ludwig, E., Kuehn, R., Moeschwitzer, U., Analysis of free amino acids in green coffee beans, Part 1, Determination of amino acids after precolumn derivatization using 9-fluorenylmethylchloroformate, *Z. Lebensm.-Forsch.* 199(1), 22, 1994. (CA121:132515y)
88. Steinhart, H., Luger, A., Amino acid pattern of steam treated coffee, *Colloq. Sci. Int. Cafe*, 16th(Vol.1), 278, 1995. (CA124:143964g)
89. Nehring, U. P., Maier, H. G., Indirect determination of degree of roast in coffee, *Lebensm.-Unters. Forsch.* 195(1), 39, 1992. (CA117:190397q)
90. Kele, M., Ohmacht, R., Determination of serotonin released from coffee wax by liquid chromatography, *J. Chromatogr. A.*, 730 (1+2), 59, 1996. (CA124:337857v)
91. Gosch, B., Montag, A., Nucleopurine content of coffee, *Dtsch. Lebensm.-Rundsch.* 91(7), 208, 1995. (German) (CA124:7543s)
92. Lehrer, S. B., Karr, R. M., Salvaggio, J. E., Analysis of green coffee bean and castor bean allergens using RAST inhibition, *Clin. Allergy*, 11, 357, 1981. (CA95:201844p)
93. Becker, C. G., Lower allergenicity and lower thrombogenicity foods, PCT Int. Appl. WO 82 01, 132. 15 Apr 1982. (CA97:54307b)
94. Berndt, W., Meier-Cabell, E., Properties of some proteins as well as acid phosphatase from green coffee, *Coll, Int, Chim, Cafes*, 7, 225, 1975. (CA85:155547n)
95. Thaler, H., Macromolecular structures in coffee, *Coll. Int. Chim. Cafe*, 7, 175, 1975.
96. Thaler, H., The chemistry of coffee extraction in relation to polysaccharides, *Food Chem.*, 4, 13, 1979. (CA90:166719z)
97. Leloup, V., Liardon, R., Analytical characterization of coffee carbohydrates, *Colloq. Sci. Int. Cafe*, 15th(vol. 2), 694, 1993. (CA121:33728p)
98. Ara, V., Thaler, H., Studies of coffee and coffee-substitute. XVIII. Dependence of the quantity and composition of a high polymer galactomannan on the coffee species and the degree of roasting, *Z. Lebensm.-Unters. Forsch.*, 161, 143, 1976. (CA85:92372d)
99. Ara, V., Thaler, H., Studies on coffee and coffee substitutes. XIX. Dependence of the quantity of a highly polymeric galactomannan on the degree of extraction of commercially prepared coffee-extracts, *Z. Lebensm.-Unters. Forsch.*, 164, 8, 1977. (CA87:51829f)
100. Gonis, J., Hewitt, D. G., Troup, G., Hutton, D. R., Hunter, C. R., The chemical origin of free radicals in coffee and other beverages, *Free Radical Res.*, 23(4), 393, 1995. (CA124:85240e)
101. Nakabayashi, T., Chemical studies on the quality of coffee. V. Changes in the sucrose content of coffee beans during roasting, *Nippon Shokuhin Kogyo Gakkaishi*, 24, 479, 1977. (CA91:209617e)
102. Sabbagh, N. K., Yokomizo, Y., Faria, J. B., The influence of roasting on the monosaccharide contents of Arabica, Robusta and Icatu hybrid coffees, *Col. Inst. Tecnol. Aliment. (Campinas Braz.)*, 8, 111, 1977. (CA89:89061d)
103. Ollroge, I., Aldoses and polysaccharides in coffee, Report 1980, Order No PB81-167264, NTIS, *Gov Rep Announce Index* (U.S.) 81, 2568, 1981. (CA95:78598g)
104. Sabbagh, N. K., Faria, J. B., Yokomizo, Y., Determination of monosaccharides in soluble Brazilian coffees, *Col. Inst. Technol. Aliment. (Campinas, Braz.)*, 8, 55, 1977. (CA89:89059j)

105. Steinhart, H., Packert, A., Melanoidins in coffee. Separation and characterization by different chromatographic procedures, *Colloq. Sci. Int. Cafe* 15th(Vol.2), 593, 1993. (CA121:33720e)
106. Wurziger, J., Drews, R., Bundesen, G., Green and roasted Arabusta coffee, *Colloq. Sci. Int. Cafe.*, 8, 101,1977. (CA92:196564d)
107. Folstar, P., Pilnik, W., De Heus, J. G., Van der Plas. H. C., The composition of the fatty acids in coffee oil and coffee wax, *Colloq. Int. Chim. Cafes.*, 7, 253, 1975. (CA85:190980v)
108. Hara, S., Okamoto, S., Totani, Y., Lipid constituents of coffee beans and their denaturation, *Seikei Daigaku Kogakubu Kogaku Hokoku*, 27, 1895, 1979. (CA91:18551u)
109. Sarra, C., The possible employment of food industry residues in animal feeding: First report on the chemical and bromatological composition of coffee grounds and suggestions for their use, *Ann. Fac. Mid. Vet. Torino*, 23, 232, 1976. (CA87:166306a)
110. Ratnayake, W. M. N., Hollywood, R., O'Grady, E., Stavric, B., Lipid content and composition of coffee brews prepared by different methods, *Food Chem. Toxicol.* 31(4), 263, 1993. (CA119:27040a)
111. Nagasampagi, B. A., Rowe, J. W., Simpson, R., Goad, L. J., Sterols of coffee, *Phytochemistry*, 10, 1101, 1971.
112. Tiscornia, E., Centi-Grossi, M., Tassi-Micco, C., Evangelisti, F., The sterol fraction of the oil extracted from coffee (Coffea arabica L.) seeds, *Riv. Ital. Sostanze Grasse*, 56, 283, 1979. (CA92:90899b)
113. Turchetto, E., Lercker, G., Bortolomeazzi, R., Oxysterol determination in selected coffees, *Toxicol. Ind. Health*, 9(3), 519, 1993. (CA121:81456v)
114. Folstar, P., Van der Plas, H. C., Pilnik, W., De Heus, J. G., Tocopherols in the unsaponifiable matter of coffee bean oil, *J. Agric. Food. Chem.*, 25, 283, 1977. (CA86:119436n)
115. Lehmann, G., Neunhoeffer, O., Roselius, W., Vitzthum, O., Protection of autoxidizable materials by addition of extract of green coffee beans, US 3,663,581, 1972. (CA77:60335n)
116. Lehmann, G., Neunhoeffer, O., Roselius, W., Vitzthum, O., Antioxidant derived from green coffee beans, Br 1,275,129, 1972. (CA77:60341m)
117. Lehmann, G., Neunhoeffer, O., Roselius, W., Vitzthum, O., Antioxidants made from green coffee beans and their use for protecting autoxidizable foods, Ger 1,668,236, 1979. (CA90: 185220w)
118. Lam, L. K. T., Sparnins, V. L., Wattenberg, L. W., Isolation and identification of kahweol palmitate and cafestol palmitate as active constituents of green coffee beans that enhance glutathione-S transferase activity in the mouse, *Cancer Res.*, 42, 1193, 1982. (CA96: 198149d)
119. Hirsbrunner, P., Bertholet, R., Saponification treatment of spent coffee grounds, US 4,293,581, 6 Oct 1981. (CA96:33641v)
120. Wurziger, J., Diterpenes in coffee oils for the evaluation of raw coffee according to type and processing, *Fette Seiffen Anstrichm.*, 79, 334, 1977. (CA88: 103392a)
121. Katan, M. B., Urgert, R., The cholesterol-elevating factor from coffee beans. *Colloq. Sci. Int. Cafe*, 16th (Vol. 1), 49, 1995. (CA124:173701m)
122. Weusten-Van Der Wouw, M. P. M. E., Katan, M. B., Viani, R., Huggett, A. C., Liardon, R., Lung-Larsen, P. G., Thelle, D. S., Ahola, I., Aro, A., et al., Identity of the cholesterol-raising factor from boiled coffee and its effect on liver function enzymes, *J. Lipid Res.*, 35(4), 721, 1994. (CA120:268552v)
123. Urgert, R., van der Weg, G., Kosmeijer-Schuil, T. G., Truus, G., van de Bovenkamp, P., Hovenier, R., Katan, M. B., Levels of the cholesterol-elevating diterpenes cafestol and kahweol in various coffee brews, *J. Agric. Food Chem.*, 43 (8), 2167, 1995. (CA123:82056t)

124. Mensink, R. P., Lebbink, W. J., Lobbezoo, I. E., Weusten-Van Der Wouw, M. P. M. E., Zock, P.I., Katan, M. B., Diterpene composition of oils from Arabica and Robusta coffee beans and their effects on serum lipids in man, *J. Intern. Med.*, 237(6), 543, 1995. (CA123:142232j)
125. Tewis, R., Montag, A., Speer, K., Dehydrocafestol and dehydrokahweol: two new roasting components in coffee, *Colloq. Sci. Int. Cafe* 15th(Vol.2), 878, 1993. (CA121:33731j)
126. Lercker, G., Frega, N., Bocci, F., Rodriguez-Estrada, M. T., High resolution gas chromatographic determination of diterpenic alcohols and sterols in coffee lipids, *Chromatographia*, 41(1/2), 29, 1995. (CA123:255201s)
127. Frega, N., Bocci, F., Lercker, G., Determination of Robusta in commercial blends with Arabica coffee, *Ind. Aliment. (Pinerolo, Italy)*, 34(339), 705, 1995. (CA123:337687u)
128. Speer, K., Fatty acid esters of the 16-O-methylcafestol, *Colloq. Sci. Int. Cafe*, 16th (Vol. 1), 224, 1995. (CA124:174201j)
129. Speer, K., Tewis, R., Montag, A., 16-O-methylcafestol: a quality indicator for coffee, *Colloq. Sci. Int. Cafe*, 14th, 237, 1991. (CA117:89129d)
130. Richter, H., Spiteller, G., A new furokaurane glycoside from green coffee beans, *Chem. Ber.*, 112, 1088, 1979. (CA91:74837d)
131. Ludwig, H., Obermann, H., Spiteller, G., Diterpenes recently found in coffee, *Colloq. Int. Chim. Cafe*, 7, 205, 1975.
132. Wahlberg, I., Enzell, C. R., Rowe, J. W., *ent*-16-Kauren-l9-ol from coffee, *Phytochemistry*, 14, 1677, 1975. (CA84:2227n)
133. Richter, H., Obermann, H., Spiteller G., A new kauran-18-oic acid glucopyranosylester from green coffee beans, *Chem. Ber.*, 110, 1963, 1977. (CA87:68579x)
134. Richter, H., Spiteller, G., A new atractyligenin glycoside from green coffee beans, *Chem. Ber.*, 111, 3506, 1978. (CA90:19037x)
135. Aeschbach, R., Kuay, A., Maier, H. G., Diterpenes of coffee. 1. Atractyligenin, *Z. Lebensm.- Unters. Forsch.*, 175, 337, 1982. (CA98:15571j)
136. Matzel, U., Maier, H. G., Atractyligenin and its glycosides in coffee, *Z. Lebensm.- Unters. Forsch.*, 176, 281, 1983.
137. Folstar, P., Van der Plas, H. C., Pilnik, W., Schols, H. A., Melger, P., Liquid chromatographic analysis of N-alkanoyl-5-hydroxytryptamine (C-5-HT) in green coffee beans, *J. Agric. Food Chem.*, 27, 12, 1979. (CA90:70640r)
138. Fontana, G., Mantia, G., Vetri, P., Venturella, F., Hopps, V., Cascio, G., Effects on the carbohydrate metabolism of "coffee atractylosides", *Fitoterapia*, 65(1), 29, 1994. (CA122:208m)
139. Hunziker, H. R., Miserez, A., HPLC determination of 5-hydroxytryptamide in coffee, *Mitt. Geb. Lebensmitt. Hyg.*, 70, 142, 1979. (CA91:122210t)
140. Folstar, P., Pilnik, W., Van der Plas, H. C., Liquid chromatographic coffee wax analysis, *Colloq. Sci. Int. Cafe*, 8, 121, 1977. (CA92:179145a)
141. Iyimen, S., Lehmann, G., Neunhoeffer, O., Vitzthum, O., Procedure for the recovery of serotonin from coffee wax, Swiss 577 470, 1976.
142. Beyeler, T., Separation of serotonin from coffee wax, Ger Offen 2,702,108. 24 May 1978. (CA89:65256v)
143. Hirsbrunner, P., Brambilla, E., Separation of serotonin from coffee wax, Ger Offen 2,532,308. 2 Dec 1976. (CA86:78671q)
144. Roselius, W., Vitzthum, O., Hubert, P., Removal of undesirable irritants from raw coffee beans, US 3,770,456, 1973. (CA80:58631z)
145. Van der Stegen, G. H. D., The effect of dewaxing of green coffee on the coffee brew, *Food Chem.* 4, 23, 1979. (CA90:166720t)
146. Mohr, E., Seiler, A., Removal of outer layers harmful to health from kernels serving as food, Ger Offen 2,455,591. 26 May 1976. (CA85:45198s)

147. Roselius, L., Kurzhals, H. A., Sylla, K. P., Hubert, P., Eliminating irritating substances from coffee, Fr Demande 2,362,592. 24 Mar 1978. (CA89:213889w)
148. Van der Stegen, G. H. D., Noomen, P. J., Mass balance of carboxy-5-hydroxytryptamides (C-5-HT) in regular and treated coffee, *Lebensm. Wiss. Technol.*, 10, 321, 1977. (CA88:103509u)
149. Rizvi, S. J. H., Jaiswal, V., Mukerji, D., Mather, S. N., Antifungal properties of 1,3,7-trimethylxanthine isolated from Coffea arabica, *Naturwissenschaften*, 67, 459, 1980. (CA93: 180195u)
150. Rizvi, S. J. H., Mukerji, D., Mather, S. N., Selective phytotoxicity of 1,3,7-trimethylxanthine between Phaseolus mungo and some weeds, *Agric. Biol. Chem.*, 45, 1255, 1981. (CA95:37021v)
151. Rizvi, S. J. H., Pandey, S. K., Mukerji, D., Mather, S. N., 1,3,7-trimethylxanthine, a new chemosterilant for stored grain pest, Callosobruchus chinensis (L.), *Z. Angew. Entomol.*, 90, 378, 1980. (CA94: 11610r)
152. Charrier, A., Variation of the caffeine content in coffee plants, *Colloq. Int. Chim. Cafes.*, 7, 295, 1975. (CA85:156639f)
153. Gilbert, R. M., Marshman, J. A., Schwieder, M., Berg, R., Caffeine content of beverages as consumed, *Can. Med. Assoc. J.*, 114, 205, 1976. (CA84:134237a)
154. de Andrage, J. B., Pinheiro, H. L. C., Lopes, A., Martins, S., Amorin, A. M. M., Brandao, A. M., Determination of caffeine in beverages by high performance liquid chromatography (HPLC), *Quim. Nova*, 18(4), 379, 1995. (Portuguese) (CA123:110346h)
155. Dong, M., Hoffmann, D., Locke, D. C., Ferrand, E., The occurrence of caffeine in the air of New York City, *Atmos. Environ.*, 11, 651, 1977. (CA88:176313k)
156. Ndjouenkeu, R., Clo, G., Voilley, A., Effect of coffee beverage extraction conditions on the concentration in methyl xanthines measured by HPLC, *Sci. Aliments.*, 1, 365, 1981. (CA95:202163c)
157. Roberts, M. F., Waller, G. R., N-methyltransferases and 7-methyl-N-nucleoside hydrolase activity in Coffea arabica and the biosynthesis of caffeine, *Phytochemistry*, 18, 451, 1979. (CA92: 18866w)
158. Schulthess, B. H., Baumann, T. W., Are xanthosine and 7-methylxanthosine caffeine precursors? *Phytochemistry*, 39(6), 1363, 1995. (CA123:165175g)
159. Mazzafera, P., Wingsle, G., Olsson, O., Sandberg, G., *S*-Adenosyl-L-methionine:theobromine 1-*N*-methyltransferase, an enzyme catalyzing the synthesis of caffeine in coffee, *Phytochemistry*, 37(6), 1577, 1994. (CA122:259411n)
160. Stadler, R. H., Fay, L. B., Antioxidative reactions of caffeine: formation of 8-oxocaffeine (1,3,7-trimethyluric acid) in coffee subjected to oxidative stress, *J. Agric. Food Chem.*, 43(5), 1332, 1995. (CA122:289398f)
161. Viani, R., Horman, I., Determination of trigonelline in coffee, *Coll. Int. Chim. Cafes* 7, 273, 1975. (CA85:190824x)
162. Vasudeva, N., Gopal, N. H., Studies on ascorbic acid in coffee plants. II. Distribution in ripe fruits and its relation with coffee quality, *J. Coffee Res.*, 4, 25, 1974. (CA85:59606k)
163. Tchetche, A. G., Quantitative determination of vitamin PP or niacin in Coffea canephora var. robusta by a microbiological method using Lactobacillus arabinosus, *Colloq. Sci. Int. Cafe*, 8, 147, 1977. (CA92:196459)
164. Oliveira, E. N. S., Blaskowski, M. M. M., Vitamin B6 in Brazilian coffees. II. Free and combined, *Arq. Biol. Tecnol.*, 22, 183, 1979. (CA93:41553w)
165. Leszczynska, T., Nitrate and nitrite content of tea, coffee and cocoa, *Bromatol. Chem. Toksykol.*, 27(4), 327, 1994. (Polish) (CA122:263903s)
166. Tsuji, S., Shibata, T., Ohara K., Okada, N., Ito, Y., Factors affecting the formation of hydrogen peroxide in coffee, *Shokuhin Eiseigaku Zasshi*, 32(6), 504, 1991. (Japanese) (CA117:68821h)

167. Fonseca, H., Guttierrez, L. E., Teixeira, A. A,. Total nitrogen in green coffee samples of different kinds of beverage, *Esc. Super Agric Luiz de Queiroz Univ. Sao Paulo*, 31, 491, 1974. (CA85:107636u)
168. Clarke, R. J., Walker, L. J., The interrelation of potassium contents of green roasted and instant coffees, *Coll. Int. Chim. Cafes*, 7, 159, 1975. (CA85: 190979b)
169. Macrae, R., Petracco, M., Illy, E., Trace metal profiles of green coffee, *Colloq. Sci. Int. Cafe*, 15th(Vol. 2), 650, 1993. (CA121:33724j)
170. Lara, W. H., Toledo, M., Takahashi, M. Y., Copper contents in roasted and ground coffee and in coffee drink, *Rev. Inst. Adolfo Lutz*, 35-36, 17, 1976. (CA88:73226e)
171. Quijano-Rico, M., Spettel, B., Determination of the content of various elements in samples of different varieties of coffee, *Colloq. Int. Chim. Cafes*, 7,165, 1975. (CA85:158131h)
172. Vergote, G., Van Zele, W., De Clerck, F., Heyndrickx, A., Fluoride intake by man from beverages, *Farm. Tijdschr. Belg.*, 56, 130, 1979. (CA91:54832v)
173. Sadowski, S., Skorkowska-Zieleniewska, J., Fluorine in selected beverages in the domestic market (Poland), *Rocz. Panstw. Zakl. Hig.*, 31, 413, 1980. (CA94:63945y)
174. Ciurea, I. C., Lipka, Y. F., Occurrence of cadmium in cocoa and coffee, *Mitt. Geb. Lebensmittelunters. Hyg.*, 83(2), 197, 1992. (CA118:21235a)
175. Kohiyama, M., Kanematsu, H., Niiya, I., Heavy metals particularly nickel, contained in cacao beans and chocolate, *Nippon Shokuhin Kogyo Gakkaishi*, 39(7), 596, 1992. (CA118:146452a)
176. Chacho, M. J., Bhat, P. K., Preliminary studies on control of Araecerus fasciculatus infesting coffee by bag impregnation, *J. Coffee Res.*, 9, 24, 1979. (CA92:89293t)
177. Jordao, B. A., Yokomizo, Y., Sartori, M. R., De Moraes, R. M., Carvalho, G. R., Medina, J. C., Establishment of levels for inorganic bromide residues in green coffee due to fumigation with methyl bromide, *Bol. Inst. Tecnol. Aliment. (Campinas Braz)*, 60, 41, 1978. (CA92:89255g)
178. Haarer, A. K., *Modern Coffee Production*, Leonard Hill, London, 1962.
179. Visweswariah, K., Jayaram, M., Venkataramaiah, G. H., Investigations on BHC residues in drinking water from coffee plantations and coffee beans, *J. Coffee Res.*, 3, 96, 1973. (CA84: 146057e)
180. Oliveira, J. C., Silva, D. M., Teixeira, A. A., Amorim, H. V., Effects of the application of insecticides to control coffee tree borers on the polyphenoloxidase activity and beverage quality of coffee, *Cientifica*, 7, 221, 1979. (CA93:184545f)
181. Holt, L., Pease, H. L., Determination of oxamyl residues using flame photometric gas chromatography, *J. Agric. Food Chem.*, 24, 263, 1976. (CA84:134161w)
182. Baker, P. G., The determination of fentin residues, *Meded. Fac. Landbouwwet. Rijksuniv. Gent.*, 45, 853, 1980. (CA94:63886e)
183. Cerutti, G., Finoli, C., Gerosa, A., Zappaviene, R., Organochlorine pesticide residues in foods and beverages, *Riv. Soc. Ital. Sci. Aliment.*, 5, 339, 1976. (CA86:104549c)
184. Blumenthal, A., Cerny, M., Organochlorine pesticide residues in tea and coffee, *Mitt. Geb. Lebensmitt. Hyg.*, 67, 515, 1976. (CA86:154106b)
185. Ribas, C., Pigati, P., Ferreira, M. S., Netto, N. D., Effect of roasting on residues of lindane and endosulfan in coffee beans, *Biologico*, 43, 208, 1977. (CA89:74390m)
186. Ribas, C., Pigati, P., Guindani, C. M. A., Dias, N. M., Effect of the period of application on lindane residues in coffee beans, *Arq. Inst. Biol. Sao Paulo*, 43, 121, 1976. (CA88:49111 t)
187. Venkataramaiah, G. H., Singh, M. B. D., Carbofuran residues in coffee bean, *J. Coffee Res.*, 6, 40, 1976. (CA86: 154114c)
188. Mithyantha, M. S., Agnihothrudu, V., Carbofuran residues in coffee beans, Comments, *J. Coffee Res.*, 7, 84, 1978. (CA89:174694g)

189. Bonilla, G. J. C., Study on the effect of fungicides recommended for use against red blight (Hemileia vastatrix Berk. and Br.), *Actas Simp. Latinoam Cafic.*, 3, 40, 1980. (CA97: 121940t)
190. Morallo-Rejesus, B., Baldos, E. P., Tejeda, A. M., Evaluation of insecticides against coffee berry borer and its residues in processed coffee, *Philipp. Entomol.*, 4, 415, 1981. (CA96:50842d)
191. Anon., Glyphosate tolerances for residues, *Fed. Regist.*, 44, 5136, 1979. (CA90:136358p)
192. Anon., Tolerances for pesticide chemicals in or on raw agricultural commodities; N,N-diethyl-2-(1-naphthalenyloxy)-propionamide, *Fed. Regist.*, 46, 47547, 1981. (CA95:202197s)
193. McCarthy, J. P., Adinolfi, J., McMullin, S. L., Rehman, W. C., Zalon, P. S., Zuckerman, L. M., Marshall, R. D., McLain, K. C., NCA survey of pesticide residues in brewed coffees, *Colloq. Sci. Int. Cafe*, 14th, 175, 1991. (CA117:46901g)
194. Anon., Aldicarb; tolerances for residues, *Fed. Regist.*, 43, 60465, 1978. (CA90:202319e)
195. Gallaz, L., Stalder, R., Ochratoxin A in Coffee, *Chem. Mikrobiol. Technol. Lebensm.*, 4, 147, 1976. (CA84:178507t)
196. Fritz, W., Buthig, C., Donath, R., Engst, R., Studies on the formation of ochratoxin A in grain and other food, *Z. Gesamte Hyg. Ihre Grenzgeb.*, 25, 929, 1979. (CA94:45683g)
197. De Palo, D., Gabucci, G., Valussi, S., Study on the possible presence of aflatoxin, sterigmatocystine and ochratoxin in green coffee, *Colloq. Sci. Int. Cafe*, 8, 539, 1977. (CA92: 162258s)
198. De Campos, M., Santos, J. C., Olszyna-Marzys, A.,K., Aflatoxin contamination in grains from the Pacific Coast in Guatamala and the effect of storage upon contamination, *Bull. Environ. Contam. Toxicol.*, 24, 789, 1980. (CA93:89863z)
199. Nartowicz, V. B., Buchanan, R. L., Segall, S., Aflatoxin production in regular and decaffeinated coffee beans, *J. Food Sci.*, 44, 446, 1979. (CA90:166747g)
200. Buchanan, R. L., Tice, G., Marino, D., Caffeine inhibition of ochratoxin A production, *J. Food Sci.*, 47, 319, 1981. (CA96:67387g)
201. Levi, C., Mycotoxins in coffee, *J. Assoc. Off. Anal. Chem.*, 63, 1282, 1980. (CA94:45623n)
202. Haberle, V., Balenovic, J., Briski, B., Aflatoxin content in imported peanuts, coffee, barley, wheat and walnuts (Yugoslavia), *Hrana Ishrana*, 19, 451, 1978. (CA90:185047v)
203. Studer-Rohr, I, Dietrich, D. R., Schlatter, J., Schlatter. C., The occurrence of ochratoxin A in coffee, *Food Chem. Toxicol.*, 33(5), 341, 1995. (CA123:8219g)
204. Studer-Rohr, I., Dietrich, D. R., Schlatter, J., Schlatter, C., Ochratoxin A and coffee, *Mitt. Geb. Lebensmittelunters.* Hyg., 85(6), 719, 1994. (CA123:54443y)
205. Milanez, T. V., Sabino, M., Lamardo, L. C. A., Comparison of two methods for the determination of ochratoxin A in green coffee beans, *Rev. Microbiol.* 26(2), 79, 1995. (CA124:173784r)
206. Koch, M., Steinmeyer, S., Tiebach, R., Weber, R., Weyerstahl, P., Determination of ochratoxin A in roasted coffee, *Dtsch. Lebensm.-Rundsch.*, 92(2), 48-51, 1996. (CA124:341185s)
207. Micco, C., Miraglia, M., Brera, C., Desiderio, C., Masci, V., The effect of roasting on the fate of aflatoxin B1 in artificially contaminated green coffee beans, *Mycotoxin Res.*, 8(2), 93, 1992. (CA118:146443y)
208. Van Rillaer, W., Janssens, G., Beernaert, H., Gas chromatographic determination of residual solvents in decaffeinated coffee, *Z. Lebensm. Unters. Forsch.*, 175, 413, 1982. (CA98:52021a)

209. Bejr, V., Extraction of caffeine from green grain coffee, Czech., 184,966, 1978. (CA94:190554v)
210. Panzer, H. P., Yare, R. S., Forber, M. R., Green [coffee] bean decaffeination employing fluorinated hydrocarbons, US 3,769,033, 1973. (CA86:70422p)
211. Kurzhals, H. A., Sylla, K. F., Decaffeinating green coffee beans, Fr. Demande 2,389,333, 1978. (CA91:122433t)
212. Katz, S.N., Gottesman, M., Decaffeinating coffee. US 4,276,315, 1981. (CA95:95801k)
213. Zosel, K., Decaffeination of coffee, US 4,260,639, 1981. (CA95:78780k)
214. Hubert, P., Vitzthum, O., Separation of caffeine from supercritical solutions, Ger. Offen. 2,637,197, 1978.
215. Roselius, L., Kurzhals, H. A., Hubert, P., Selective extraction of caffeine from plant materials, Ger. Offen. 2,727,191, 1978. (CA90:85545n)
216. Jones, G. V., Coogan, J. F., Removing caffeine from coffee, Ger. 2,641,146, 1977. (CA87:4323b)
217. Werkoff, P., Hubert, P., Decaffeination of green coffee, Ger. Offen. 2,853,169, 1980.(CA93: 130967b)
218. Anon., Composition for improving the taste of coffee, Neth. Appl. 74 08,455, 1975.(CA85: 107677h)
219. Zeitlin, B. R., Levenson, H. S., Pritchard, A. B., Methylxanthine antagonism, Can. 1,043,156, 1978. (CA90:102245j)
220. Anon., Antagonizing the stimulating effects of methylxanthines in foods, Neth. Appl. 76 03,263, 1977. (CA89:22560x)
221. Motoda, T., Color improvement of cacao and coffee beans with polyphenoloxidase, Jpn. Kokai Tokkyo Koho 79,143,561, 1979. (CA92:109427v)
222. Anon., Deoxygenator for roasted and powdered coffee storage, Jpn. Kokai Tokkyo Koho JP 81,130,223, 1981. (CA96:50986d)
223. Anon., Thermoplastic sheets for absorption of carbon dioxide, Jpn. Kokai Tokkyo Koho 80,158,933, 1980. (CA:157990m)
224. Takamori, K., Coffee bean oxidation inhibition with sodium sorbate, Jpn. Kokai 77 72,861,1977. (CA166371t)
225. Gopal, N. H., Venkataramanan, D., Effect of ethrel on carbohydrate fractions of Coffea arabica L. fruits, *Turrialba*. 27, 101, 1977. (CA87:97235n)
226. Bose, P. K., Chatterjee, T. K., Das, S. P., Roy, B. R., Detection of cashew nut shells admixed in tea, coffee and chicory, *J. Indian Acad. Forensic Sci.*, 15, 42, 1976. (CA86:184037x)
227. Lee, D. H., Lee, Y. J., A study on the microdetermination of nicotine in contaminated beverage by thin-layer chromatography, *Saengyak Hakhoe Chi (Hanguk Saengyak Hakhoe)*, 10, 23, 1979. (CA92:92812s)
228. Adachi, K., Mass fragmentographic determination of polymethylbiphenyl in foods contaminated with petroleum products, *Bull. Environ. Contam. Toxicol.*, 26, 737, 1981. (CA95: 113485s)
229. Grob, K., Artho, A., Biedermann, M., Caramaschi, A., Mikle, H., Batching oil on sisal bags used for packaging foods: analysis by coupled LC/GC, *J. AOAC Int.* 75(2), 283, 1992. (CA117:88985t)

General references

Clarke, R. J., Macrae, R., Eds., *Coffee Volume 1: Chemistry*, Elsevier Applied Science, London, 1985.
Illy, A., Viani, R., Eds., *Espresso Coffee: The Chemistry of Quality*, Academic Press, London, 1995.
Viani, R., The composition of coffee, in *Caffeine, Coffee, and Health*, Garattini, S., Ed., Raven Press, New York, 1993, 17.

Chapter 7

Methylxanthine Composition and Consumption Patterns of Cocoa and Chocolate Products

Joan L. Apgar and Stanley M. Tarka, Jr.

CONTENTS

0-8493-2647-8/98/$0.00+$.50

I. INTRODUCTION

Foods derived from cocoa beans have been consumed by humans since at least 460 to 480 AD. The source of cocoa beans, the species *Theobroma*, contains a variety of biologically active components. These include the purine alkaloids theobromine, caffeine, and theophylline. Structurally, they are methylated xanthines and, thus, are often referred to as methylxanthines. Theobromine (3, 7-dimethylxanthine) is the predominant purine alkaloid in cocoa and chocolate. Caffeine (1, 3, 7-trimethylxanthine), the major purine alkaloid found in coffee and tea, is found in cocoa and chocolate at about one eighth the concentration of theobromine. Only trace amounts of theophylline (1, 3-dimethylxanthine) are detected in cocoa and chocolate products.

Over the years there has been a concern over the presence of natural toxicants in our food supply. Much work has been reported on the pharmacological and toxicological effects of caffeine and coffee. This includes the FDA commissioning the Select Committee on GRAS Substances to evaluate the safety of caffeine as an added food ingredient.[1] For many years, little attention was paid to the effects of theobromine, cocoa, and chocolate products, presumably due to the long-term consumption of cocoa-related products with no major health effects. In 1982, a comprehensive literature review on cocoa and the methylxanthines identified the need for scientific investigations.[2] Over the last 15 years, the major worldwide producers of chocolate and cocoa have sponsored a detailed research program to determine the effects of theobromine, cocoa, and chocolate products. Two of the most recent animal studies showed no evidence of reproductive toxicity or carcinogenicity in rats from chronic dietary exposure to a reference cocoa powder.[3,4]

This chapter defines the methylxanthine composition of raw and processed cocoa, as well as various chocolate foods and beverages. Patterns of consumption for cocoa and chocolate products are discussed and dietary intakes of caffeine from chocolate products are reported.

II. HISTORICAL ASPECTS

The cacao tree is believed to have originated more than 4,000 years ago in the forests of the Amazon and Orinoco.[5,6] Historical evidence indicates that the cacao tree was cultivated by the Aztec Indians of Mexico and the Maya Indians of Central America since at least 460 to 480 AD. Whatever the exact origin of cacao, no reference has been found in the literature of any civilization other than America prior to 1502. In that year, Christopher Columbus, during his fourth voyage to America, intercepted an agricultural trading ship off the Yucatan coast and brought the first specimen of cacao beans to Spain. Since the custom of using cacao was not yet known in Europe at that time, no value was placed on this discovery.

During the 1519 Spanish conquest of the Aztec empire, Cortez discovered that cacao beans could be roasted, ground, and mixed with maize or spices to prepare a thick bitter drink called "chocolatl" (from the Aztec word "choco" meaning warm and "atl" meaning drink). Realizing the commercial possibilities for the development of cacao, Cortez studied the cultivation and preparation methods from the Aztecs. In 1528, he returned to Spain and introduced "chocolatl" to the Spaniards, who found it too bitter for their taste and improved the palatability by adding sugar. The cultivation of cocoa spread to other Spanish colonies in the Caribbean in order to supply the growing European market, but the methods of preparation were kept a closely guarded secret for almost 100 years.

In 1606, chocolate was introduced into Italy by Antonio Carlotti, who also was instrumental in bringing it to France during the reign of Louis XIII. The French began cultivation of cacao in Martinique in 1660, with the first crop shipped to the mother country in 1679. The custom of drinking chocolate quickly spread to England, where the development of "chocolate houses" became popular. Chocolate remained a luxury during the seventeenth and eighteenth centuries largely due to the high duties that were imposed on the beans and liquor. In addition to supplying the demands of a luxury trade in drinking chocolate, cacao became popular as a medicinal agent. The use of chocolate as a stimulating agent was recorded in Germany as early as 1640, as evidenced by price lists from apothecaries' shops.[5]

The first important technical development in the chocolate manufacturing process occurred when water-powered mills superseded the use of manual labor to grind cocoa beans. This led to the establishment of many chocolate factories from 1804 to 1840. Early production consisted entirely of a type of chocolate beverage that was somewhat indigestible since none of the cocoa butter was removed during processing. In 1828, the Dutch firm of Van Houten invented the cocoa press, which facilitated the production of cocoa powder by partial removal of the cocoa butter from beans.

The second major technical development occurred in 1876, when milk chocolate was invented in Switzerland by M. D. Peter. This process provided a new stimulus to the cacao trade. Milk chocolate powder and cocoa butter were later combined to make an eating chocolate that formed the backbone of the chocolate industry today.

III. BOTANY AND AGRICULTURE OF CACAO

General information on the botany and husbandry of cacao is documented in several references.[5-7] For the purposes of this text, material on these topics has been limited to a brief overview.

A. Classification

Linnaeus, in his writings of 1720, named the cocoa tree *Theobroma cacao* from the Greek "Theos" meaning god and "broma" meaning food, thus conveying the early meaning "food of the gods". At least 20 species of *Theobroma* are presently known. The fruits of various uncultivated species are eaten by natives of the Amazon Basin; however, *T. cacao* is the most important commercial type.[8, 9] The clear identity of this species is not known and the genetic influence of other species, such as *T. pentagona, T. leiocarpa*, and *T. bicolor*, must be recognized.

For commercial purposes, the varieties developed through breeding and cultivation are more important than the species of *Theobroma*. These varieties are often classified into three or four broad categories: Criollo, Forastero, Trinitario, and Nacional. This segregation is not based on botanical purposes, but on the sharp distinction in the kind of flavor and color they exhibit in the manufacturing process.

Criollo (meaning "native") was probably cultivated first in the region from southern Mexico. It is believed that this is the type of cocoa that was grown by the Aztecs and Mayas.[6] Forastero (meaning foreign) has its origins in the upper Amazon basin area of northern Brazil, eastern Venezuela, Colombia, and Ecuador. There is no indication that Forastero was cultivated until the Spaniards extended planting into South America. A partial explanation for the early preference of Criollo may be that a palatable drink could be obtained with little or no preliminary fermentation, while Forastero cocoa requires several days of fermentation. Trinitario ("of Trinidad") is a cross between Criollo and Forastero which probably occurred naturally when the Spaniards introduced Forastero to the area. Finally, Nacional (or Arriba) is scientifically a Forastero, but is classified separately due to its distinctive aromatic floral nature.[6] Today, widespread crossbreeding has made segregation of cacao varieties difficult. As a result, beans are often classified today by country of origin or even port of shipment.

B. Tree Morphology

The cacao tree, with its distinctive brown-gray bark, customarily attains a height of 15 to 25 ft at maturity (in about 10 years), although height will vary with shade and other conditions. The cacao tree is an evergreen, and while it sheds leaves throughout the year, it is never without its brilliant dark green foliage.

The cacao tree is a "cauliflorous" plant in that the flowers grow on the old wood of the trunk and main branches. Trees may produce 10,000 or more flowers in a year; however, only 10 to 50 eventually develop into ripe pods 4 to 6 months later. Two standard crops are harvested each year although fruits in various stages of development may be continually on the tree. Cacao trees begin to bear significant amounts of fruit when they are 4 to 8 years old, and continue to do so for 50 years or more.

The mature fruit consists of a pod usually 6 to10 in. long containing 20 to 40 seeds or beans covered by a white, mucilaginous pulp. The beans are dicotyledonous, oval-shaped, and about 1 to 1 1/2 in. long with colors varying from white to shades of purple.

C. Cultivation

T. cacao is cultivated at low altitudes within 1000 ft of sea level. Cacao grows exclusively between the latitudes 20°N and 20°S with 75% of the world's crop grown within 8° of the equator. Cacao requires a warm and humid climate and thrives best at shade temperatures of 65° to 95°F, although the tree has flourished under conditions of 105°F and almost 100% humidity found in areas of West Africa. Minimum rainfall requirements are an evenly distributed 40 in. per year with 60 to 80 in. desirable.

Cacao seedlings are usually planted 7 to 10 ft apart and require special attention against weeds and pests during the early stages of development. The cacao tree is usually grown under the shade provided by the foliage of larger trees so that soil does not dry out from the intense rays of the tropical sun. Leguminous shade trees often are used to retain the nitrogen value of the soil.

After the ripe pods are harvested, they are cut open and the beans and adhering pulp are removed for fermentation. It is during the process of fermentation that cacao acquires much of its characteristic flavor and aroma. Fermentation soon occurs due to the high sugar content of the pulp and the presence of microorganisms. The sugars are converted to alcohols and finally to acetic acid, which drains off. The acetic acid and heat formed

TABLE 1

Composition of Unfermented and Fermented Cacao Beans (Percent by Weight)

	Beans (17 varieties)		Unfermented Ghana Beans		Fermented Ghana beans		
	Original	Dry fat-free	Original	Dry fat-free	Original	Dry fat-free	Fermented Indian beans
Water	2.72	—	3.65	—	2.13	—	5.23
Fat	50.12	—	53.05	—	54.68	—	50.32
Ash							
total	3.32	7.04	2.63	6.07	2.74	6.34	3.12
Nitrogen							
Total nitrogen	2.38	5.05	2.28	5.27	2.16	5.00	—
Protein nitrogen	—	—	1.50	3.46	1.34	3.10	—
Theobromine	1.04	2.21	1.71	3.95	1.42	3.29	1.66
Caffeine	0.40	0.86	0.08	0.20	0.07	0.15	—
Carbohydrates							
Glucose	—	—	0.30	0.69	0.10	0.23	—
Sucrose	—	—	Nil	Nil	Nil	Nil	—
Starch	8.07	17.10	6.10	14.09	6.14	14.22	—
Pectins	—	—	2.25	5.20	4.11	9.52	—
Fiber	2.64	5.61	2.09	4.83	2.13	4.93	—
Cellulose	—	—	1.92	4.43	1.90	4.39	—
Pentosans	—	—	1.27	2.93	1.21	2.80	—
Mucilage/gums	—	—	0.38	0.88	1.84	4.26	—
Tannins							
Tannic acid	—	—	2.24	5.17	1.99	4.61	2.54
Cacao-purple and cacao-brown	—	—	5.30	12.26	4.16	9.63	—
Acids							
Acetic (free)	—	—	0.014	0.032	0.136	0.315	—
Oxalic	—	—	0.29	0.67	0.30	0.70	—
Reference	10		11		11		12

during fermentation penetrate the skin or shell of the bean where they cause the death of the bean and initiate the chemical changes necessary for flavor development.

With the death of the bean, cellular structure is lost, allowing the mixing of water-soluble components that normally would not come into contact with each other. The complex chemistry that occurs during fermentation is not fully understood, but certain cocoa enzymes such as glycosidase, protease, and polyphenol oxidase are active. In general, proteins are hydrolyzed to smaller proteins and amino acids, complex glycosides are split, polyphenols are partially transformed, sugars are hydrolyzed, volatile acids are formed, and purine alkaloids diffuse into the bean shell. The chemical composition of both unfermented and fermented cocoa beans is compared in Table 1.

TABLE 2

World Production of Raw Cocoa in Thousands of Metric Tons

	1970/71	1975/76	1980/81	1985/86	1990/91	1995/96[a]
Africa	*(73.2)*[b]	*(66.2)*	*(59.9)*	*(56.5)*	*(56.7)*	*(65.6)*
	1,098	1000	995	1,109	1,432	1,811
Cameroon	112	96	120	118	107	120
Ghana	392	397	258	219	293	390
Ivory Coast	180	231	403	585	819	1,125
Nigeria	308	216	156	110	170	150
America	*(21.2)*	*(27.1)*	*(31.8)*	*(30.2)*	*(24.5)*	*(15.9)*
	318	410	528	593	617	438
Brazil	182	258	349	376	377	219
Colombia	21	26	39	48	52	51
Ecuador	61	63	81	96	106	93
Mexico	25	33	30	39	43	35
Venezuela	19	15	14	10	16	16
West Indies	*(2.6)*	*(2.7)*	*(2.7)*	*(2.7)*	*(2.0)*	*(2.4)*
	39	41	45	53	50	65
Dominican Republic	25	30	32	40	42	55
Asia and Oceania	*(2.9)*	*(4.0)*	*(5.5)*	*(10.6)*	*(16.7)*	*(16.1)*
	44	60	92	209	422	446
Indonesia	2	3	8	35	145	290
Malaysia	4	17	43	125	224	105
New Guinea	29	32	28	32	33	34
World total	1,499	1,511	1,660	1,964	2,521	2,760
Reference	13	13	14	14	15	15

[a] Forecasted production.

[b] Percent of total world production.

During fermentation and subsequent drying, the unfermented wet beans lose about 65% of their weight. The reduction of moisture halts the enzymatic processes. Drying is complete when the moisture content reaches about 6% and the beans readily break into pieces called nibs.

D. World Production

In 1895, the worldwide production of raw cocoa or unroasted cocoa beans was about 75,000 metric tons. One hundred years later, raw cocoa production has increased almost 40-fold to the forecasted 1995–1996 production of 2,760,000 metric tons (Table 2).[15] The majority of today's world cocoa supply comes from Ghana, Nigeria, Ivory Coast, and the Republic of Cameroon even though cacao is not indigenous to east Africa. Although Africa historically has been and still is the largest producer of the world's cocoa supply, the relative quantities produced within African countries has shifted. While Ghana was the highest cocoa producer from 1946 to as recently as 1975, the Ivory Coast now leads production. It is also interesting to note that the production of cocoa in Asia and Oceania has been increasing steadily.

IV. METHYLXANTHINE COMPOSITION

A. Raw Materials and Semifinished Products

1. Bean

Although low levels of methylxanthines have been detected in the leaves and flowers of *T. cacao*, the primary storage location is within the seed or bean.[16] The cocoa bean is the major natural source of the methylxanthine theobromine, but contains only small amounts of caffeine. Theophylline has been detected in cacao beans, but at such low concentrations that its presence generally is ignored. Together, theobromine and caffeine account for up to 99% of the alkaloid content of *T. cacao* beans. Alkaloid content is affected by genetic makeup, maturity of beans at harvest, and fermentation process. Analytical methodology also is partially responsible for some of the disparity in methylxanthine values since many early methods were unable to separate theobromine and caffeine.

In live cocoa seeds, the methylxanthines are localized in polyphenolic storage cells. Bean death, which occurs 24 to 48 h after initiation of fermentation, triggers diffusion of the methylxanthines from the nib to the shell. The early studies of Humphries state that cacao cotyledons lose about 40% of their theobromine during fermentation.[17] According to Knapp and Wadsworth, the loss of theobromine and caffeine becomes significant on the third day when the methylxanthines begin to diffuse into the shell.[18] This migration continues until the concentration of the methylxanthines in nibs and shell are almost equal.

Timbie followed the changes in theobromine concentration in whole beans, nibs, and shells during growth and fermentation.[19,20] Theobromine synthesis was especially active at the end stage of pod growth and the early stages of ripening. During the 7-d fermentation period, theobromine concentration in the whole bean did not change appreciably. However, theobromine in the nibs gradually decreased by about 27% from approximately 31 to 22 mg/g. Shell theobromine content increased 75% from about 12 mg/g to about 21 mg/g. Obviously, the same migration of theobromine from nib to shell occurred as reported in earlier studies. In contrast, Sotelo and Alvarez reported no significant difference in theobromine and caffeine content between unfermented and fermented cacao beans.[9]

TABLE 3

Concentration of Theobromine, Caffeine, and Theophylline in *Theobroma* Beans (mg/g)

Species/ variety	Sample description	Theo-bromine	Caffeine	Theo-phylline	Theo-bromine/ caffeine ratio	Ref.
T. cacao						
Criollo	Defatted	12.4	11.3	—	1.10:1	20
	Dried, fermented	14.7	9.2	3.7	1.6:1	9
Trinitario	Defatted	33.2	6.3	—	5.27:1	20
Nacional	Defatted	35.4	2.4	—	14.8:1	20
Forastero	Defatted	36.2	1.3	—	27.8:1	20
Costarrica	Dried, fermented	20.2	1.8	3.6	11.2:1	9
T. cacao	Dried fermented	16.6	—	—	—	12
T. cacao	Fresh mass	11.1	1.1	—	10.1:1	8
T. speciosum	Fresh mass	0.1	—	—	—	8
T. mariae	Fresh mass	23.5	1.2	—	19.6:1	8
T. bicolor	Dried, fermented	1.1	0.1	0.2	11.0:1	9
T. angustifolium	Dried, fermented	0.3	0.03	0.08	10.0:1	9

The methylxanthine content of beans is influenced by the species, varietal type, and hybrid.[8,12,19-21] Table 3 lists the methylxanthine content of several *Theobroma* species and varieties. In analyses of 10 hybrids from four varieties of *T. cacao*, total alkaloids in dry, fat-free beans varied from a low of 23.7 mg/g to a high of 49.7 mg/g.[19] The average for the 10 hybrids was 37.0 mg/g. The contribution of theobromine to total alkaloid content ranged from a low of 52.3% in a Criollo clone to 99.1% in a Amazon Forastero bean, with a mean for the 10 samples of 87.0%. Although the Criollo bean had the lowest concentration of total alkaloid, its caffeine content was the highest. Trinitario beans also had relatively high caffeine levels. Methylxanthine content can also vary within clones of the same varietal type. The combined theobromine/caffeine content of four Trinitario clones ranged from 29.8 to 49.7 mg/g of defatted shell-free bean.

Asamoa and Wurziger tabulated the caffeine content of a variety of cocoa beans.[22] The mean concentration (percentage in fat-free samples) in Amelonado and Amazonas beans, respectively, after 5 d of fermentation at various stages of maturity were: green beans 0.06, 0.19; yellow 0.09, 0.18; orange 0.08, 0.23; and black 0.10, 0.22. These results confirmed significant differences between the two varieties and also the low caffeine content of Forastero-type beans. The caffeine content of 16 other samples of various origins ranged between 0.07 and 1.70%, suggesting the following classification: African cocoa and Brazilian "Bahia" as Amelonados; Para, Arriba, and Jamaica cocoa (caffeine, 0.42%) as Amazonas; Samoa and Maracaibo cocoa (1.42 and 1.70%) as pure Criollos flavor cocoa; and Guinea (0.53%), Caracas (0.60 to 0.63%), and Puerto Cabello (0.78%) as Criollo-Forastero hybrids. In a compilation of literature data, Hadorn reported a mean total alkaloid (theobromine and caffeine) content of 3.11 ± 0.69% for 44 samples of cocoa beans of known variety and origin.[23]

After fermentation, cacao beans are dried and then transported to the factory for roasting. The ultimate purpose of roasting is to develop desirable bean flavor and aroma, as well as the necessary texture for later grinding. As shown in Table 4, the methylxanthine content of cacao beans was not found to change significantly during the roasting process.[5, 24-26]

2. Liquor

Chocolate liquor is the solid or semiplastic food prepared by finely grinding the nib of the cacao bean. It is commonly called baking chocolate, unsweetened chocolate, or bitter chocolate and, in Europe, is frequently referred to as chocolate mass or cocoa paste. Chocolate liquor is essentially the starting point from which all chocolate products are produced. Table 5 lists the theobromine and caffeine content of 22 various chocolate liquor samples determined by high pressure liquid chromatography (HPLC). The liquors averaged 1.22% theobromine and 0.214% caffeine.[27, 28] The ratio of theobromine to caffeine ranged from 2.5:1 to 23.0:1.

3. Cocoa Powder

Cocoa powder, or simply cocoa, is prepared by pulverizing the material remaining after a portion of the fat (cocoa butter) is removed from the liquor. Cocoa powder is the basic flavoring ingredient in many chocolate foods, including cookies, cakes, and ice cream. Theobromine and caffeine are components of the cocoa solids or nonlipid portion of the chocolate liquor; therefore, cocoa has a higher concentration of theobromine and caffeine than liquor. Cocoa can be prepared from a single liquor type or from blends of various liquors, thus, influencing the theobromine and caffeine levels.

According to Schutz, it is well known that cocoa contains about 2.5% by weight of theobromine and caffeine.[29] Although the presence of theophylline has been demonstrated, its concentration is so low that it is generally ignored. In a summary of the literature values for 27 commercial cocoa powders and cocoa masses, Hadorn found that the mean total alkaloid content was 3.36 ± 0.48%.[23] Theobromine and caffeine content of several cocoa powders is shown in Table 6. HPLC analyses by DeVries et

TABLE 4

Changes in Cacao Nib Composition Due to Roasting (Percent by Weight)

	Beans, not specified		Accra		Grenada		St. Thomes		Trinidad	
	Raw	Medium roast	Raw	Roast	Raw	Roast	Raw	Low Roast	Raw	Low Roast
Moisture	5.13	3.71	4.90	3.20	4.80	2.90	4.70	3.46	5.58	3.89
Fat	54.22	53.63	53.90	55.10	53.40	54.40	53.76	53.26	50.64	50.64
Ash	1.46	1.51	2.24	2.50	2.03	2.23	2.52	2.64	2.60	2.86
Starch	7.31	7.70	—	—	—	—	8.89	8.94	9.55	9.29
Protein	11.99	12.01	12.88	13.00	12.16	12.13	11.18	11.43	11.62	11.00
Theobromine	1.09	1.06	1.36	1.33	1.07	0.75	0.89	0.99	0.74	0.64
Caffeine	0.44	0.43	—	—	—	—	0.08	0.22	0.38	0.34
Reference	24	24	25	25	25	25	26	26	26	26

TABLE 5

Theobromine and Caffeine Levels in Chocolate Liquor

Liquor origin	Theo-bromine (%)	Caffeine (%)	Theo-bromine: caffeine ratio	Ref.
Liberia	1.26	0.075	16.8:1	28
San Thome	1.19	0.062	19.2:1	28
Ghana sample #1	1.73	0.159	10.9:1	27
Ghana sample #2	1.23	0.137	9.0:1	27
Fernando Po	1.47	0.064	23.0:1	27
Guatemala	1.25	0.205	6.1:1	28
Haiti	1.26	0.105	16.8:1	28
Costa Rica	1.14	0.385	2.7:1	28
Venezuela	1.23	0.416	3.0:1	28
Belize	0.97	0.258	3.8:1	28
Brazil sample #1	1.25	0.206	6.0:1	28
Brazil sample #2	1.21	0.183	6.6:1	27
Ecuador sample #1	1.07	0.234	4.6:1	28
Ecuador sample #2	1.33	0.289	4.6:1	28
Tobago	1.41	0.113	12.5:1	27
Trinidad	1.24	0.233	5.3:1	27
Dominican Republic sample #1	1.57	0.177	8.9:1	27
Dominican Republic sample #2	1.25	0.261	4.8:1	27
New Guinea sample #1	0.82	0.329	2.5:1	27
New Guinea sample #2	0.93	0.330	2.8:1	27
Malaysia sample #1	1.05	0.252	4.2:1	27
Malaysia sample #2	1.01	0.228	4.4:1	27
Mean ± SD	1.22 ± 0.21	0.214 ± 0.099	7.9:1	

TABLE 6

Theobromine and Caffeine Concentration in Cocoa Powder

Description	N	Theo-bromine(%)	Caffeine (%)	Total alkaloid (%)	Theo-bromine: caffeine ratio	Ref.
Natural cocoa	8	2.56 ± 0.19	0.26 ± 0.08	2.82 ± 0.16	11.8:1	30
Red dutched cocoa	10	2.69 ± 0.11	0.16 ± 0.07	2.86 ± 0.08	19.6:1	30
Commercial cocoa	8	1.89 ± 0.46	0.21 ± 0.59	2.10 ± 0.50	10.9:1	28
	1	2.03	0.31	2.34	6.5:1	31
	—	3.3				32
	5	2.60	0.25	2.85	10.4:1	33
Cocoa, dutched	—	2.5				32

al. resulted in a total methylxanthine content (theobromine plus caffeine) on a moisture-free basis of 2.82 ± 0.16% for natural cocoa and 2.85 ± 0.08% for red dutched or alkalized cocoa.[30] Zoumas et al. reported 1.89% theobromine and 0.21% caffeine in eight commercial brands of cocoa powder.[28] Results were not calculated on a moisture-free basis as were the data in the DeVries study, partially explaining the lower values reported by Zoumas et al.

4. Cocoa Butter

Cocoa butter is the fat obtained from subjecting chocolate liquor to pressure. Since the alkaloids are sparingly soluble in fat, only trace amounts of theobromine and caffeine in cocoa butter have been reported. The theobromine and caffeine content of four cocoa butter samples averaged 0.008% and 0.038%, respectively.[33]

B. Finished Products

The combination of ground cocoa beans and sugar produces a very hard substance with an unpleasant mouthfeel. However, the addition of extra cocoa butter results in a product that melts easily in the mouth. Additionally, the production of cocoa butter results in a lower fat cocoa powder which can be used more readily in both beverages and foods. As the amounts of cocoa butter and other fats, milk solids, sugar, and other ingredients increase, the amount of theobromine and caffeine in the final product decreases.

1. *Beverages*

The methylxanthine content of beverages has been reported in numerous studies. Most hot cocoa beverages are prepared from ready-to-use mixes that include both sugar and dry milk in addition to the cocoa, so that only the addition of hot water is required. Label directions can vary considerably, resulting in a wide range of reported methylxanthine values for hot cocoa and chocolate milk-based beverages.[27,28,32,34-37] Lack of documentation regarding preparation and source, incorrect references to early literature, differences in analytical methodology, and use of different reference volumes (e.g., "cup" size) all contribute to the variation in reported methylxanthine contents. Some studies failed to report the cup size and, when it was reported, it ranged from 87 to 250 ml.[34]

Two chocolate beverages made from unsweetened cocoa contained 228 and 284 mg theobromine per serving.[32] Burg reported 272 mg theobromine and 6 mg caffeine per cup of beverage made from African cocoa, and 232 mg theobromine and 42 mg caffeine for a similar beverage made with South American cocoa.[34] Both beverages were prepared according to manufacturer's directions.

Bunker and McWilliams found that two beverages prepared from instant cocoa (with Dutch process cocoa) contained 10 to 17 mg caffeine per cup.[37] Table 7 lists the theobromine and caffeine concentration of hot cocoa and chocolate milk prepared from instant mixes. Zoumas et al. analyzed five commercial hot cocoa mixes and reported an average of 65 mg per serving of theobromine and 4 mg per serving of caffeine.[28] Similar results were reported by Blauch and Tarka.[36]

Chocolate milk samples prepared from sweetened cocoa powders averaged 58 mg per serving of theobromine and 5 mg per serving of caffeine.[28] Analysis of a "home-style" recipe resulted in higher methylxanthine values — 94 mg theobromine and 10 mg caffeine per serving. However, the authors noted that this recipe also had a stronger chocolate flavor. The lower values reported by Zoumas et al. and Blauch and Tarka compared to others was attributed to the inability of older methods to separate theobromine and caffeine, and the lack of precision and accuracy of the older methods. A compendium of theobromine and caffeine values reported for chocolate beverages from both published and unpublished studies has been compiled in Table 8.

2. *Foods*

It is necessary to determine the methylxanthine content of chocolate foods, as well as beverages, in order to obtain an accurate assessment of the total amount of theobromine and caffeine that is ingested via the diet. This area of analysis has received little attention, and only scant published data exist on the methylxanthine content of chocolate foods.

TABLE 7

Theobromine and Caffeine Concentration in Hot Cocoa and Chocolate Milk Prepared From Instant Mixes

	Theobromine (mg/serving)	Caffeine (mg/serving)	Ref.
Hot cocoa (brand)[a]			
A	65	2	
B	71	2	
C	60	5	
D	77	2	
E	54	7	
Mean ± SD	65 ± 9	4 ± 2	28
Hot cocoa (brand)[b]			
A	48	4	
B	40	1	
C	54	2	
D	68	6	
E	73	6	
F	78	3	
G	80	3	
H	64	8	
I	56	6	
Mean ± SD	62 ± 14	4 ± 2	36
Home recipe[c]	94	10	28
Chocolate milk[a]			
A	99	7	
B	36	6	
C	64	5	
D	35	2	
Mean ± SD	58 ± 30	5 ± 2	28

[a] Amount per 5-oz hot cocoa or 8-oz chocolate milk prepared as directed from mixes.

[b] Serving equivalent to one individual packet of instant mix.

[c] Beverage was prepared from a home recipe using cocoa powder instead of instant mix.

Most chocolate is consumed in the form of chocolate confectionery. Sweet chocolate is produced from chocolate liquor with the addition of sugar and cocoa butter. Sometimes called dark chocolate, sweet chocolate must contain at least 15% chocolate liquor, but may contain as much as 50%. Semisweet or bittersweet chocolate consists of a minimum of 35% chocolate liquor. The chocolate liquor content results in sweet and semisweet chocolate containing the highest amount of theobromine and caffeine per serving of any type of chocolate confectionery (Table 9). Within brands of sweet chocolate, there is wide variation in the methylxanthine

TABLE 8

Theobromine and Caffeine Concentration in Chocolate Beverages

Beverage	Theo-bromine (%)	Caffeine (%)	Ref.
Chocolate milk			
Instant mix	0.024	0.002	28
Prepared	0.012	0.002	38
commercially	0.016	0.001	33
Hot Cocoa			
Instant mix	0.043	0.003	28
Instant mix	0.042	0.003	36
Malted preparation	0.052	0.002	36
Chocolate beverage	0.026	0.001	39
Chocolate drink	0.044	0.003	39
Chocolate drink	0.021	0.002	38
Chocolate diet soda	0.003	0.017	38
Diet creme soda	0.003	0.001	38
Chocolate milk shake (commercial)	0.015	0.003	38

content due to the amount of chocolate liquor and other factors previously discussed. Analysis of eight brands of commercial sweet chocolate showed a range in methylxanthine content from 0.359 to 0.628% for theobromine and from 0.017 to 0.125% for caffeine.[28] Based on analytical data, an average 40-g sweet chocolate bar contains about 185 mg theobromine and 30 mg caffeine.

Consumption of sweet chocolate in the U.S. is low. The majority of chocolate consumed is milk chocolate produced from chocolate liquor, sugar, cocoa butter, and milk solids. Because most milk chocolate produced in the U.S. contains 10 to 12% chocolate liquor, differences in methylxanthine content among commercial milk chocolate are due more to the varieties and blends of cocoa bean (Table 9). Based on analytical data from seven brands of commercial milk chocolate, a typical 40-g milk chocolate bar contains approximately 65 mg theobromine and less than 10 mg caffeine.[28] Milk chocolate bars containing other ingredients, such as peanuts, almonds, and confectionery fillings, obviously contain less methylxanthines. In a survey of 49 marketed chocolate and confectionery products, theobromine concentrations ranged from 0.001 to 2.598% and caffeine content from 0.001 to 0.247%.[33]

The theobromine content of chocolate foods prepared from home recipes using common chocolate sources — cocoa, semisweet baking choco-

TABLE 9

Theobromine and Caffeine Concentration in Commercial Chocolate Confectionery Products

	N	Theo-bromine (%)	Caffeine (%)	Ref.
Unsweetened baking chocolate	2	1.30	0.155	31
	4	1.31	0.098	35
	5	1.39	0.164	33
Sweet/dark chocolate	8	0.463	0.069	28
	4	0.460	0.050	35
	2	0.441	0.054	31
	1	0.320	0.044	40
	1	0.417	—[a]	41
	5	0.474	0.076	33
Semisweet chocolate chips	3	0.565	0.062	31
	5	0.487	0.077	33
Milk chocolate	7	0.160	0.025	28
	4	0.190	0.017	35
	6	0.188	0.019	31
	2	0.140	0.025	40
	2	0.132	—[a]	41
	5	0.197	0.022	33
Milk chocolate w/almonds	5	0.161	0.016	33
Milk chocolate w/rice	5	0.150	0.018	33
Milk chocolate chips	2	0.150	0.026	33
White chocolate	2	0.005	0.006	40

[a] Not measured.

late, and syrup — can be calculated on a per-serving basis by using the average methylxanthine concentrations of the various chocolate sources. Derived estimates for some typical home recipes are shown in Table 10.[42]

Chemical analysis of the finished food product is a more accurate determination of the methylxanthine content. In studies performed at Hershey Foods Corporation, the methylxanthine content of a large variety of commercially available chocolate foods was measured by HPLC methods.[38] These results have been compiled together with other literature values in Table 11. Large methylxanthine variations can be seen among the chocolate foods, as well as within different brands of the same item.

Due to the wide range of values in the scientific literature for the caffeine content of foods, Barone and Roberts suggested the following

TABLE 10

Calculated Methylxanthine Content Per Serving of Chocolate Foods Prepared from Home Recipes

Food	Source of chocolate for recipe	No. of servings	Serving size (g)	Theobromine (mg/serving)	Caffeine (mg/serving)
Chocolate cake	Cocoa	12	80	58	6
Chocolate cake with frosting	Cocoa	12	61	58	6
	Cocoa	12	73	69	7
Dark chocolate	Cocoa	20	60	78	8
cake with frosting	Cocoa	20	93	130	13
Chocolate cupcakes	Cocoa	18	40	39	4
Chocolate frosting	Semisweet chips	12	35	69	11
Chocolate cheesecake	Cocoa	9	123	77	7
Chocolate chip cookies	Semisweet chips	60	20	28	4
Chocolate cookies	Cocoa	48	15	14	1
Chocolate chocolate chip cookies	Cocoa Semisweet chips	60	22	39	6
Chocolate pudding	Cocoa	4	145	98	9
Chocolate mousse	Semisweet chips	9	90	92	15
Chocolate cream pie	Semisweet chips	8	186	207	33
Chocolate brownies	Cocoa Semisweet chips	24	42	78	10
Chocolate brownies	Cocoa Syrup	36	30	42	4
Chocolate brownies	Cocoa	36	30	43	4
Fudge	Semisweet chips	18	25	69	11

From Hershey Foods Corporation Technical Center, Nutrition Group, Unpublished data, 1996. With permission.

TABLE 11

Theobromine and Caffeine Concentration in Chocolate Foods

Food[a]	N	Theo-bromine (%)	Caffeine (%)	Total alkaloids (%)	Ref.
Chocolate brownie[b]	2	0.046	0.013	0.059	38
	6	0.142	0.014	0.156	31
Chocolate cake[b]	6	0.086	0.007	0.092	38
	1	0.137	0.016	0.153	43
	8	0.162	0.016	0.178	31
Chocolate cupcakes	6	0.116	0.026	0.141	38
	3	0.150	0.018	0.168	31
Chocolate frosting	4	0.131	0.020	0.152	38
Chocolate cookies	4	0.106	0.014	0.120	38
Chocolate chip cookies	2	0.070	0.014	0.085	38
Chocolate-covered doughnut	1	0.106	0.015	0.121	38
Chocolate pies	2	0.056	0.016	0.072	38
Chocolate puddings (canned)	4	0.131	0.019	0.150	38
	2	0.062	0.005	0.067	31
Chocolate ice cream	3	0.051	0.005	0.056	38
	3	0.062	0.003	0.065	31
Chocolate fudge ice cream bar	1	0.032	0.002	0.034	38
Chocolate-covered ice cream bar	1	0.034	0.005	0.039	38
Chocolate syrups/toppings	3	0.123	0.010	0.133	38
	—	0.240	0.014	0.254	44
	6	0.195	0.014	0.209	31
	5	0.240	0.019	0.259	33
Chocolate fudge	1	0.655	0.065	0.720	31
Chocolate cereal	4	0.079	0.012	0.091	38
	3	0.070	0.007	0.077	31
Chocolate breakfast bar	1	0.136	0.012	0.148	31

[a] All items were purchased at commercial retail stores or were prepared from commercial mixes were indicated.
[b] Prepared from commercial mix.

standard values for the U.S.: cocoa/hot chocolate, 4 mg/5 oz; chocolate milk, 4 mg/6 oz; and chocolate candy, 1.5 to 6.0 mg/oz.[45] In order to gain a better insight into the amount of methylxanthines consumed via the diet, more studies on the methylxanthine content of chocolate foods, as well as beverages, are needed.

V. CONSUMPTION OF COCOA AND CHOCOLATE PRODUCTS

A. Cocoa Consumption

It is difficult to compare consumption of cocoa and chocolate products among countries. Not all countries collect data, methods to measure consumption differ, and definitions of food products may vary. Regardless of these differences, we know that the consumption of cocoa increased steadily after 1828 when the technology became available to extract fat from cocoa beans and, again, after 1876 when the production of milk chocolate began. Today, cocoa consumption parallels cocoa supply for the most part. In fact, cocoa consumption is often estimated from raw cocoa production data that has been adjusted for imports and exports. Other factors, including cocoa and sugar prices, general economic conditions, and demographics also influence consumption throughout the world.

The peak of cocoa consumption occurred during the early to mid-1960s, a time period in which the crucial consumption-determining factors were favorable. During the mid- to late 1970s, cocoa consumption leveled off, and even declined in some countries.[46] The major contributing factor to the poor consumption of cocoa during the late 1970s was the high price of cocoa beans and resulting products. During this period, the prices were the highest ever achieved in the industry.

The consumption of cocoa in the major consuming countries for the last 25 years is summarized in Table 12. From this data, it can be seen that the U.S. has been the leading consumer for many years. In 1995–1996, the largest consumption (in thousands of metric tons) occurred in the U.S. (560), followed by Germany (245), the Russian Federation (187), and the U.K. (184).

Per capita consumption of cocoa also is shown in Table 12. Switzerland repeatedly had the highest per capita intake, with average intakes ranging from 3.4 to 5.1 kg per capita. Per capita consumption in Austria, Belgium, and Germany were also high with similar intakes. Consumption in the U.S. was lower than in these European countries, ranging from 1.4 kg in 1980–1981 to 2.2 kg in 1990–1991.

TABLE 12

Cocoa Consumption in Major Cocoa-Consuming Countries[a]

	1969/70	1975/76	1980/81	1985/86	1990/91	1995/96[b]
Australia	19.8 *(1.6)*	18.1 *(1.3)*	23.0 *(1.6)*	27.7 *(1.8)*	32.5 *(1.9)*	33.2 *(1.8)*
Austria	11.8 *(1.6)*	17.4 *(2.3)*	22.6 *(3.0)*	24.2 *(3.2)*	27.8 *(3.6)*	25.0 *(3.1)*
Belgium	24.3 *(2.5)*	30.0 *(3.1)*	30.0 *(2.9)*	31.4 *(3.1)*	47.2 *(4.6)*	52.2 *(5.0)*
Canada	36.7 *(1.7)*	32.5 *(1.5)*	34.4 *(1.4)*	45.3 *(1.8)*	51.0 *(1.7)*	60.0 *(2.2)*
France	76.7 *(1.5)*	93.9 *(1.8)*	103.8 *(1.9)*	106.3 *(1.9)*	146.2 *(2.6)*	156.5 *(2.7)*
Germany	156.2 *(2.6)*	158.5 *(2.6)*	157.8 *(2.6)*	177.8 *(2.9)*	231.4 *(3.7)*	244.7 *(3.0)*
Japan	47.3 *(0.5)*	63.1 *(0.6)*	53.9 *(0.5)*	75.5 *(0.6)*	109.5 *(0.9)*	112.7 *(0.9)*
Netherlands	36.7 *(2.8)*	36.3 *(2.7)*	31.7 *(2.2)*	17.6 *(1.2)*	23.0 *(1.5)*	18.9 *(1.2)*
U.K.	114.4 *(2.1)*	101.9 *(1.8)*	92.0 *(1.6)*	128.9 *(2.3)*	161.8 *(2.8)*	184.0 *(3.1)*
Italy	33.2 *(0.6)*	32.4 *(0.6)*	42.3 *(0.6)*	64.0 *(1.1)*	65.0 *(1.1)*	85.4 *(1.5)*
Switzerland	22.3 *(3.6)*	21.6 *(3.4)*	24.2 *(3.8)*	25.9 *(4.0)*	34.2 *(5.1)*	24.6 *(3.5)*
U.S.	346.6 *(1.8)*	215.6 *(1.5)*	316.6 *(1.4)*	452.0 *(1.9)*	540.0 *(2.2)*	560.1 *(2.1)*
USSR/Russian Federation	111.0 *(0.5)*	167.3 *(0.7)*	135.1 *(0.5)*	216.3 *(0.8)*	134.2 *(0.5)*	187.3 *(1.1)*
Ref.	14	14	47	48	49	49

[a] Consumption represents cocoa bean grindings adjusted by net imports or exports of cocoa products and chocolate converted into bean equivalents in thousands of metric tons (*per capita, kg*).

[b] Forecasted consumption.

B. Chocolate Confectionery

Chocolate has been identified in several studies as the single most craved food. It has been suggested that chocolate cravings may have a biological basis or simply eaten for the sensory gratification. In a study of 75 individuals who identified themselves as "chocoholics", subjects consumed an average of 12.5 (range 1 to 70) chocolate bars per week where a bar was defined as a standard block of 60 g.[50] Although the majority of subjects preferred solid chocolate (42%) and chocolate bars (38%), chocolate was also eaten in a variety of other forms including cakes, biscuits, desserts, ice cream, and beverages.

Nuttall estimated that 15 to 20% of chocolate is eaten on its own, i.e., in candy form.[51] The remainder is used to coat other foods including ice cream or confectionery products. According to the same source, nearly all people in highly industrialized countries have eaten confectionery at some time, and over 90% of the population may buy it on a regular basis. The author viewed confectionery as one of the first "convenience" foods, leading to the popularity of chocolate as a snack food.

On the basis of United States Department of Commerce Shipment data, Americans consumed about 5 kg per person of chocolate confectionery products in 1993.[52] Of this quantity, enrobed and molded chocolate products comprised 53%, solid chocolate products with or without inclusions were 22%, and panned or assorted chocolate products made up the remaining 23%. Per capita consumption of chocolate confectionery products in 1993 increased 4.3% over the previous year and 0.7 kg per person since 1983.

Data based on 3-d intakes of commonly used foods and food groups by individuals have been reported by the United States Department of Agriculture (USDA). The USDA conducted three Continuing Surveys of Food Intakes by Individuals (CSFII) during 1989–1990, 1990–1991, and 1991–1992. Food and beverage intake of all individuals residing in a survey household was measured over a 3-d period by using a 24-h recall followed by a 2-d dietary record. Based on combined data from the three CSFII surveys, 12% of the population consumed chocolate confectionery at least once in three days.[53] Less than 1% consumed chocolate candy on all three survey days, and the average intake of users was 50.5 g on days when consumed. Analysis of the dietary data also showed that chocolate consumption patterns in the U.S. varied with geographic region, season, ethnic group, time of day, gender, and age.

C. Other Foods

Consumption of various categories of chocolate foods was also calculated, using CSFII data, and summarized in Table 13.[53] Approximately

TABLE 13

Consumption Data for Selected Chocolate Beverages and Foods from the USDA Continuing Surveys of Food Intakes by Individuals, 1989-1992[a]

Food source	Total individuals using food (%)		Average quantity consumed per day (g)		Average quantity consumed per eating occasion(g)	
	All Ages	5-6 Yr	All Ages	5-6 Yr	All Ages	5-6 Yr
Chocolate candy	12.2	9.7	50	30	45	27
Chocolate milk	4.7	11.2	322	268	295	247
Chocolate cookies/ brownies[b]	9.6	15.4	53	41	47	36
Chocolate chip cookies	9.6	21.5	36	31	31	26
Chocolate cakes and cupcakes	6.8	9.4	87	93	80	92

[a] USDA data analyzed using *TAS International Diet Research Systems*.[42] Data represent users who consumed the food at least once in 3 days; number of individuals with complete 3-day records was 11,912.

[b] Includes chocolate cookies other than chocolate chip cookies.

11% of children aged 5 to 6 years consumed chocolate milk at least once in three days compared to 5% of the total population. Chocolate chip cookies were consumed by 20% of children aged 5 to 6 years. The primary dietary source of chocolate (on a gram per day basis) was chocolate milk.

D. Methylxanthine Consumption From Chocolate Products

Significant scientific attention has focused on caffeine and its health effects. However, limited data are available for the actual dietary consumption of caffeine or theobromine from individual foods. Even less data exist on the contribution of cocoa and chocolate foods to methylxanthine intake.

In 1977, the National Academy of Sciences assessed dietary caffeine intakes by Americans. Based on this data, Graham estimated that 82% of people over 18 years consumed caffeine on a daily basis.[54] Dietary caffeine was consumed almost entirely in beverages, with coffee as the major source among adults, and tea and coffee the primary contributor for children aged 1 to 17 years.

Caffeine intake of children has been investigated in several studies (Table 14). Morgan et al. quantitated the amount and dietary sources of

TABLE 14

Average Caffeine Consumption Per Day and Per Body Weight

Reference/Subjects	Source of Data	Caffeine mg/d	Caffeine mg/kg/d
Morgan et al.[55]			
All ages	7-d food diaries	37.4	0.9
9-10 yr olds		24.7	0.8
Arbeit et al.[56]			
All 10-yr olds	24-h dietary recall	61.4	1.7
White 10-yr old boys		57.5	2.8
White 10-yr old girls		62.1	2.7
Black 10-yr old boys		22.0	0.6
Black 10-yr old girls		21.8	0.9
Ellison et al.[57]			
All children (7-10 yr)	3-day food diaries	16.0	0.5
Boys (7-10 yr)		14.4	0.4
Girls (7-10 yr)		16.0	0.5
Barone & Roberts[45]			
All ages	14-d menu census	—[a]	1.9
6-11 yr olds		—[a]	0.7

[a] Not reported.

caffeine and saccharin intake from a nationwide, 7-d food consumption survey.[55] Among individuals 5 to 18 years of age, approximately 98% of those sampled consumed caffeine at least once during the survey week. The 7-d average intake of caffeine was 37 mg; however, there was considerable variation in caffeine intake and some individuals consumed as much as 250 mg/d. On days when dietary caffeine was consumed, the average intake for all ages was 48 mg. The intake level of caffeine increased with increasing age. When data were expressed on the basis of milligram per kilogram body weight, caffeine intake was 0.9 mg/kg and generally was constant across age groups. However, children aged 5 to 6 years had significantly higher intakes (1.1 mg/kg/d) than children aged 7 to 8 years (0.9 mg/kg/d). By comparing the 7-d caffeine averages from different dietary sources, it was found that the major source of caffeine for these children was tea, followed by carbonated beverages (Table 15). Chocolate candy and other chocolate foods contributed an average of 6.4 mg or 17% of the total caffeine intake. Similar consumption patterns were reported by Burg who also identified tea, followed by soft drinks, as the major source of dietary caffeine in children and teenagers.[34]

Sources of caffeine intake also were assessed in a biracial sample of 1284 children aged 6 months to 17 years during 1973 to 1982 of the Bogalusa Heart Study.[56] Overall, mean intakes of caffeine were higher

TABLE 15

Average Daily Consumption of Caffeine in Children by Food and Beverage Source

	Morgan et al.[55]		Ellison et al.[57]	
	7-d average (mg)	Contribution (%)	3-d average (mg)	Contribution (%)
Carbonated beverages	9.8 ± 12.6	26.4	8.9 ± 11.7	54.5
Tea	12.8 ± 25.8	34.2	1.3 ± 5.8	7.6
Coffee	8.3 ± 54.5	22.1	0	0
Chocolate foods/beverages	6.4 ± 9.8	17.3	6.2 ± 5.5	37.9

than those reported by Morgan et al. and almost double when compared on a body weight basis. The average caffeine intake in the Bogalusa study for 10- to 17-year-olds was 1.5 mg/d. On a body weight basis, 2- and 3-year-old children consumed the largest amounts of caffeine (2.5 to 7.8 mg/kg/d), about two to four times the caffeine consumed by adolescents (0.6 to 2.8 mg/kg/d). From ages 2 to 15 years, the most popular sources of caffeine were chocolate-containing foods, consumed by 57 to 77% of children surveyed. However, the major source of caffeine in the diet was carbonated beverages. Among 10-year-olds, about 32% consumed chocolate milk beverages, puddings, or ice creams. Arbeit also noted racial differences in consumption patterns in that white children consistently consumed more caffeine than blacks. Caffeine intakes among 2-year-olds were 35 to 37 mg/d in black children and 63 to 95 mg/d in white children. Among 13-year-olds, caffeine intake was 26 to 39 mg and 121 to 138 mg in black and white children, respectively.

Ellison et al. examined caffeine intake among young children in the Framingham Children's Study.[57] Foods containing caffeine were classified into six categories: soft drinks, tea, baked goods, dairy beverages, candy, and dairy desserts. Analysis of 3-d food diaries indicated an average caffeine intake of 16 mg/d. Children 10 years of age consumed an average of 24.8 mg/d. Boys consumed slightly more caffeine than girls (17.1 and 14.4 mg/d, respectively). As in previously reported studies, caffeine intake tended to increase with age. Approximately 38% of the caffeine intake (6.2 mg/d) was obtained from chocolate foods and beverages, 17% from baked products, 11% from dairy beverages, 5% from candy, and 5% from dairy desserts. Ellison's results were more similar to those of Morgan et al. than those from the Bogalusa study. In particular, the authors noted that the subjects reported limited tea and no coffee consumption. This observation suggests that there may be regional patterns of use of caffeine-containing foods.

Results of the 1989 Marketing Research Corporation of America survey suggested that the mean daily caffeine intake in the U.S. for all ages and all sources was 1.9 mg/kg, and 0.7 mg/kg for children aged 6 to 11 years.[45] The 14-d average caffeine intake from chocolate-containing foods was 0.06 mg/kg for all ages and 0.12 mg/kg for children 6 to 11 years. The authors also estimated caffeine intakes based on the "standard" caffeine content of products and dietary consumption data from the 1987–1988 USDA Nationwide Food Consumption Survey (NFCS). The estimated average caffeine intake using NFCS data was 3.7 mg/kg from coffee, 1.0 mg/kg from tea, 0.6 mg/kg from soft drinks, and 2.8 mg/kg from coffee, tea, and soft drinks combined. Contribution of caffeine from chocolate foods was not included.

In the U.K., only 12% of the population reported regular consumption of chocolate beverages. These chocolate beverages provided 1 mg or less of caffeine per day, or less than 0.4% of the daily caffeine intake from all beverage sources.[39] Caffeine intake from chocolate foods was not calculated in Scott's study.

VI. SUMMARY

This chapter has compiled and evaluated information on the methylxanthine composition of cocoa and various chocolate foods and beverages, as well as the consumption pattern for these commodities. Cacao is the major natural source of the xanthine base theobromine. Small amounts of caffeine are present in the bean along with trace amounts of theophylline. Numerous factors, including varietal type and fermentation process, influence the methylxanthine content of beans.

Chocolate liquor is a semifinished product commonly called "baking" or unsweetened chocolate. The average theobromine and caffeine content of liquors has been reported at 1.2% and 0.21%, respectively. Cocoa powder, which is prepared after partial removal of the cocoa butter, contains about 1.9 to 2.7% theobromine and 0. 16 to 0.26% caffeine. Milk chocolate averages 0.168% theobromine and 0.022% caffeine, thus providing about 65 mg of theobromine and less than 10 mg of caffeine in a 40-g serving. The methylxanthine content of chocolate foods has received only slight attention in the literature, yet is necessary in order to obtain an accurate assessment of the total amount of theobromine and caffeine that is ingested via the diet.

Foods derived from cocoa beans have been consumed by humans since at least 460 to 480 AD, presumably with no major health effects. Most chocolate is consumed in the form of chocolate confectionery. On the basis of USDA dietary survey data, 12% of the population consumed chocolate confectionery at least once in three days with an average intake of 50.5 g on days when consumed. Chocolate confectionery consumption patterns in the U.S. varied with geographic region, season, ethnic group, time of day, gender, and age. Approximately 5% of the total population and 11% of children aged 5 to 6 years consumed chocolate milk at least once in three days. Chocolate chip cookies were consumed by 20% of children aged 5 to 6 years.

Comparison of the 7-d caffeine averages from different dietary sources showed that the major source of caffeine for children was tea, followed by carbonated beverages. Chocolate candy and other chocolate foods contributed an average of 6.4 mg or 17% of the total caffeine intake. Another study indicated that the most popular sources of caffeine among children were chocolate-containing foods, consumed by 57 to 77% of children surveyed. However, the major source of caffeine in the diet was carbonated beverages. These studies also suggest that there may be regional patterns of use of caffeine-containing foods. The amount and dietary sources of caffeine intake have been quantitated in several studies. Results of the 1989 Marketing Research Corporation of America survey suggested that the mean daily caffeine intake in the U.S. from chocolate-containing foods was 0.06 mg/kg for all ages and 0.12 mg/kg for children 6 to 11 years.

Significant scientific attention has focused on caffeine and its health effects. However, limited data is available for the actual dietary consumption of caffeine or theobromine from individual foods. Even less data exists on the contribution of cocoa and chocolate foods to methylxanthine intake. In children and teenagers, the major dietary source of caffeine was found to be tea, followed by soft drinks and coffee, respectively. Although chocolate foods and beverages ranked the lowest of these dietary sources to provide caffeine, they do constitute the major source of dietary theobromine. In order to gain a better insight into the amount of methylxanthines consumed via the diet, more studies on the methylxanthine content of chocolate foods, as well as beverages, are needed.

REFERENCES

1. Evaluation of health aspects of caffeine as a food ingredient: SCOGS-89 Report, prepared by the Life Sciences Research Office of the Federation of American Societies for Experimental Biology and Medicine for the Bureau of Foods, FDA, US Dept. of Health, Education and Welfare, Washington, DC, 1978.
2. Tarka, S., The toxicology of cocoa and methylxanthines: A review of the literature. *CRC Crit. Rev. Toxicol.*, 9, 275, 1982.
3. Hostetler, K. A., Morrissey, R. B., Tarka, S. M., Jr., Apgar, J. L., Shively, C. A., Three-generation reproductive study of cocoa powder in rats, *Food Chem. Toxicol.*, 28, 483, 1990.

4. Tarka, S. M., Jr., Morrissey, R. B., Apgar, J. L., Hostetler, K. A., Shively, C. A., Chronic toxicity/carcinogenicity studies of cocoa powder in rats, *Food Chem. Toxicol.*, 29, 7, 1991.
5. Chaat, E., *Cocoa*, Interscience, New York, 1954.
6. Cook, R., *Chocolate Production and Use*, Books for Industry, New York. 1972, chap. 3-4.
7. Cobley, L., *An Introduction to the Botany of Tropical Crops*, 2nd ed., revised by Steele, W., Longman, New York, 1970, 207.
8. Marx, F., Maia, J. G. S., Purine alkaloids in seeds of *Theobroma* species from the Amazon, *Z. Lebensm. Unters. Forsch.*,193, 460, 1991.
9. Sotelo, A., Alverez, R. G., Chemical composition of wild *Theobroma* species and their comparison to the cacao bean. *J. Agric. Food Chem.*, 39, 1940, 1991.
10. Meyers, E., Graham, A., Finnegan, E., Kreiser, W., Chocolate and cocoa products, in *Encyclopedia of Industrial Chemical Analysis*, vol 9, John Wiley & Sons, New York, 1970, 534.
11. Knapp, A., *Cacao Fermentation*, Bale, Sons and Curnow, London, 1937.
12. Malini, E., Puranaik, J., Shivashankar, S., Nambudiri, E. S., Physical and chemical composition of Indian cocoa (*Theobroma cacao* L.) beans, *J. Food Sci. Technol.*, 24, 96, 1987.
13. Gill, Duffus, Cocoa Market Report No. 287, Gill & Duffus Group, September 3, 1979.
14. Gill, Duffus, Cocoa Market Report No. 332, Gill & Duffus Group, November 15, 1988.
15. Gill, Duffus, Cocoa Market Report No. 356, E D & F Man Cocoa, Ltd., September 12, 1996.
16. Somorin, D., Caffeine distribution in *C. acuminata*, *T. cacao* and *C. arabica*, *J. Food Sci.*, 39, 1055, 1974.
17. Humphries, E., Changes in fat and theobromine content of the kernel of the cocoa bean during fermentation and drying, *Rep. Cocoa Res. Trinidad*, 8, 34, 1939.
18. Knapp, A., Wadsworth, R., Cocoa fermentation, *J. Soc. Chem. Ind.*, 43, 1247,1924.
19. Timbie, D., Studies on the protein and purine alkaloids of cocoa beans, Ph.D. thesis, The Pennsylvania State University, 1977.
20. Timbie, D., Sechrist, L., Keeney, P., Application of high pressure liquid chromatography to the study of variables affecting theobromine and caffeine concentrations in cocoa beans, *J. Food Sci.*, 43, 560, 1978.
21. Moores, R., Campbell, H., Determination of theobromine and caffeine in cocoa materials, *Anal. Chem.*, 20, 40, 1948.
22. Asamoa, Y., Wurziger, J., Caffeine content of cocoa beans, *Gordian*, 76, 138, 1976.
23. Hadorn, H., Theobromine-, caffeine- and total alkaloid contents of cocoa mass, *CCB Rev. Chocolate Confectionery Bakery*, 5, 26, 1980.
24. Winton, A. L., Winton, K. B., *Structure and Composition of Food*, vol IV, Wiley, New York, 1936.
25. Jensen, H. R., *The Chemistry, Flavouring and Manufacture of Chocolate, Confectionery and Cocoa*, Churchill, London, 1931.
26. Lecoq, R., *Cacao*, Vigot, Paris, 1926.
27. Kreiser, W., Martin, R., Cacao products — high pressure liquid chromatographic determination of theobromine in cocoa and chocolate products, *J. Assoc. Off. Anal. Chem.*, 61, 1424, 1978.
28. Zoumas, B., Kreiser, W., Martin, R., Theobromine and caffeine content of chocolate products, *J. Food Sci.*, 45, 314, 1980.
29. Schutz, G. P., Prinsen, A. J., Pater, A., The spectrophotometric determination of caffeine and theobromine in cocoa and cocoa products, *Rev. Int. Choc.*, 25, 7, 1970.

30. DeVries, J., Johnson, K., Heroff, J., HPLC determination of caffeine and theobromine content of various natural and red dutched cocoas, *J. Food Sci.*, 46, 1968, 1981.
31. Craig, W. J., Nguyen, T. T., Caffeine and theobromine levels in cocoa and carob products, *J. Food Sci.*, 49, 302, 1984.
32. Martinek, R., Wolman, W., Xanthines, tannins and sodium in coffee, tea, and cocoa, *JAMA*, 158, 1030, 1955.
33. Kiefer, B. A., Martin, R. A., Determination of theobromine and caffeine in chocolate products by HPLC. Unpublished data, 1987.
24. Burg, A., How much caffeine in the cup, *Tea Coffee Trade J.*, 1, 40, 1975.
35. Kreiser, W., Martin, R., High pressure liquid chromatographic determination of theobromine and caffeine in cocoa and chocolate products: collaborative study, *J. Assoc. Off. Anal. Chem.*, 63, 591, 1980.
36. Blauch, J., Tarka, S., HPLC determination of caffeine in theobromine in coffee, tea, and instant hot cocoa mixes, *J. Food Sci.*, 48, 745, 1983.
37. Bunker, M., McWilliams, M., Caffeine content of common beverages, *J. Am. Diet. Assoc.*, 74, 28, 1979.
38. Hershey Foods Corporation Technical Center, Analytical Research Laboratory, unpublished data.
39. Scott, N. R., Chakraborty, J., Marks, V., Caffeine consumption in the United Kingdom: a retrospective survey, *Food Sciences Nutrition* 42F, 183, 1989.
40. Love, J. L., Caffeine, theophylline, and theobromine in New Zealand foods, *Food Technol. New Zealand*, 24, 29, 1989.
41. Brereton, P., Hague, M., Wood, R., The determination of theobromine in cocoa and chocolate products, *J. Assoc. Publ. Analysts*, 30, 23, 1994.
42. Hershey Foods Corporation Technical Center, Nutrition Group, unpublished data, 1996.
43. Terada, H., Sakabe, Y., High performance liquid chromatographic determination of theobromine, theophylline and caffeine in food products, *J. Chromat.*, 291, 453, 1984.
44. Zoumas, B. L., Finnegan, E.J., Chocolate and cocoa, in *Kirk-Othmer's Encyclopedia of Chemical Technology*, vol 6, 3rd ed., John Wiley & Sons, New York, 1979.
45. Barone, J. J., Roberts, H. R., Caffeine consumption, *Food Chem. Toxicol.*, 34, 119, 1996.
46. Gill, Duffus, Cocoa Market Report No. 306, Gill & Duffus Group, March 30, 1983.
47. International Cocoa Organization, Quarterly Bulletin of Cocoa Statistics, London, 11 (3), June 1985.
48. International Cocoa Organization, Quarterly Bulletin of Cocoa Statistics, London, 15 (1), December 1988.
49. International Cocoa Organization, Quarterly Bulletin of Cocoa Statistics, London, 12 (3), June 1996.
50. Hetherington, M. M., Macdiarmid, J. I., "Chocolate addiction": a preliminary study of its description and its relationship to problem eating, *Appetite*, 21, 233, 1993.
51. Nuttall, C., Chocolate marketing and other aspects of the confectionery industry worldwide, in *Industrial Chocolate Manufacture and Use*, Beckett, S. T., Ed., Van Nostrand Reinhold, New York 1988, chap. 18.
52. Bureau of Census, U.S. Department of Commerce Economics and Statistics Administration, Current Industrial Reports, Confectionery, U.S., Department of Commerce, Washington, D.C., 1994.
53. Apgar, J. L., Seligson, F. H., Consumer consumption patterns of chocolate and confectionery, *Manuf. Confectioner*, 75, 31, 1995.

54. Graham, D., Caffeine - its identity, dietary sources, intake and biological effects, *Nutr. Rev.*, 36, 97, 1978.
55. Morgan, K., Stults, V., Zabik, M., Amount and dietary sources of caffeine and saccharin intake by individuals ages 5 to 18 years, *Regul. Toxicol. Pharmacol.*, 2, 296, 1982.
56. Arbeit, M. L., Nicklas, T. A., Frank, G. C., Webber, L. S., Miner, M. H., Berenson, G. S., Caffeine intakes of children from a biracial population: the Bogalusa Heart Study, *J. Am. Diet. Assoc.*, 88, 466, 1988
57. Ellison, R. C., Singer, M. R., Moore, L. L., Nguyen, U. D. T., Garrahie, E. J., Marmor, J. K. Current caffeine intake of young children: amount and sources, *J. Am. Diet. Assoc.*, 95, 802, 1995.

Chapter 8

MATÉ

Harold N. Graham

CONTENTS

I. INTRODUCTION

Maté is the beverage prepared from the leaves of *Ilex paraguariensis*, a member of the holly family. The leaves from a number of other members of the *Ilex* genus are sometimes used along with those from *paraguariensis*. The species exists in several varieties and, like *Camellia sinesis*, there is a divergence of opinion concerning their identity and nomenclature.

0-8493-2647-8/98/$0.00+$.50

Maté contains caffeine and, for a group of people in Argentina, Brazil, Paraguay, Uruguay, and Chile, it constitutes the primary source of methylxanthines in the diet.[1,2] World production of maté is in excess of 200,000 t. Table 1 shows approximate production levels in the several countries where it is grown.

A significant quantity of Brazilian and Paraguayan production is exported to Argentina, Chile, and Uruguay.

TABLE 1

Approximate Annual Production of Maté (t)

Country	Amount	Ref.
Argentina	100,000	3
Brazil	100,000	4
Paraguay	60,000	4

II. OCCURRENCE AND HISTORY

Maté is native to the area of South America between 18° and 25° S latitude and from the Atlantic Ocean to the Paraguay River. This area takes in a portion of southern Brazil and Paraguay. The plant was used for beverage purposes by the indigenous populations of the area long before the first Spanish colonists arrived early in the sixteenth century. Its use was taken up by the colonists who found it so desirable that the governor of Paraguay gave settlers the right to enforce the collection of the leaves and, in effect, enslaved the Indian population for this purpose.[1]

Jesuit priests who arrived in the middle of the century gradually took over control of most of the producing areas and began the cultivation of selected varieties to ensure supply. Portuguese invaders from Brazil brought back Indian prisoners with their knowledge of the use of the plant as a beverage, which facilitated the spread of its use in many parts of Brazil.

Virtually all of Argentinian and Brazilian production is now cultivated. Much of Paraguayan production is derived from wild plants.

III. BOTANY

Ilex paraguariensis var. *genuina* is an evergreen tree that grows to a height of 20 to 30 m unattended but under cultivation is kept at 4 to 6 m. The leaves are oval or elliptical, 3 to 20 cm in length, 2 to 9 cm in width, dark green in color. Flowers form in the leaf axils and at the base of the small branches. They bear four or five petals and produce a small fruit in racemes that usually contain four seeds.[1]

IV. AGRICULTURE

The tree is started from seed that is planted in raised beds in rich soil containing an abundance of humus. Irrigation and the prevention of soil caking are essential. Plants may be moved to larger beds when appropriate and then to fields with a planting rate of 800 to 1,000 trees per hectare.

TABLE 2

Variation of Caffeine With Leaf Age

Leaf age	Percent caffeine (dry wt.)
Young, growing	2.0 –2.2
Adult–1 year	1.6
Old–2 years	0.68

Annual pruning to regulate height and conformation of the tree is carried out for a few years. Harvesting begins after 3 to 5 years depending on variety and growing conditions and then takes place at intervals of 1 to 3 years. Full productivity is achieved in about 10 years and continues for an additional 10 years. The harvesting procedure consists of cutting off the smaller branches. The leaves at the extremities of the larger branches are allowed to remain in order to maintain photosynthesis and respiration.[2]

A. Methylxanthines

Maté has been extensively analyzed to determine the content of the methylxanthines, which is largely the basis for its use as a beverage. Reported caffeine levels vary from 0.9% to 2.2%.[5, 6] Age of leaf is an important determinant of caffeine composition, as shown in Table 2.[7]

As is true for other caffeine containing beverages, analytical procedures are often inadequate to cope with interfering components resulting in much conflicting data. In addition, the fact that some 60 species of plant are often found in "maté" along with *I. paraguariensis* leads to significantly different caffeine levels depending on the source of leaf.[6]

Theobromine and theophylline also occur in maté, although several investigators have failed to find these dimethylxanthines.[8] Likely levels of these substances in the dried product are: theobromine, 0.3%; theophylline, 0.004%.[5]

TABLE 3

Components of Maté

Component	Amount (% dry wt. of leaf)	Ref.
Sucrose	3.33	15
Raffinose	0.44	15
Glucose	0.27	15
Fructose	0.16	15
Amino acids	?	16
Trigonelline	0.50	17
Choline	15 mg/g	18
Thiamine	1 mg/g	7
Riboflavin	trace	7
Ascorbic acid	20 mg/g	7
Folic acid	16 mg/g	19
Total extractable ash	5.99	20

B. Other Components

Polyphenolic compounds are present in maté. Flavanols, at least in significant quantities, are absent.[9] The major phenolic compounds are chlorogenic acid and its oxidation products referred to as "resinotanol", which are formed during the manufacturing process.[10] The chlorogenic acid may be a mixture of three different isomers.[11]

Perioxidase and polyphenolase are found in the fresh leaf.[12,13]

Additional components that have been reported in maté beverage are shown in Table 3.

V. MANUFACTURE

A. Traditional Processing

The trees are cleared of vines and smaller branches are cut off. These leaf-bearing branches are "toasted" momentarily over an open fire to reduce the moisture content, but with the avoidance of "blackening". The process is known as "supeco".[1] Further drying is carried out by heating over a platform of poles suspended over an open fire for 12 to 24 h. An alternative procedure involves the use of a dome-shaped structure (barbaqua) over which the toasted branches are spread. Hot air is conducted through a tunnel from a fire some distance away. This procedure avoids direct smoke deposition on the leaf. The latter process requires 5 to 15 h.

Threshing separates leaf from bark and twigs. Further grading by sifting is carried out and the product is packed in 30 to 60 kg bags and aged. Additional grading and blending is practiced to provide greater uniformity.

B. Modern Processing

The toasting step is now frequently carried out by passing the branches through a perforated rotating metal cylinder in an inclined position over an open fire. The cylinders used are about 2 to 2.5 m in diameter and 4 m in length. Dwell time is very short. The process is called "sepecadora".

The barbaqua step may be carried out in a specially constructed room with a frame above the floor to contain the leaves that are dried with hot air conducted from a fire. Leaf temperatures reach 80 to 100°C. Some caffeine is lost at the higher temperature.

Further grinding and sifting is carried out and many different grades of maté are made available. Aging is extremely important to produce a palatable beverage. This may take place over a period of 6 to 18 months.

VI. THE BEVERAGE

The traditional way to prepare the beverage is to pour boiling water over the leaves in a gourd. The latter was known as a "maté," which is the origin of that term now used to designate the leaf and beverage. A reed or metal straw with a bulb-shaped strainer over the end is used to drink maté. Many brews are made from the same leaf by successive additions of boiling water. Teapots are now used to a great extent. About 40 to 50 g of maté is used for a liter of water. Since additional water is added, an accurate leaf:water ratio cannot be specified. Sugar and lemon are frequently added to maté. The beverage is also served cold.[4] Caffeine level in the beverage has been reported to be 25 mg per 150 ml as normally consumed.[20]

REFERENCES

1. Porter, R. H., Maté–South American or Paraguay tea, *Econ Bot,* 4, 37, 1950.
2. Cheney, R. H., The biology and economics of the beverage industry, *Econ Bot* , 1, 243, 1947.
3. Argentine Trade Commission, New York, NY.
4. Minetti, C., A South American drink: Maté, *Industrie Alimentari* 9, 103, 1970.
5. Michl, H. and Haberla, F., Determination of purines in caffeine-containing drugs. *Monatsschrift* 85:779, 1954.
6. de Sigueria, R., Pechnik, E. and Cruz, A., The chemistry and pharmacology of maté, *Tribuna Farm* 21, 1, 1953.
7. Descartes de Garcia, Paula R., Alkaloids in Brazilian maté *(Ilex paraguarieneis). Rev Brasil Quim* 54, 492, 1962.
8. deSoldi, F. and Luz, C., Separation of the alkaloids in Paraguay tea *Ilex paraguarieneis)* by chromatography and electrophoretic techniques. *Rev Fac Agric Univ Nac La Plata* 48, 1, 1972.
9. Roberts, E. A. H., The chlorogenic acid of tea and maté, *Chem Ind,* 985, 1956.
10. Descartes de Garcia, Paula R., Tannins of maté. *Rev Brasil Quim,* 42, 202, 1956.
11. Scarpati, M. L. and Guiso, M., Caffeoyl-quinic acid from coffee and maté, *Ann Chim* (Rome) 53, 1315, 1963.
12. Panek, A. D., Peroxidase in leaves of *Ilex paraguariensis, Bol Inst Quim Agric,* 39, 7, 1955.
13. Chlamiac, E. B., Polyphenol oxidase in *Ilex paraguariensis. Bol Inst Quim Agric,* 39, 13, 1955.
14. Chlamtac, E. B., *Bol Inst Quim Agric,* 38, 17, 1955.
15. Cascon, S. C., Amino acids in *Ilex parag:uariensis, Bol Inst Quim Agric,* 38, 7, 1955.
16. Corria, D., Existence of trigonelline in yerba maté, *Arq Biol Tecnol Inst Biol Pesquisas Tecnol,* 2, 265, 1947.
17. Barrelo, R. C. R., Microbiological determination of choline in herba maté, *Rev Quim Ind,* 25:, 2, 1956.
18 Martelli, H. L., Folic acid determination in mate, *Anais Assoc Brasil Quim,* 18, 83, 1959.
19. Ceccon, O., Berner, R. and Wendler, O., Maté *(Ilex paraguariensis).* II. Inorganic salts in aqueous extracts, *Arq Biol Tecool Inst Biol Pesquisas Tecnol* , 8, 407, 1953.
20. Cortes, F. F., Amount of caffeine in coffee, tea, and maté, *Arq Bromatol,* 1, 47, 1953.

Chapter 9

CAFFEINE CONSUMPTION

Lisbet S. Lundsberg

CONTENTS

0-8493-2647-8/98/$0.00+$.50

I. INTRODUCTION

Caffeine has been extensively researched as a chemical contained in many foods and beverages and is considered the world's most popular drug.[1] Caffeine can be found in over 60 species of plants.[2] As a naturally occurring compound, caffeine has long been consumed in one form or another by mankind. Origins of the coffee bean are traced back for centuries, tea has been the beverage consumed most frequently in many parts of Asia, kola nuts have long been used in Africa as food and a form of currency, and cocoa beans in South and Central America were noted by Spanish conquerors in the 16th century.

This chapter will cover the production of coffee, tea, and cocoa, which comprise the primary crops that account for the majority of worldwide caffeine consumption. Caffeine-containing crops and products comprise a large share of the international market and are primary commodities for many national economies.[3,4] Trade of such products is also important in the understanding of availability, market demand, and overall exposure to caffeine from various sources. Information is presented to a lesser degree for soft drinks, many of which do contain caffeine and are consumed primarily in the industrialized nations. Another source of caffeine exposure which contributes less than any beverages and foods under consideration are prescription and non-prescription medications, which are described in lesser detail.

Caffeine consumption is primarily due to coffee, tea and soft drinks. In the U.S., it is estimated that coffee contributes to 75% of the total caffeine intake, tea is 15%, and soda with caffeine accounts for 10%;[5] chocolate and other caffeine-containing foods and medications contribute relatively little to overall caffeine exposure. Caffeine also varies by sources: tea leaves contain 1.5 to 3.5% caffeine; kola nuts contain 2% caffeine; and roasted coffee beans contain 0.75 to 1.5% caffeine.[6] Coffee varies in caffeine content; some analyses have estimated that caffeine may range from 0.8 to 1.8%, depending on the type of coffee.[7] Crops of coffee, tea, and cocoa are very similar in their production periods and their useful life in production. Typically coffee, tea, and cocoa trees can be productive with crops every 5 years for a total period of 40 years,[8] or an estimated 8 yields per tree.

Table 1 describes several of the most common sources of caffeine, their region of origin, how they are used and consumed, and the variability in caffeine content.[1]

II. COFEE

Coffea arabico L. (arabica) and *Coffea canephora* (robusta) are the primary types of coffee produced and consumed in the world.[9] Arabica coffee is

TABLE 1

Sources of Caffeine

Source	Origin	Country producing	Consumed form	Caffeine content (% total weight)
Coffee bean				
Coffea arabica	Seed, fruit	Brazil, Colombia	Coffee	1.1
Coffea robusta	seed	Indoneasia	Coffee	2.2
Coffea liberica	Seed	Regions in Africa	Coffee	1.4
Tea				
Camellia sinensis	Leaf	China, India	Tea	3.5
Kola nut				
Cola acuminata S.	Seed	West Africa	Soft drinks, chewing nuts	
Cola nitida			Kola tea	1.5
Cocoa pod/cocoa beans				
Theobroma cocoa L	Seed	Brazil, West Africa	Cocoa, chocolate	0.03–1.7

From Gilbert, R.M., *The Methylxanthine Beverages and Foods: Chemistry, Consumption, and Health Effects,* Spiller, G., Ed., Alan Liss, Inc., 1984, 185–193. With permission.

typically grown in equatorial warm climates. Robusta coffee can be produced at colder climates; however, the beans are not amenable to temperatures below 0°C where permanent frost damage can occur, restricting their geographical diversity. Arabica coffee accounts for the majority of coffee produced and consumed (70%). Green raw beans of Robusta coffee are higher in caffeine content, 2.2% of dry matter, while arabica has 1.2% caffeine.[9] Coffee beans are produced from 40 different species of trees in the genus *Coffea.*[10] Three main ones that are commercially grown are *Coffea arabica, Coffea liberica* and *Coffea robusta.* Optimal conditions for growing the beans require an average temperature of 70°F (20°C) and 40 to 70 in. of rainfall during the year.

Raw coffee is also referred to as green coffee. This is the form of the bean as grown, containing 8 to 12% water.[9] Roasting not only dessicates the bean but also changes the chemical composition. After roasting, some coffee is further processed to make soluble, or instant, coffee. Different forms of coffee can also be described in terms of volume and weight, depending on their form: 1 lb of roasted coffee is the equivalent of 1.19 lb green coffee; 1 lb of soluble coffee is produced from 2.52 lb of roasted coffee, or 3 lb of green coffee.[8] The proportion of the roasted bean comprised of caffeine, however, is not dramatically altered. Arabica beans have been analyzed as 1.3% caffeine and robusta beans as 2.4% caffeine.[9]

Other processes beyond the high temperature roasting do not dramatically affect the bean, and with the exception of the decaffeination process, the caffeine content is relatively stable.

A. Coffee Production

Worldwide production of coffee has actually shown a decrease from 1990 (Table 2).[11-16] In 1990, the total world production was 6.3 million metric tons, which has fallen to 5.4 million metric tons as of 1994. While these figures are up from 1980, the general trend has been an overall decline. Brazil is by far the largest producer of coffee; in 1994, 1.3 million metric tons were produced, the equivalent of 23% of world-wide production. Brazil's production is larger than all African nations combined and more than double of the next leading producer, Colombia. African nations, particularly Ethiopia, Uganda, and Cameroon, produced approximately 20% of the world's coffee beans in 1994. North and Central American countries including Mexico, Guatemala, El Salvador, and Costa Rica produced 18%. Several regions in Asia including Indonesia, India, and the Philippines combined to contribute 18.7% of worldwide coffee production in 1994. Recent production statistics indicate that 99.9% of coffee production occurs in developing nations.[16]

B. Coffee Trade

Coffee is a crop that is primarily exported from producing countries, with only a small proportion retained for domestic consumption among the larger producing nations. In 1990, 80% of all coffee produced was exported, which is significantly different from other crops under consideration, particularly tea. Total exports of coffee have increased from 3.7 million metric tons in 1980 to 5.1 million metric tons in 1990 (Table 3).[17-22] South America has been the predominant exporter of coffee, contributing nearly 40% of all coffee exports in international trade. Brazil and Colombia are by far the largest exporting nations in the world; Brazil accounted for nearly 20% of all exports in 1990. Recent trends up to 1993 have shown that overall coffee exports have stabilized, if not slightly declined. After 1990, the total coffee exports have varied between 4.8 and 5.0 million metric tons up to 1993.

Table 4 shows worldwide imports of coffee, listing the primary importing nations.[17-22] Since 1980, there has been an increase in overall coffee trade. Coffee imports have risen from 3.8 million metric tons overall to 4.9 million in 1993. Trends in coffee exports are reflecting in the patterns and volume of coffee imports. After a dramatic increase during the 10 year period from 1980 to 1990, there has been an apparent stabilization from

TABLE 2

World Production of Green Coffee: 1980–1994 (1000 metric tons)

	1980	1981	1982	1983	1984	1985	1986	1987	1988	1989	1990	1991	1992	1993	1994
Africa	1140	1269	1206	1216	1158	1254	1360	1257	1226	1269	1259	1162	1051	987	1067
Ethiopia	187	202	202	220	240	178	225	186	170	200	206	158	NA	180	198
Uganda	110	145	155	192	204	210	195	156	184	174	129	180	110	141	180
N/Central America	917	933	923	1025	997	1027	974	1058	1031	1119	1263	1088	1167	1138	995
Costa Rica	109	120	113	123	137	155	128	138	145	157	151	158	168	148	138
El Salvador	165	161	143	155	162	161	141	148	120	122	156	149	162	165	146
Guatemala	163	173	162	153	177	152	156	182	190	193	202	195	205	215	168
Mexico	208	217	234	313	240	269	278	318	283	343	440	299	360	336	240
South America	2042	3315	2096	2752	2399	2872	2046	3178	2492	2546	2647	2679	2768	2680	2284
Brazil	1061	2038	1003	1665	1420	1877	1004	2203	1352	1530	1463	1497	1294	1278	1257
Columbia	724	808	840	816	694	676	708	652	780	664	845	870	1146	1080	684
Asia	649	662	654	582	624	718	753	776	748	1108	1045	1096	996	1023	1018
India	150	119	155	130	105	190	120	192	125	215	118	173	180	162	170
Indonesia	295	315	266	236	331	311	399	358	384	401	411	408	421	442	400
Phillipines	145	160	160	139	117	133	137	140	142	156	134	113	128	124	120
World	4799	6032	4934	5628	5225	5293	5188	6332	5569	6113	6282	6088	6032	5890	5430

Data from References 11 through 16.

TABLE 3

Coffee Exports 1980–1993 (metric tons)

	1980	1981	1982	1983	1984	1985	1986	1987	1988	1989	1990	1991	1992	1993
Africa	899796	972438	1055530	947576	900042	1009931	1075443	906846	964084	1011673	1105336	876038	911390	839471
Ivory Coast	207862	231288	270400	223073	187708	266300	230002	165135	235000	129562	243000	198504	220400	230500
Uganda	110000	130000	172000	1444274	133200	152300	140600	145000	150000	1765453	141489	124819	119006	114134
N/Central America	737818	719617	668951	848859	821660	864176	836733	897601	802207	916309	940521	886918	860457	993280
Costa Rica	71733	96293	95000	108533	113001	122400	93583	138624	120500	130454	139880	144698	110901	142000
El Salvador	146786	131600	114500	159000	160970	148092	123195	145575	123034	82957	141277	123049	124738	171028
Guatemala	128710	103261	82443	142860	127247	158928	154843	138000	134000	199205	20041	173376	193985	220579
Mexico	130019	121839	125758	185133	172686	192904	208345	223040	169187	271925	20925	221311	194770	195844
South America	1550306	1464057	1550919	1618771	1764947	1754931	1351708	1836202	1618634	1802441	1875850	1984037	2125402	1901971
Brazil	784465	825443	887379	939690	1031931	1014171	477913	987609	904356	943374	853324	1095026	1020511	964524
Colombia	660078	535941	531509	539452	598895	5894940	666645	661631	567726	NA	NA	740167	968241	788033
Asia	375425	389190	419315	428994	507984	531657	560214	509425	556590	667091	751109	700653	655785	743007
Indonesia	238678	210595	226985	241237	294471	292909	298174	286304	298972	357477	421831	380666	269350	349903
Europe	106084	121872	126301	141906	164867	202185	209205	232303	264661	303912	318386	353313	374731	418886
Germany	40580	47584	55921	62943	75425	80795	87030	101831	117124	136665	140023	137508	137269	135987
World	3720886	3714806	3862514	4038917	4210442	4403770	4086867	4447532	4251302	4785950	5054887	4846173	4983561	4957543

Data from References 17 through 22.

TABLE 4

Coffe Imports: 1980–1993 (metric tons)

	1980	1981	1982	1983	1984	1985	1986	1987	1988	1989	1990	1991	1992	1993
Africa	106075	125794	95709	145020	127394	132408	82075	157737	125597	171426	121467	170568	117469	155545
Algeria	65192	84228	49600	92659	70547	79575	35890	110931	71000	104308	63438	106949	48436	88201
South Africa	14782	15961	15000	19475	18148	17000	17000	17000	15000	16113	17013	16812	20144	22000
N/Central America	1213744	11311663	1175943	1112739	1197682	1251515	1287714	1324657	1057852	1295188	1312645	1279342	1449484	1232591
U.S.	1107094	1005739	1061192	998108	1080057	1136499	118245	1208777	943686	1181604	1186244	1145916	1311986	1095040
Canada	83340	98602	88464	90967	97504	96098	98756	110245	107490	108043	120955	126162	117897	129538
South America	37194	40181	48631	43640	49923	50423	37644	40609	44567	38831	38572	43943	55373	49251
Argentina	30457	33390	40214	36062	41090	42500	32756	33658	34372	29966	30067	33744	39756	35733
Asia	244010	277985	319281	389444	402209	407466	414789	426576	454221	433228	489749	515413	551695	555646
Japan	174853	175290	185828	204199	223244	231392	243014	271534	265495	286206	293969	302955	295502	315212
Singapore	7035	20865	30394	37446	58162	45537	71946	41749	23591	15839	57846	57000	82333	78354
Europe	2107455	2161186	2176398	2236750	2185143	2299951	2333042	2506989	2503085	2594767	2816879	2682532	2831786	2824915
France	327218	326041	331018	332319	306062	312791	311101	327155	335150	339029	349306	364214	368370	350880
Germany	552021	567070	613255	597105	581944	597388	643226	694045	716713	753736	766998	769670	807555	833752
Italy	220762	225452	2245965	246697	224664	284215	254119	264725	257709	268852	306945	270566	267678	326639
World	3799351	3817217	3907650	4005635	4049088	4237385	42374105	4550870	4282480	4689399	4885332	4799744	5107788	4940867

Data from References 17 through 22.

TABLE 5

U.S. Imports of Green Coffee: 1994–1995

	1994 1,000 GBE	1994 Millions U.S.$	1995 1,000 GBE	1995 Millions U.S.$
Total	15,913	2,272	15,886	2,985
Country of origin				
Brazil	2,850	422	2,302	419
Mexico	2,516	320	2,887	569
Columbia	2,372	442	2,485	524
Guatemala	1,403	225	1,637	318
Ecuador	969	182	745	117
Thailand	676	50	770	120
Venezuela	295	30	89	13
Peru	249	52	621	106
Vietnam	255	32	975	145

Note: GBE = Green bag equivalent (in 60 KG bags).

Data from Reference 23.

1990 to 1993. European nations account for the majority of all coffee imports, at nearly 60%. However, the U.S. is the largest single importing country, with 1.1 million metric tons imported in 1993. The proportion of imports attributable to the U.S. accounts for nearly one fifth of all coffee trade internationally. Comparatively, very little coffee is traded to South American nations, with the exception of Argentina which is not a leading coffee producer.

Figures from 1994 and 1995 show that coffee is primarily imported to the U.S. in its green, unroasted form (Table 5).[23] The U.S. imported nearly $2.3 billion worth of green coffee beans in 1994 and the total amount increased to close to $3 billion in 1995. The top three exporters of green coffee to the U.S. during 1994 and 1995 were Brazil, Mexico, and Columbia, accounting for 48% of the total volume of green coffee imported in 1995. While the U.S. is not considered a coffee-producing country, green coffee is imported not only for domestic consumption but also processed and exported elsewhere in the world.

Roasted coffee is imported by the U.S., however to a lesser degree. Industrialized nations of Sweden, Canada, and Italy are the primary sources of imported roasted coffee that comes to the U.S. (Table 6), contributing 69% of all roasted imports.[23] Sweden is by far the larger exporter to the U.S., generating over $40 million in revenue. While the total dollars spent on roasted coffee imports has increased by 20% from 1994 to 1995, the actual volume of roasted coffee has decreased by 16%, indicating not only a dramatic reduction of roasted coffee imports but a steep increase in the unit cost.

TABLE 6

U.S. Imports of Roasted Coffee: 1994–1995

	1994 1000 GBE	1994 Millions U.S.$	1995 1000 GBE	1995 Millions U.S.$
Total	350	81	295	98
Country of origin				
Sweden	117	28	120	40
Canada	41	12	55	19
Italy	35	10	30	12
Germany	20	5	23	7
Columbia	19	4	14	4
Ecuador	45	5	13	3
Brazil	5	1	8	3

Note: GBE = Green bag equivalent (in 60 KG bags).

Data from Reference 23.

Export values of coffee were $195.9 million in 1995 in green bean equivalent,[23] an increase from 1994. The majority of coffee exports from the U.S. were from roasted coffee, showing a dramatic increase of 52% in 1995. Roasted exports were primarily to Canada, Japan, and Korea, valued overall at $135 million. The U.S. imported $3.3 billion worth of coffee in 1995.[23] Sweden accounted for the largest share of imported roasted coffee, Mexico supplied the most green coffee to the U.S. and Brazil produced the most instant coffee for the U.S. In 1995, the average price per pound of roasted coffee was $4.02, an increase of 18% from 1994, at $3.40. It is expected that coffee prices will soar early in 1997 due to environmental and labor related issues in major producing countries.

In the U.S., sales of regular (nonsoluble) coffee have decreased over the past 10 years; however, overall revenue has increased. In 1985, 977 million pounds of coffee were sold by U.S. manufacturers, generating nearly $2.8 billion. Coffee sales decreased to 890 million pounds in 1993 and to an estimated 845 million pounds in 1994 (generating $2.2 and $2.8 billion, respectively). Soluble coffee sales have dropped by 50% during the years of 1979 to 1994, when sales were only 94 million pounds. Combined coffee sales reached a peak in 1986 in absolute revenue from sales, at $4.9 billion. In 1995, roasting of green coffee beans in the U.S. declined by 7% from 1991 levels.[23]

There are also dramatic differences in prices for coffee, according to the New York market. Figures for 1995 indicate that Colombian mild arabicas had the highest market price per pound ($1.58), followed by other mild arabicas ($1.49) and Brazilian arabicas ($1.46).[23] Robustas in general were less than arabicas at $1.27 per pound. However, these prices can fluctuate dramatically, mediated by factors that influence the international coffee market. Coffee has suffered from a combination of overproduction, leaving extra crops that are unused, and overall underconsumption. Coffee crops and commercial interests are also threatened by climatic conditions and other environmental problems.

The latest reports of coffee prices and trends have predicted that coffee prices will be increasing in 1997 due to several factors. Several of the larger coffee producers are projected to have crops cut by 20% due to labor and environmental factors: Brazil's coffee exports would be kept down by a strike and crops in Columbia have been damaged by rains. Mexico and Nicaragua have also projected a reduction in crops due to freezing temperatures and severe drought.[24] Resulting prices reported on the Coffee Sugar and Cocoa Exchange have shown a dramatic increase that is projected to affect consumers within the upcoming months.

III. TEA

Tea leaves have been grown and utilized as a crop for over 4000 years[25] and tea is the most popular beverage consumed in the world. Tea leaves are harvested from the plant *Thea sinensis,* indigenous to many regions in Asia. Tea is a crop which is more versatile in the geography of production than coffee or cocoa beans. Tea leaves are harvested from trees every few years and will be used as one of two principal types of tea: black or green tea.[8] Warm climatic conditions and temperatures ranging from 50 to 90°F (10 to 32°C) are preferred for growth, with 90 to 200 in. of rain annually. Tea crops are sensitive to weather conditions, which may be extreme in the major producing nations. Drought and flooding in India and parts of Asia have often taken an unfavorable toll on tea leaf crops.

By weight, tea leaves have double the caffeine as coffee beans;[25] however, the caffeine content is greatly diluted during preparation. Caffeine in tea has been reported to range from 2.7 to 4.1% in selected varieties of tea,[7] comparable with an estimate of 4% caffeine content in tea.[26] While tea is the most commonly consumed caffeinated beverage, the caffeine content is only one third to one half that of coffee, contributing less to overall caffeine exposure than coffee.

A. Tea Production

As shown in Table 7, tea produced in Asia contributed to over 80% of the worldwide crop in 1994.[16] China and India are the primary growers of tea leaves and they not only export but retain much of the tea for domestic consumption. African production is only 13% of the worldwide production and South American production was 72,000 metric tons in 1994.

TABLE 7

World Tea Production: 1980–1994 (1000 metric tons)

	1980	1981	1982	1983	1984	1985	1986	1987	1988	1989	1990	1991	1992	1993	1994
Africa	197	198	211	219	243	275	267	265	278	304	325	335	298	340	340
Kenya	90	91	96	119	116	147	140	156	164	181	197	204	188	211	209
Asia	1480	1482	1539	1604	1733	1810	1789	1938	2029	1930	2004	2049	2015	2142	2122
China	328	368	421	425	438	455	486	535	566	557	562	566	580	621	600
India	572	561	564	588	645	657	628	674	710	684	715	730	704	757	720
Sri Lanka	191	210	188	179	208	214	211	213	227	207	238	241	179	232	240
Indonesia	106	109	92	90	126	132	121	156	144	141	149	158	163	169	174
World	1866	1864	1951	2036	2192	2313	2296	2430	2487	2428	2533	2576	2439	2645	2623

Data from References 11 through 16.

Overall tea production between 1990 and 1994 has increased only 4%, which is down from the dramatic rise in production of 30% during the years of 1980 to 1989.[11-14] As a widely consumed beverage, the percentage exported from all tea produced was 49% in 1990 and 46% in 1991.[15] This pattern indicates that tea, compared to coffee and cocoa, is often domestically produced and consumed. Most worldwide production (91.4%) in 1991 occurred in developing countries.[15]

B. Tea Trade

Great Britain imports more tea than any other nation. In 1993, imports of tea to the U.K. were 193,837 metric tons (the equivalent of over $340,000), which represents 56% of all imports to Europe.[22] Most imports of tea to the U.K. come from Malawi and India.[27] Pakistan is the second largest importer of tea, followed by the U.S.

China is the single largest exporter of tea, exporting 206,659 metric tons in 1993.[22] Exports of tea from Asia account for 65% of worldwide export trade in this commodity. Approximately 170,000 metric tons of tea were exported from India in 1993 and 188,390 tons from Kenya in the same year.

London auction prices for tea in 1995 reflect the lowest price per pound since 1975 at 74.5 cents.[23] Lower market prices of tea are primarily due to the reduced quality of tea and record production; prices for tea were 83.7 cents per pound in 1991, down 8.5 cents from the previous year. The highest price was recorded in 1984 ($1.56 per pound), which has since fallen to the recent levels. Trade in imports and exports of tea (bag and instant) in the U.S. has been growing since 1990. While iced tea products are increasingly popular in the U.S., they are in direct competition with soft drinks which tend to dominate the cold beverage market.

IV. COCOA

Cocoa is produced in tropical environments; however, it is primarily exported for consumption in industrialized regions.[8] Exports of cocoa may be the cocoa beans as well as other semi-processed materials from cocoa including cocoa paste, cocoa powder, chocolate, cocoa butter, and other cocoa-containing products. Similar to coffee, cocoa production and trade are sensitive to environmental and climatic changes in producing regions. Factors may include drought, labor related issues, harvesting and crop maintenance, stock prices, and monetary changes. The International Cocoa Agreement in 1973[8] was designed to protect the cocoa market for producing countries with respect to exports as well as consumer nations. The International Cocoa Organization oversees much of the production, trade, and stocks of cocoa on the international market.

A. Cocoa Production

Cocoa production has dramatically increased since 1980, from worldwide production of 1.6 million metric tons to 2.6 in 1994, a 60% increase (Table 8).[11-16] There does appear to be somewhat of a leveling in production since 1990 when 2.5 million metric tons of cocoa beans were produced. Africa is the largest producer of cocoa, contributing over 50% of the total worldwide production. The Ivory Coast is the single largest national producer, with 809,000 metric tons in 1994 (32% worldwide production).

Figures for 1994 and forecasts for 1995 through 1996 show that the Ivory Coast is by far the largest producer of cocoa beans,[23] accounting for 36% of the market in 1994–1995, and estimates are close to 40% in 1995–1996. In 1994–1995, the largest producers of cocoa beans were: Ivory Coast (873,000 metric tons), Ghana (315,000 metric tons), Indonesia (275,000 metric tons) and Brazil (234,000 metric tons). African production of cocoa beans in that year accounted for 60% of worldwide production. Forecasts of cocoa production are at record highs for 1995 and 1996,[23] with an estimated 2.7 million metric tons of cocoa beans being produced. Brazil, one of the largest producers of cocoa, has recently been importing cocoa to produce some of the cocoa products that contribute to their economy, such as chocolate. The Ivory Coast is the major producer of cocoa beans, and the largest supplier of imported cocoa beans to the U.S. Nearly all cocoa produced worldwide originates in developing nations.[16]

B. Cocoa Trade

In 1990, 74% of all cocoa produced was exported.[21] This figure does not include semi-processed cocoa products, including cocoa paste, cocoa butter, cocoa powder, and chocolate. However, it demonstrates that cocoa is not a crop of domestic consumption within the major producing nations. Similarly to coffee, cocoa contributes to the economy of several large producing nations.

Cocoa beans and related cocoa product imports (liquor, paste, powder) to the U.S. all declined in 1995; however, cocoa butter and chocolate rose in total imports. U.S. exports of cocoa have a large market in neighboring countries of Canada and Mexico; together they account for 51% of all cocoa products exported by the U.S., or $316.8 million in value.[23]

Cocoa bean prices have been relatively low during the past 10 years.[23] Prices on the New York stock market peaked in 1977 at $1.72 per pound and have fallen since then. The lowest market price was registered in 1993 at 46.7 cents per pound and has only risen slightly in recent years.

TABLE 8

World Cocoa Production: 1980–1994 (1000 metric tons)

	1980	1981	1982	1983	1984	1985	1986	1987	1988	1989	1990	1991	1992	1993	1994
Africa	984	1016	979	808	1049	1070	1061	1181	1442	1378	1357	1275	1288	1324	1361
Cameroon	120	115	105	108	121	115	120	131	124	126	99	95	90	97	100
Ghana	250	230	203	160	173	212	240	184	289	300	295	295	312	240	270
Ivory Coast	400	445	465	360	550	580	520	664	820	725	750	710	697	804	809
Nigeria	155	160	153	123	150	110	125	150	160	160	150	115	145	135	135
South America	4565	445	512	489	440	613	626	464	539	560	588	570	513	513	523
Brazil	319	304	351	380	330	420	459	329	375	393	355	345	329	340	344
Ecuador	91	80	97	45	49	131	100	50	85	83	147	136	94	83	84
Asia	50	59	84	97	134	146	176	258	298	355	409	459	416	485	531
World	1621	1640	1711	1524	1748	1963	2002	2044	2440	2460	2528	2455	2373	2493	2564

Data from References 11 through 16.

V. CAFFEINE CONSUMPTION

Caffeine occurs naturally in coffee beans, tea leaves, and cocoa and is added to many beverages, foods, and medications. The most prevalent exposure to caffeine is from tea drinking; however, coffee drinking accounts for the most caffeine that is consumed. Coffee is higher in caffeine content than tea by approximately 60 to 70%. Alternative sources of caffeine include soft drinks, which are increasingly popular in the industrialized nations. While decaffeinated sodas are produced as a caffeine-free alternative, these beverages account for a small percentage of all soft drinks. Only about 5% of all sodas sold in 1994 were caffeine-free versions.[28] Caffeine is found not only in coffee, tea, and soda but also in an estimated 2,000 other products that are consumed[2] including medications, chocolate, chocolate-containing foods and confectioneries, and other foods.

Other dietary factors that may influence overall caffeine consumption include foods that contain cocoa or chocolate, such as candies and sweets. These products do not contribute as much caffeine as either coffee or tea; however, their contribution to caffeine exposure should be recognized. Caffeine may also be in foods and beverages as an additive, which the Food and Drug Administration monitors and requires to be labeled on the product.

As shown in Table 9, the caffeine content of coffee, tea, and other products can vary dramatically.[5,29-33] Caffeine content in a cup of coffee has been reported as 74 mg for percolated coffee and 112 mg for automatic drip coffee, showing substantial differences according to preparation.[34] Instant coffee is significantly less at 66 mg and caffeine from decaffeinated coffee is negligible (1 to 3 mg caffeine).

One source of caffeine that is often overlooked is medications, both prescription and nonprescription. It was estimated in 1980 that there were several thousand over-the-counter and prescription medications containing caffeine.[28] Selected medications that contain caffeine are listed in Table 10. The primary indications for caffeine-containing medications include pain relief, drugs used for alertness, diet or weight loss, cough or cold, and diuretics.[5,31,33,35,36] Some of the stronger medications may contain up to 200 mg of caffeine per tablet (approximately equal to two 5-oz cups of coffee). However, overall use of these medications in the general population does not approach coffee and tea drinking as the primary exposure to caffeine.

A. International Coffee Consumption

Recent analysis of 1989 coffee consumption[37] determined that annual coffee drinking was the highest per kilogram per person in Scandinavia: consumption, expressed as green coffee equivalents, in Finland was 12.6

TABLE 9

Caffeine Content of Varous Beverages and Foods

Beverage	Serving/volume	Caffeine (mg)
Coffee		
Automatic drip/brewed	5 oz	115 (80–175
Percolated	5 oz	80 (40–170)
Instant	5 oz	60 (46–71)
Expresso	1.5–2 oz	100
Cappuccino	6 oz	60–120
Decaffeinated	6 oz	<1
Tea	6 oz	30–80
Iced	12 oz	70
Brewed, imported	7 oz	60
Brewed, U.S.	7 oz	40
Chocolate		
Chocolate milk	8 oz	2–8
Hot chocolate	8 oz	10
Milk chocolate candy	1 oz	6
Dark chocolate	1 oz	20
Chocolate cake	1 slice	20–30
Soft drinks		
Jolt	12	100
Mountain Dew	12	54.0
Mello Yellow	12	52.8
Coca-cola	12	45.6
Dr. Pepper	12	39.6
Pepsi	12	38.4
RC Cola	12	36.0
Diet Rite	12	36.0

Data from References 5 and 29 through 33.

kg/pp/yr, followed by Sweden at 10.9 kg, Denmark at 10.7 kg, and Norway at 10.2 kg. The 10 top consumers of coffee were all European nations. Consumption in Costa Rica was 6 kg per year, 4.7 kg in the U.S., 4.6 kg in the Dominican Republic, and 4.4 kg in Italy.

The U.S. is responsible for consuming the most coffee overall in the world; in 1991, it was estimated that each person consumed nearly 27 gallons (101.4 liters) of coffee.[10] Decaffeinated coffee is consumed less frequently in the U.S., at levels of 24% in 1987 to 15% in 1993.[10] Table 11 shows that the U.S. by far consumed the most coffee in weight than any other nation in the world, nearly double that of Germany as the second highest consumer.[38] Estimates for the U.S. up to the early 1990s did not show a great increase in total consumption, but rather a stabilization that is consistent with coffee trade to and from the U.S.

In Scandinavian countries, it is primarily Arabica coffee that is imported and consumed[37] which is 1.1% caffeine; in other countries, the mix

TABLE 10

Selected Prescription and Non-Prescription Medications Containing Caffeine

Medications	Dose	Caffeine (mg)
Analgesics/pain relief		
Excedrin	2 tablets	130
Anacin	2 tablets	64
Midol	2 tablets	64
Midol, Max Strength	1 tablet	60
Cafergot	1 tablet	100
Darvon	2 tablets	60
Fioricet with codeine	1 tablet	40
Fiorinal	1 tablet	40
Norgesic	1 tablet	30
Norgesic Forte	1 tablet	60
Vanquish	1 tablet	33
Decongestant		
Dristan decongestant	2 tablets	32
Stimulant		
NoDoz	1 dose	200
Vivarin	1 dose	200
Weight loss		
Dexatrim	1 dose	200

Data from References 5, 31, 33, 35, and 36.

between Arabica and Robusta coffee, 2.2% caffeine, will amount to a higher average caffeine exposure. In Italy, for example, where 52% of the coffee consumed is Arabica and 48% is Robusta, the caffeine percentage is intermediate at 1.63%. Brewing methods will also affect the caffeine exposure (primarily espresso and mocha in Italy compared to filter and boiling methods used in Scandinavia) as well as cup size (20 to 50 ml in Italy and 50 to 190 ml in Scandinavia). Brewing methods are especially important due to the fact that extraction efficiency will vary dramatically depending on the preparation method. Variation in cup size can be even greater; a typical cup in Canada has been estimated to be 225 ml, ranging from 25 to 330 ml.[28]

Total caffeine consumption will vary with a number of factors that are often difficult to disentangle. For caffeine exposure attributable to coffee, this includes brewing method and preparation; type of coffee (Arabica, Robusta, instant), averaging to 1.3% caffeine for roasted beans;[39] brand of coffee; size of coffee cup; and the volume of added ingredients, such as milk, cream sweeteners, and syrups. There are several different brewing or preparation techniques by which coffee can be prepared. Most notably, they differ in their final extraction of caffeine depending on the process. Filter coffee or automatic drip coffee results in approximately 97 to 100% caffeine extraction;[37] however, regional differences in the volume of coffee

TABLE 11

Coffee Consumption (in thousands of 60 kg): 1986–1992

	1986	1987	1988	1989	1990	1991[a]	1992[a]
U.S.	17572	18197	17889	18544	18974	19891	17909
Germany	8707	9572	9677	9881	9079	10477	10771
France	5067	5404	56384	5290	5203	5557	5614
Italy	4168	4308	4216	4314	4859	4228	4130
Japan	4506	4963	5087	5100	5236	6038	5272
Netherlands	2342	2560	2447	2244	2553	2486	2547
Spain	2224	2106	2312	2592	2713	2652	3044
U.K.	2282	2355	2331	2177	2348	2342	2516
Canada	1786	1800	1814	1822	1974	2068	NA
World	64530	70294	69474	72668	71241	72000	72000

[a] Estimates.

Data from Reference 38.

used in preparation will yield different concentrations of caffeine in the cup. Percolated coffee recirculates water through ground coffee and achieves 85% total caffeine extraction. Espresso uses a smaller total volume of water and coffee for preparation, and caffeine extraction is estimated at 80%. Another type of coffee boils the ground coffee in water and is consumed without filtering; this method achieves 75% caffeine extraction.[37]

While percolators were long used and the most common method of coffee preparation up to 1975 (51%), automatic drip machines have steadily increased to be the method used for nearly half of all coffee prepared in 1981,[41] as compared to only 7% automatic drip in 1975. This trend does impact caffeine exposure, as the different preparation methods have differential extraction of caffeine from the coffee that is used.

There are other ways to also describe coffee, including varietals (where the coffee was cultivated), styles or types of roasting, and blends. One of the primary distinctions for coffee is that of origin and type of bean, specifically Arabica and Robusta. The main consideration is the difference not only in taste and preference among consumers, but the caffeine content. Green coffee is roasted to bring out the aromatic compounds that make it an attractive beverage for consumers, particularly the oil caffeol.[10] The roasting process may also affect the caffeine content of coffee beans. Roasting tends to destroy caffeine, so that darker roasted beans will, in effect, have less caffeine. If coffee is decaffeinated, only about 3% of the caffeine remains after this process.[10] In the U.S., methylene chloride is used for direction extraction of caffeine from coffee. Steam extraction of caffeine is also used in the decaffeination process of coffee beans.

While overall consumption of coffee may be highest in the U.S., per capita caffeine intake is greater in several other industrialized nations,

TABLE 12

Worldwide Consumption of Coffee[a]: 1990–1994 (kg per person)

	Average 1990–1994	1990	1991	1992	1993	1994
Finland	12.7	13.0	12.1	12.3	13.0	13.4
Sweden	11.4	11.8	11.2	11.3	11.2	11.5
Denmark	10.4	10.1	10.5	11.0	10.3	10.3
Norway	10.4	10.3	10.5	10.4	9.7	11.2
Netherlands	10.2	10.3	10.1	11.5	10.1	9.0
Iceland	9.7	9.1	10.1	10.2	10.2	9.1
Austria	9.5	11.1	9.6	9.1	9.6	7.8
Costa Rica	8.3	5.8	5.1	11.1	9.9	9.8
Germany	7.8	8.4	7.5	7.8	8.1	7.4
Switzerland	7.6	8.1	7.8	7.5	7.3	7.1
France	5.9	5.8	6.0	6.0	6.1	5.6
Lebanon	5.1	3.9	5.7	6.9	5.0	4.1
Italy	4.7	5.0	4.4	4.3	5.1	4.9
Dominica	4.5	4.5	5.0	4.2	4.2	4.3
Canada	4.4	4.2	4.2	4.4	4.7	4.7
U.S.	4.3	4.5	4.4	4.2	4.3	4.1
Slovenia	4.0	NA	NA	3.3	4.4	4.4
Spain	3.8	3.8	3.8	4.0	3.7	3.7
Haiti	3.6	4.1	3.8	2.7	3.5	3.8
Bolivia	3.5	2.9	3.8	3.4	3.6	3.7
World	1.1	1.1	1.1	1.0	1.0	1.0

[a]Green coffee and coffee products.

Data from Reference 40.

including Denmark[28] and Sweden, where the primary source of caffeine is coffee. Coffee is the most popular drink in several European countries, including Finland and Switzerland.[37] In the U.K., 95% of a surveyed population consumed a caffeinated beverage over a period of one week,[28] however, the primary beverage was tea (81%).

Table 12 shows the patterns of coffee consumption among selected countries.[40] Finland was the country with the highest per capita coffee consumption during the years of 1990 to 1994. In this country, individuals consumed on average 12.7 kg of coffee, nearly 12 times the worldwide average consumption of coffee. The highest consumption recorded in 1994 was 13.4 kg per person in Finland. Many of the Scandinavian countries had heavy coffee consumption, most over 10 kg of coffee per person each year. Nine of the ten heaviest coffee drinking nations are European, reflecting distinct regional patterns of coffee consumption. Trends of coffee consumption in Canada and the U.S. are similar to one another, with average per capita consumption of 4.4 and 4.3 kg, respectively. Over the 4-year period, there has been an increasing trend in coffee consumption in

Canada, while consumption has declined in the U.S. Worldwide consumption, 1.1 kg per person annually over the 4-year period, has shown a slight decline as well.

B. Domestic Coffee Consumption: United States

The Winter Drinking Study has found in the past few years that the population drinking coffee in the U.S. has decreased from 52% in 1990 to 51% in 1991, 47% in 1995, and 49% in 1996.[42] Among the whole population, this amounts to 1.7 cups per day in 1990, 1.8 cups per day in 1991, and 1.7 cups per day in 1995 and 1996. This is a reduction from an earlier survey[41] in 1980, where the average daily coffee consumption was 2.0 cups per person.

Long term trends show dramatic changes in coffee drinking in the U.S. over the past 40 years.[41] In 1955, over 75% of the population was drinking coffee. A dramatic decline in coffee consumption occurred between 1960 and 1980. In 1962, 74.7% of the population was drinking coffee, yet in 1980, 56.6% were drinking coffee. During that time, the reduction in overall coffee consumption was attributable primarily to the reduction in regular (ground) coffee of 21%. Soluble coffee, although consumed less frequently, showed a marginal reduction of 0.3% over the same time period. The number of cups consumed decreased by 16%, from 4.2 cups per drinking individual in 1962 to 3.4 cups in 1981.[41]

Decaffeinated coffee appears to be consumed less frequently, however there are interesting trends over the past few decades. In the early 1960s, 4% of the U.S. population drank decaffeinated coffee, which increased dramatically to 13.1% in 1980.[41] More recently, 15% of all coffee consumption in 1990 was from decaffeinated coffee, which fell to 11% in 1996.[42] Women are more likely to be drinking decaffeinated coffee as compared to men (12% vs. 9% in 1996) and older adults drink more decaffeinated coffee (24% in ages 60 and over) compared to younger age groups: 11% in ages 30 to 59 and 3% among ages 20 to 29 years. Decaffeinated coffee has increased in popularity since 1981, when it accounted for 6% of coffee consumption.[41]

In the early 1960s, coffee was the primary beverage consumed in the U.S.,[41] more common than the consumption of milk (54%), juice (41%), tea (25%), or soft drinks (33%). The Winter Coffee Drinking Study found that while coffee drinking decreased over the next 20 years, the proportion of the population drinking tea increased to 33% and soft drinks became the more popular beverage at 52%. Between the 1960s and 1980s, coffee drinking declined by a large margin.[43] Several factors have likely contributed to the reduction in coffee drinking, including price sensitivity, economic environments, and alternative beverages, both with and without caffeine.

Health concerns about the effects of coffee are also an important consideration in coffee drinking trends. While many health issues have not been systematically and thoroughly evaluated, these concerns have undoubtedly contributed to consumption patterns. However, the most significant changes in coffee consumption occurred prior to scientific research and knowledge of health effects due to caffeine exposure.

Coffee is now sold and marketed from a wide variety of distributors and vendors. These include delis, coffee stores and cafes, discount retailers, mail order and catalog companies, gift stores, and markets. The Specialty Coffee Association of America has compiled statistics about the retail value of coffee sales over the past 30 years.[44] In 1969, the value of specialty coffee sales were $44 million. By 1979, this grew to $763 million and nearly doubled to $1.5 billion by 1989.

As the trends have shown that coffee drinking has stabilized and even declined in recent years, the specialty coffee market has replaced much of the standard coffee typically consumed. Currently, it has been estimated that there are 8,000 outlets selling coffee in the U.S. today.[45] One of the largest chains is Starbuck's, which may grow to 2,000 outlets by the turn of the century. It has been predicted that there will be a significant increase in the continuing popularity of specialty coffee outlets (coffee houses, coffee bars, shops brewing and selling coffee beverages and items) over the next few years. According to the Specialty Coffee Association of America, the number of coffee shops in the country had grown from 200 in 1989 to 4,500 in 1994,[46] with projections running to 10,000 coffee shops and outlets by the turn of the century. As an alternative providing more varieties of blends and coffee bean types, the specialty beverages and their revenues have been estimated at $1.9 billion in 1993 and may reach $3 billion by the year 2000.

C. Tea Consumption

Table 13 shows that the highest tea-consuming nations have a wide geographical distribution.[40] Uruguay has the highest per capita tea consumption at 6.3 kg per year on average during 1990 to 1994. Sudan (5.9 kg), Argentina (5.4 kg), Seychelles (4.0 kg), and Ireland (3.2 kg) are also among the highest tea drinking nations. In the U.K., tea drinking is at 2.5 kg per person. Certain nations that consume a high volume of tea have reduced per capita consumption during recent years, including Libya, Mongolia, and Gambia. Both Canada and the U.S. consume less tea than the worldwide average, 0.5 kg and 0.3 kg per person compared to 0.6 kg, respectively.

Caffeine content varies not only with the type of tea but with the brewing time (steeping time) as well. In general, more caffeine is extracted

TABLE 13

Worldwide Consumption of Tea: 1990–1994 (kg per person)

	Average 1990–1994	1990	1991	1992	1993	1994
Uruguay	6.3	4.8	5.0	7.8	6.3	7.4
Sudan	5.9	4.3	5.5	6.2	6.0	7.4
Argentina	5.4	4.6	4.7	4.9	6.3	6.6
Seychelles	4.0	3.6	4.3	3.7	4.3	4.1
Ireland	3.2	3.3	3.1	3.2	3.2	3.2
Libya	2.9	3.8	3.7	2.9	2.0	2.1
U.K.	2.5	2.5	2.5	2.5	2.5	2.6
Mongolia	2.2	3.2	1.8	1.6	2.5	1.7
Kuwait	2.2	1.9	2.2	1.9	2.4	2.6
Gambia	2.1	2.0	2.2	2.7	2.2	1.2
Syria	2.0	1.7	2.3	2.2	1.6	2.2
Canada	0.5	0.5	0.5	0.5	0.5	0.5
U.S.	0.3	0.3	0.3	0.3	0.3	0.4
World	0.6	0.6	0.6	0.5	0.5	0.6

Data from Reference 40.

the longer the tea is brewed. Black tea tends to have a higher caffeine content than Oolong tea, depending on preparation method. Variability in a single serving of tea can range from 18 mg/180 ml to 107 mg caffeine/180 ml liquid.[47] Other research found that tea had the same large range of variability[34] and a median caffeine content of 27 mg.

D. Cocoa Consumption

The consumption of cocoa, similarly to coffee, is highest among the European nations (Table 14).[40] Cocoa consumption per capita is highest in Dominica at 4.7 kg per year on average during 1990 to 1994. Consumption in Iceland (4.0 kg per person), Belgium-Luxembourg (3.8 kg per person), Denmark (3.3 kg per person), and Germany (3.2 kg per person) are all far above the world average consumption of cocoa and cocoa products (0.5 kg per person). Consumption in the U.S. is 2.4 kg per person, while it is slightly lower in Canada, at 2.1 kg per person. Similar to coffee, cocoa consumption shows the same patterns as coffee, with higher rates of consumption in industrialized nations in Europe and North America.

VI. SUMMARY

Table 15 shows the trends in consumption of various beverages in the U.S. during the period of 1980 to 1992.[38] The patterns that are most apparent include the reduction in per capita coffee consumption, a slight in-

TABLE 14

Worldwide Consumption of Cocoa: 1990–1994 (kg per person)[a]

	Average 1990–1994	1990	1991	1992	1993	1994
Dominica	4.7	5.7	5.6	4.8	4.8	2.9
Iceland	4.0	3.9	4.2	4.2	3.8	3.9
Belgium-Lux	3.8	3.0	3.4	3.1	3.2	6.2
Denmark	3.3	2.7	3.2	3.4	3.5	3.5
Germany	3.2	3.0	3.3	2.9	3.5	3.3
France	2.9	2.7	2.9	3.0	2.8	2.9
Austria	2.9	3.1	3.1	2.9	2.8	2.7
U.K.	2.7	2.6	3.1	2.9	2.4	2.5
Norway	2.5	2.6	2.8	2.5	2.1	2.5
U.S.	2.4	2.4	2.4	2.3	2.4	2.4
Grenada	2.4	1.2	1.8	2.4	3.0	2.3
Malta	2.3	0.9	2.5	2.7	3.0	2.3
Canada	2.1	1.7	1.8	2.4	2.2	2.2
Spain	2.1	2.1	2.1	2.1	2.3	2.1
World	0.5	0.5	0.5	0.4	0.4	0.5

[a] Includes cocoa and cocoa products.

Data from Reference 40.

TABLE 15

Per Capita Consumption of Various Beverages in the U.S.: 1980–1991 (gallons)

	1970	1980	1985	1990	1991	1992
Coffee	35.7	27.2	26.8	26.4	26.5	26.1
Tea	5.2	7.3	7.3	7.0	6.7	6.8
Soft drinks	22.7	34.2	40.8	47.7	47.8	48.0

Data from Reference 38

crease in tea consumption, and a dramatic increase in the consumption of soft drinks. Estimates of dail caffeine exposure have been made at approximately 3 mg/kg for all U.S. adults and 4 mg/kg for adults consuming products with caffeine, equaling 177 mg for a 120-pound female and 231 mg for a 170-pound male. However, this is not just an issue for adults; many children consume high levels of caffeine from soda, iced tea, and chocolate-containing foods and candy, which can easily climb to levels above 200 mg caffeine per day.[2] In fact, one can of caffeinated soda, approximately 50 mg of caffeine, for a child may have the same biologic and physiologic effects as 2 cups of coffee (200 milligrams or more) in a grown adult.[48]

TABLE 16

Coffee Consumption in the U.S.: 1980–1993 (cups per person/day)

Year	Regular	Soluble	Decaffeinated	Total
1980	1.39	0.62	0.34	2.02
1981	1.38	0.54	0.33	1.92
1982	1.33	0.56	0.38	1.90
1983	1.31	0.53	0.39	1.85
1984	1.44	0.54	0.44	1.99
1985	1.39	0.42	0.42	1.83
1986	1.37	0.36	0.41	1.74
1987	1.37	0.37	0.43	1.76
1988	1.31	0.34	0.38	1.67
1989	1.43	0.32	0.40	1.75
1990	1.42	0.29	0.36	1.73
1991	1.46	0.27	0.32	1.75
1993	1.61	0.25	0.28	1.87

Data from Reference 38.

It is also important to recognize the trends in caffeine consumption, and the various contributing sources. The primary source of caffeine in the U.S. and many other industrialized nations is coffee. Table 16 shows the reduction in coffee consumption over the past two decades, with an apparent decline in all three forms of coffee: regular, soluble, and decaffeinated coffee.[38] Recent declines in coffee consumption may perhaps be explained by a number of factors. There is currently more concern about the health effects of caffeine, reflected in the increasing number of scientific investigations and epidemiological studies. Increasing competition from other beverages also affects the coffee market. More beverages are available, particularly soft drinks and iced tea in the U.S., and are consumed at increasing rates. All of these factors will affect the overall exposure to caffeine, which has shown variation across different geographical regions and over time.

REFERENCES

1. Gilbert RM. Caffeine consumption. In: *The Methylxanthine Beverages and Foods: Chemistry, Consumption, and Health Effects.* Ed: Gene Spiller. Alan Liss, Inc. 1984: 185-193.
2. Clay D. The caffeine controversy. *The Philadelphia Tribune.* September 12, 1995.
3. Lucier, Richard L. *The International Political Economy of Coffee: From Juan Valdez to Yank's Diner.* Praeger Publishers, New York: 1988.

4. Marshall CF. *The World Coffee Trade: A Guide to the Production, Trading and Consumption of Coffee.* Woodhead-Faulkner Ltd, Cambridge: 1983.
5. Schardt D, Schmidt S. Caffeine: *The Inside Scoop. Nutrition Action Health Letter.* Vol 23 (10): December 1996. Center for Science in the Public Interest, Washington, D.C.
6. Bianchine JR. Caffeine. *Colliers Encyclopedia.* Vol 5. 1996.
7. Kaplan E, Holmes JH, Sapeika N. Caffeine content of tea and coffee. *S Afr Med J.* 1974;48:510-11.
8. Singh, Shamsher, Vries JD, Hulley JCL, Yeung P. *Coffee, Tea, and Cocoa: Market Prospects and Development Lending.* World Bank Paper, No. 22. Johns Hopkins University Press, Baltimore:1977.
9. Viani, Rinantonio. The Composition of Coffee. In: *Caffeine, Coffee, and Health.* Ed S. Garattini. Raven Press, Ltd. New York. 1993.
10. Cheney RH. Coffee. *Colliers Encyclopedia.* Vol 6. 1996.
11. Food and Agriculture Organization of the United Nations. FAO Production Yearbook 1982. Vol. 36, No. 47.
12. Food and Agriculture Organization of the United Nations. FAO Production Yearbook 1984. Vol. 38, No. 61.
13. Food and Agriculture Organization of the United Nations. FAO Production Yearbook 1986. Vol. 40.
14. Food and Agriculture Organization of the United Nations. FAO Production Yearbook 1989. Vol. 43, No. 94.
15. Food and Agriculture Organization of the United Nations. FAO Production Yearbook 1991. Vol. 45, No. 104.
16. Food and Agriculture Organization of the United Nations. FAO Production Yearbook 1994. Vol 48, No. 125.
17. Food and Agriculture Organization of the United Nations. FAO Trade Yearbook 1980. Vol. 47.
18. Food and Agriculture Organization of the United Nations. FAO Trade Yearbook 1982. Vol. 36, No. 49.
19. Food and Agriculture Organization of the United Nations. FAO Trade Yearbook 1985. Vol. 39, No. 72.
20. Food and Agriculture Organization of the United Nations. FAO Trade Yearbook 1988. Vol. 42, No. 91.
21. Food and Agriculture Organization of the United Nations. FAO Trade Yearbook 1991. Vol. 45, No. 109.
22. Food and Agriculture Organization of the United Nations. FAO Trade Yearbook 1993. Vol. 47.
23. United States Department of Agriculture. *Tropical Products: World Markets and Trade.* Foreign Agriculture Service. Circular Series. FTROP 1-96.
24. Adivan P. Coffee, soy, oil prices soar while copper falls. *Reuters Business Report.* January 29, 1997.
25. Cheney RH. Tea. *Colliers Encyclopedia.* Vol 22. 1996.
26. Graham DM. Caffeine - It's identity, dietary sources, intake and biological effects. *Nutrition Reviews.* 1978;36(4):97-102.
27. United States Department of Agriculture. *World Tea Situation.* Foreign Agriculture Service. Circular Series FTEA 3-92.
28. Barone JJ, Roberts HR. Caffeine consumption. *Food Chemical Toxicology.* 1996;34(1):119-129.
29. Beason HW. Nutrition: pay attention to caffeine content of every-day foods. *Gannett News Service.*
30. Lecos C. Caffeine Jitters: Some safety questions remain. *FDA Consumer.* December 1987-January 1988.

31. Lecos C. The Latest Caffeine Scorecard. *FDA Consumer.* March 1984.
32. Bunker ML, McWilliams. Caffeine content of common beverages. *J Am Diet Assoc.* 1979;74:28-32.
33. Wickens B, Wood C. Grounds for debate. *Macleans.* Vol 107, 1994, p 48.
34. Gilbert RM, Marshman JA, Schwieder M, Berg R. Caffeine content of beverages as consumed. *Can Med Assoc J.* 1976;114:205-8.
35. *Physicians' Desk Reference for Nonprescription Drugs.* Medical Economics Company, Montvale, New Jersey: 1996.
36. *Physicians' Desk Reference.* Medical Economics Company, Montvale, New Jersey: 1997.
37. D'Amicis Amleto and Viani, Rinantonio. The Consumption of Coffee. In: *Caffeine, Coffee, and Health.* Ed S. Garattini. Raven Press, Ltd. New York. 1993.
38. United States Department of Agriculture. *World Coffee Situation.* Foreign Agriculture Service. Circular Series, FCOF 1-93.
39. Wolman W. Instant and decaffeinated coffee. *JAMA.* 1955;159:250.
40. Food and Agriculture Organization, United Nations. FAOSTAT Commodity Balance Sheets. France, 1994.
41. International Coffee Organization. Summary of National Coffee Drinking Study, Winter 1981. London, 1981.
42. National Coffee Association. Winter Drinking Study, 1996 (personal communication).
43. James JE. Caffeine, health and commercial interests. *Addiction.* 1994;89:1595-99.
44. Andrews MC. Avenues for Growth: A 20-year review of the US Specialty Coffee Market. Specialty Coffee Association of America.
45. Reese J. Starbucks inside the coffee cult. America's red-hot caffeine peddler gives new meaning to "addiction," "precision," and "barista." If you doubt that coffee means business, consider: a latte a. *Fortune.* December 9, 1996. pp. 190.
46. Raloff J. For coffee drinkers, a shift in the daily grind. Tufts University Diet and Nutrition Letter. July 1, 1994. Vol 12, pp 4.
47. Groisser DS. A study of caffeine in tea. *Am J Clin Nutr.* 1978;31:1727-31.
48. Engels F. Caffeine dependency 'brewing.' Tufts University Diet and Nutrition Letter, November 11, 1995.

Chapter 10

Basic Metabolism and Physiological Effects of the Methylxanthines

Gene A. Spiller

CONTENTS

I. INTRODUCTION

This chapter is intended as a brief overview of the basic metabolism and physiological effects of caffeine and other methylxanthines. It is designed in a form to make possible easy access to key points on each topic, rather than as an in-depth discussion and review. In the spirit of a book

0-8493-2647-8/98/$0.00+$.50

intended to cover caffeine and related compounds in human nutrition, the focus will be on absorption, disposition, gastrointestinal, cardiovascular, renal, and endocrinological and neurophysiological effects as an introduction to other chapters in this book where specific points are discussed in detail such as the effect of coffee on serum cholesterol or performance. The aim of this chapter is to offer a quick, easily accessible guide to key points as they may be useful to the nutritionist, physician, or other health professional rather than to the research biochemist or physiologist.

II. BASIC METABOLISM[1-3]

1. Caffeine increases the metabolic rate. This is a very early finding dating back to 1917. This calorigenic effect is probably the reason for the desire for caffeine beverages in cold climates. This effect is true in lean as well as obese subjects.
2. Caffeine and other methylxanthines are essentially non-ionized under physiological conditions.
3. Caffeine and other methylxanthines easily cross biological membranes; pH affects the rate of absorption.
4. After 20 min the percentage absorbed is 9% at pH 2.1, 14% at pH 3.5, and 22% at pH 7.0. These values refer to the pH of the caffeine solution as it enters the stomach of subjects.
5. The percentage of binding to plasma protein is low for caffeine (35%) and theobromine (15 to 25%), but fairly high for theophylline (55 to 67%). This higher binding of theophylline should be considered when it is used as a prescription drug.
6. The key metabolites of caffeine (a trimethylxanthine) found in plasma, are the dimethylxanthines paraxanthine, theophylline, and theobromine; the monomethylxanthine 1-methylxanthine; the C-8 oxidized monomethylxanthine 1-methyluric acid; and the ring oxidized uracil: 5-acetyl-amino-6-amino-3-methyluracil.
7. The catabolism and the amount remaining in the body of males and females is given in Table 1. Females on oral contraceptives have more caffeine left in the body than females not on contraceptives in all periods, but this is especially noticeable in the 12- to 24-h period.
8. Free fatty acids and glycerol rise in the plasma following caffeine and methylxanthine administration, showing a major effect on adipose tissues.
9. Caffeine can mobilize calcium from cells.
10. Various factors affect the pharmacokinetics of caffeine:
    a. Cigarette smoking increases clearance.
    b. Liver failure slows clearance.

TABLE 1

Catablism of Caffeine by Humans Administered 5 mg/kg per os

Observation period (h)	Rate of catabolism (μg/min/kg)	Amount catabolized (μg/kg)	Cumulative amount catabolized (μg/kg)	Amount remaining in body (μg/kg)	Cumulative amount excreted (μg/kg)
Males					
0-1	11.1	645	645	4,294	18
1-3	7.2	867	1,512	3,427	45
3-5	6.9	829	2,341	2,598	57
5-8	4.8	860	3,201	1,738	63
8-12	3.8	922	4,123	816	70
12-24	1.1	744	4,867	42	82
Females					
0-1	17.3	1,021	1,021	3,979	19
1-3	6.7	806	1,827	3,173	44
3-5	6.1	727	2,554	2,446	54
5-8	4.6	828	3,382	1,618	58
8-12	3.1	732	4,114	886	63
12-24	1.0	736	4,850	150	66
Females on oral contraceptives					
0-1	7.2	434	434	4,497	28
1-3	3.4	391	825	4,106	50
3-5	4.6	541	1,366	3,687	65
5-8	3.5	611	1,977	3,076	81
8-12	3.5	812	2,789	2,264	99
12-24	1.6	1,144	3,933	1,120	116

From Yesair, S.W., Branfman, A.R., and Callahan, M.M., Human disposition and some biochemical aspects of methylxanthines, in *The Methylxanthine Beverages and Foods: Chemistry, Consumption and Health Effects,* Spiller, G.A., Ed., Alan R. Liss, New York, 1984, 215. With permission.

c. Premature and full-term newborns have slow elimination.

d. In the second and third trimester of pregnancy clearance is decreased.

e. Genetic factors seem to contribute, probably due to variation in the acetylation of N-acetyltransferase, and there seems to be a bimodal distribution: some people are *fast* and others are *slow acetylators.*

III. BASIC PHYSIOLOGICAL EFFECTS

A. Neuro- and Endocrine Physiology[3-5]

1. The primary use of caffeine is that of a central nervous system (CNS) stimulation.

2. There is overwhelming evidence that the methylxanthines at average consumption levels act by blocking the effects of the neuromodulator adenosine. Thus, the primary mechanism of action of caffeine taken at food or beverage levels (rather than pharmacological levels) is that of adenosine receptor antagonism. This is probably a main reason for the stimulating effect of caffeine on the CNS.
3. The body responds to chronic presence of caffeine by increasing the number of adenosine receptor sites. This may be one of the reasons for the increased tolerance (and decreased efficacy as a stimulant) to caffeine in heavy coffee and tea drinkers.
4. Caffeine stimulates secretion of serotonin in the cerebral cortex and cerebellum.
5. Caffeine in high doses induces stress-like effects in the pituitary-adrenal axis.
6. Caffeine and theophylline affect cerebral circulation, most likely through their effect as adenosine antagonists.
7. The often severe headaches, common in caffeine withdrawal, appear to be caused by vasodilation of cerebral blood vessels. This action is probably mediated by the action of the methylxanthines on adenosine receptors.

B. Cardiovascular System[3,6-8]

1. Caffeine and other methylxanthines affect cardiovascular function by directly modifying contractility of the heart and blood vessels and, indirectly, by influencing neurotransmission in the CNS and peripheral nervous system.
2. In nonhabitual coffee users, caffeine may cause a small rise in blood pressure that usually returns to pre-ingestion levels after 3 to 4 h.
3. Caffeine causes a rise in plasma epinephrine and norepinephrine in subjects unused to caffeine beverages.
4. This blood pressure and the plasma epinephrine and norepinephrine (2 and 3 above) effect of caffeine disappear after a few days, even if heavy coffee consumption continues.
5. Extremely heavy coffee drinkers often have tachycardia and extrasystoles.
6. Some effects of caffeine on the cardiovascular system may be related to modification of the Ca^{2+} content of the cells or its distribution within the cell.
7. Electrophysiological changes take place in the human heart even under the influence of limited doses of caffeine.
8. Caffeine and theophylline increase the conduction velocity in the heart.

9. Heavy coffee drinking raises the levels of plasma homocysteine, a risk for heart disease. The dose response of plasma homocysteine to coffee appears stronger than the association to serum cholesterol levels. Heavy coffee consumption was found to cause an increase of about 2 mmol/L.
10. Possible effects of coffee on blood coagulation factors need further study, even though possible links may exist.

Chapter 14 covers the effects of coffee and caffeine on serum cholesterol.

C. Gastrointestinal System[3,9]

1. Individual sensitivity to coffee drinking may or may not be related to its caffeine content. Other compounds found in coffee are probably responsible, as the same individuals can often drink tea without adverse gastrointestinal effect.
2. In some studies, over 60% of participants reported adverse gastrointestinal effects of coffee, such as acid indigestion, heartburn, abdominal pain, and symptoms due to gas or constipation.
3. Heartburn is probably the major reason for people discontinuing the use of coffee.
4. Caffeine stimulates gastric secretion. Other factors in coffee besides caffeine also cause increase gastric secretion. This is probably the most striking effect of coffee on the gastrointestinal tract.
5. Coffee can produce emesis.
6. Methylxanthines affect gastric and intestinal motility, but probably not the mouth-to-cecum transit time.
7. Coffee stimulates gall bladder contraction.
8. Caffeine and theophylline stimulate pancreatic hormone secretions even in normal doses.
9. Liver metabolism is affected by methylxanthines. In high doses, theophylline and caffeine increase the level of cyclic AMP. Very high levels of methylxanthines decrease the level of branched chain and aromatic amino acids in plasma. Coffee appears to have little effect on ethanol metabolism.

D. Respiratory System And Skeletal Muscle[3,10]

1. Caffeine stimulates respiration and has been used in apneic spells in premature infants.
2. The neurotransmitters dopamine and serotonin are the likely mediators of this effect.

3. Theophylline causes relaxation of tracheal smooth muscle.
3. Theophylline is used pharmacologically to manage asthma. Therapeutic effect is seen at concentrations in plasma above 10 mg/L. At 20 mg/L, adverse effects limit the usefulness of theophylline.
5. Methylxanthines, especially caffeine, affect skeletal muscle contractility.
6. Tremor is a frequent side effect of caffeine or theophylline consumption and tremulousness is often attributed to caffeine by the public.
7. Caffeine increases the effect of acetylcholine or cholinesterase inhibitors.

E. Renal System[3,6]

1. The diuretic effect of the methylxanthines is well known. Theophylline is the most potent diuretic, followed by caffeine and theobromine.
2. The major cause of the diuretic effect is an increase in renal blood flow and glomerular filtration rate.
3. Theophylline and caffeine enhance renin release from the kidneys.
4. Most likely the major action of methylxanthines as adenosine antagonist is the reason for these effects on the renal system.

ACKNOWLEDGMENTS

The author wishes to acknowledge the chapters of Drs. Kenneth Hirsh; David W. Yesair, Alan R. Branfman and Marianne M. Callahan; Bertil B. Fredholm; and Eliot Spindel in *The Methylxanthine Beverages and Foods: Chemistry, Consumption and Health Effects* (Alan R. Liss, 1984) that have been a valuable resource in writing this chapter.

REFERENCES

1. Yesair, D. W., Branfman, A. R., and Callahan, M. M., Human disposition and some biochemical aspects of methylxanthines, in *The Methylxanthine Beverages and Foods: Chemistry, Consumption and Health Effects*, Spiller, G. A., Ed., Alan R. Liss, New York, 1984, 215.
2. Arnaud, M. J., Metabolism of caffeine and other components of coffee, in *Caffeine, Coffee, and Health*, Garattini, S., Ed., Raven Press, New York, 1993, 43.
3. Milon, H., Guidoux, R., and Antonioli, J. A., Physiological effects of coffee and its components, in *Coffee, Vol. 3: Physiology*, Clarke, R. J. and Macrae, R., Elsevier Applied Science, London, 1988, 81.

4. Hirsh, K., Central nervous system pharmacology of the dietary methylxanthines, in *The Methylxanthine Beverages and Foods: Chemistry, Consumption and Health Effects*, Spiller, G. A., Ed., Alan R. Liss, New York, 1984, 235.
5. Spindel, E., Action of the methylxanthines on the pituitary and pituitary-dependent hormones, in *The Methylxanthine Beverages and Foods: Chemistry, Consumption and Health Effects*, Spiller, G. A., Ed., Alan R. Liss, New York, 1984, 355.
6. Fredholm, B. B., Cardiovascular and renal actions of methylxanthines, in *The Methylxanthine Beverages and Foods: Chemistry, Consumption and Health Effects*, Spiller, G. A., Ed., Alan R. Liss, New York, 1984, 303.
7. Daly, J. W., Mechanism of action of caffeine, in *Caffeine, Coffee, and Health*, Garattini, S., Ed., Raven Press, New York, 1993, 97.
8. Nygård, O., Refsum, H., Ueland, P. M., Stensvold, I., Nordrehaug, J. E., Kvåle, G., and Vollset, S. E., Coffee consumption and plasma total homocysteine: The Hordaland Homocysteine Study, *Am J Clin Nutr*, 65, 136, 1997.
9. Fredholm, B. B., Gastrointestinal and metabolic effects of methylxanthines, in *The Methylxanthine Beverages and Foods: Chemistry, Consumption and Health Effects*, Spiller, G. A., Ed., Alan R. Liss, New York, 1984, 331.
10. Fredholm, B. B., Effects of methylxanthines on skeletal muscle and on respiration, in *The Methylxanthine Beverages and Foods: Chemistry, Consumption and Health Effects*, Spiller, G. A., Ed., Alan R. Liss, New York, 1984, 365.

Chapter 11

CAFFEINE AS AN ERGOGENIC AID

Roland J. Lamarine

CONTENTS

0-8493-2647-8/98/$0.00+$.50

The arrival of the Centennial Olympic games in Atlanta, Georgia, during the summer of 1996, marked the convergence of a great athletic competition with the home of perhaps the world's favorite soft drink, Coca Cola. This soft drink company, a leading sponsor of the games, provides a legal product that supplies a significant amount of a psychoactive and a purported ergogenic drug, caffeine. This chapter will explore the evidence surrounding the topic of caffeine as an ergogenic aid.

Caffeine may have been first used by athletes in strength related competitions prompting the International Olympic Committee (IOC) to list caffeine as a restricted substance until the 1972 Munich games by which time research had suggested caffeine's lack of efficacy as an ergogenic aid in competition requiring strength.[1] Caffeine's absence from the IOC restricted list was short-lived when subsequent research provided strong evidence that it may significantly enhance endurance performance.[2,3]

I. METHODOLOGICAL WEAKNESSES IN CAFFEINE RESEARCH

The literature regarding caffeine's potential ergogenicity offers a number of inconsistent findings and some that are clearly contradictory. A lack of standardization of research protocols probably contributes to some of the confusion. Problems encountered include the extrapolation of research findings from caffeine naive test animals to caffeine tolerant humans; lack of standardized experimental protocols including variations in the intensity and duration of work performed; differences in caffeine dosages and in time of administration; physiological and somatic differences in test subjects, including athletic conditioning and ratio of muscle fiber types; subjects' habituation to caffeine; and variations in the test environments employed for the research.[4,5]

II. MECHANISMS OF ACTION

Ideally, to establish a causal relationship between caffeine and improved athletic performance, evidence would be obtained from epidemiological population studies, followed by careful, double-blind, placebo controlled experimental protocols isolating the purported etiological agent (caffeine), and eventually culminating with strong laboratory findings explaining the previously identified ergogenic effects in humans in terms of physiological mechanisms of action.

Caffeine's ergogenicity has been suggested by a number of sometimes controversial laboratory experiments which will be examined later in this chapter. In a somewhat peculiar situation, research on caffeine as an ergogenic agent is unusually abundant; however, the picture that has emerged is anything but clear.

Three major mechanisms of action have dominated as possible explanations for the ergogenic potential of caffeine in the enhancement of exercise performance. These three mechanisms involve (1) the mobilization of intracellular calcium from the sarcoplasmic reticulum of skeletal muscle, (2) the increase of cyclic-3′,5′-adenosine monophosphate (cAMP) by the inhibition of phosphodiesterases in muscles and adipocytes, and (3) the competitive antagonism of adenosine receptors, primarily in the central nervous system (CNS).[6-9]

A. Mobilization Of Intracellular Calcium

For over three decades, laboratory research has shown caffeine to be effective at mobilizing calcium in skeletal muscle. *In vitro* experiments have amply demonstrated that caffeine lowers the excitability threshold and extends the length of muscular contractions via calcium release from the sarcoplasmic reticulum.[10-12] Caffeine also inhibits calcium reuptake by the sarcoplasmic reticulum, perpetuating calcium availability for muscle work.[13-16] Also, caffeine promotes increased twitch tension development in muscles.[17,18]

Despite the apparent promise for this line of research to explain caffeine's potential ergogenicity, the doses of caffeine necessary to produce significant calcium shifts are midway between toxic and lethal levels when transposed to *in vitro* situations.[5] These dosage requirements suggest that the mobilization of intracellular calcium is not a viable explanation for caffeine's potential ergogenic effects in live human subjects.

B. Increased Cellular cAMP Levels

cAMP has been identified as significant in the control of glycogen metabolism and peripheral lipolysis.[19,20] Caffeine inhibits cyclic nucleotide phosphodiesterase's activity blocking the enzymatic breakdown of cAMP. This action increases lipolysis via increased cAMP levels leading to increased levels of free fatty acids (FFAs) during exercise and yielding a glycogen sparing effect during prolonged endurance activity.[9]

Once again, however, an attractive mechanism identified in the laboratory encounters problems of external validity when transposed into an *in vivo* setting. The dosages of caffeine needed to inhibit phosphodiesterases are at toxic levels for living subjects suggesting a lack of pragmatic utility for this particular explanation.[21-23]

C. Adenosine Receptor Inhibition

The most promising mechanism of action, which may account for some of caffeine's potential ergogenic effects, involves its demonstrated ability as a competitive antagonist of the depressant effects of adenosine analogs in the central nervous system. Adenosine and its derivatives have been shown to inhibit neuronal electrical activity, the release of neurotransmitters, and to interfere with synaptic transmission.[19,24-27]

Caffeine is also effective in the antagonism of peripheral adenosine (type I) receptors, which are known to inhibit lipolysis by subduing adenylate cyclase activity.[28] The appeal of this mechanism of action is that the majority of the pharmacological effects of adenosine on the central nervous system can be inhibited by doses of caffeine that are well within physiologically non-toxic levels comparable to only a couple of cups of coffee.[5]

III. STRENGTH/ANAEROBIC POWER

The absorption pattern of caffeine throughout the body parallels the distribution of water in the body, leading to its heaviest concentrations in muscle tissue yet most research suggests no ergogenic effects on strength performance under anaerobic conditions.[29,30] Ergogenic effects attributable to caffeine have been absent in examinations of the magnitude of endurance during high intensity exercise and in the ability of the body to generate peak power.[31]

Although research has been suggestive of caffeine modulated increases in muscular contractions leading to hand tremor, it is more likely that the hand tremor response is the result of caffeine's effects on the central nervous system.[32] There is even evidence that moderate doses of caffeine may actually diminish muscle tone.[32]

A. Laboratory Studies

Somewhat of a dichotomy exists in the research literature pertaining to caffeine's ergogenic potential to enhance short-term, intense exercise. In general, laboratory research (*in vitro/in situ*) has consistently demonstrated positive results related to caffeine's ability to generate increased muscular force. Human studies have consistently been suggestive of no significant effects on short-term, high intensity performance. There have been a number of studies, some dating as far back as 1942, indicating that caffeine could enhance power output in fatigued human subjects.[33] Caffeine has been shown to enhance neural transmission, which could be instrumental in elevating motor neuron recruitment.[34] Caffeine has been associated with increased muscle contractility.[35] Some studies have indicated that caffeine potentiates twitch tension in muscle *in vitro* and *in situ*,[35-37] and increases muscle contractility *in situ*.[35]

Caffeine was found to significantly increase muscular force output at low frequencies of electrical stimulation (10 to 50 Hz), but at high frequencies (100 Hz) there was no significant increase in maximal voluntary contractions or endurance.[38] Such results may suggest that at high intensity, the sympathetic response may negate the effects noted at low intensity.[39]

B. Human Studies

Collomp and colleagues[40] found significant increases in swimming velocity in highly trained swimmers compared to untrained occasional swimmers following ingestion of 250 mg of caffeine. Anselme and coworkers[41] also noted positive effects on maximal anaerobic power in a 6-s cycle sprint, following ingestion of 250 mg of caffeine by a group of recreational athletes.

Wiles and associates[42] found that caffeine decreased the time needed to complete a 1500-m run and that it increased the velocity of the "finishing burst" among well-trained, middle distance runners. Jacobson and colleagues[43] examined 20 elite, strength-trained athletes to determine the effects of caffeine on knee extensors and flexors. They found increases in voluntary strength and power output in this group of well-trained athletes.

Numerous studies have suggested that caffeine produces no significant effects on power or fatigue during cycle ergometry,[31] no significant differences in grip strength,[37] no significant improvement in isokinetic strength of untrained subjects,[44-46] no significant effect on power output,[47] and no effect on work capacity.[48,49]

Perkins and Williams[50] found no significant effects of caffeine on time to exhaustion during high intensity exercise on a bicycle ergometer. Williams and colleagues[51] also failed to detect significant effects on maximal handgrip strength using untrained subjects. In a subsequent study[31] of short term, high intensity exercise on a cycle ergometer, they found that caffeine induced no significant improvements in delayed fatigue, peak power, and total work.

Collomp and associates,[52] using a Wingate Anaerobic Test, found that caffeine did not affect maximal anaerobic capacity or power in six untrained subjects. Bond et al.[29] found no differences in peak anaerobic power among 12 trained athletes, while other researchers have detected no ergogenic effects associated with the use of caffeine on performance in the shot put, long jump, or 100-m dash.[5]

IV. SUMMARY OF CAFFEINE'S EFFECTS ON STRENGTH

Jacobson et al.[43] suggested that some of the disagreement in results among studies of caffeine's effects on strength may be related to (1) greater dosages used for *in vitro* research, (2) differences in experimental protocols, (3) nutritional variations among subjects (i.e., high carbohydrate diets may inhibit the ergogenic effects of caffeine),[53] (4) delay of muscular fatigue, (5) differences in fiber type ratios of subjects, (6) the use of highly conditioned vs. untrained subjects, and (7) altered perceived exertion levels and improved attitude towards exercise.

Some researchers reject the explanation that caffeine inhibits glycogen depletion during short term exercise[54] but there is an increasing abundance of research supporting the notion of variable sensitivity to caffeine by muscle type. Muscles with higher ratios of type I fibers appear more sensitive than type II fibers, both in animal[55,56] and human models.[57]

In their study of untrained vs. trained swimmers, Collomp et al.[40] suggested that specific training may be the catalyst that stimulates caffeine's ergogenic effects during high intensity, anaerobic activity. The results of many studies have also suggested that only well-trained athletes derive significant benefits from caffeine due to the athletes' previously stimulated lipolytic activity and the increased size and density of their mitochondria.[40,52,58,59]

There is no consensus in the literature concerning caffeine's ergogenic potential to enhance anaerobic power but the most recent work is suggestive of little or no anaerobic benefits. Williams[60] concludes that the "effects of caffeine on muscular endurance and fatigue are at present equivocal", while Conlee[39] surmises "it appears that caffeine does not increase...maximal force output" and provides "little benefit to power activities". Conlee also makes the excellent point that the reality of caffeine's ineffectiveness as an anaerobic ergogenic aid contrasts vividly with many athletes' perceptions of its ergogenicity. Purported benefits could be related to previous training, muscle fiber type ratios, or to a placebo effect.

V. ENDURANCE PERFORMANCE

A series of studies conducted in the late 1970s at Ball State University's Human Performance Laboratory by Costill and associates[61-63] has established caffeine as an effective ergogenic aid for the enhancement of endurance in "prolonged exhaustive exercise". Many studies have attempted to replicate the outcomes of these early investigations with mixed results. As the research has become more sophisticated, the results have indicated a complex relationship between caffeine and endurance performance, a relationship that is possibly mediated by a variety of intevening variables.

A. Endurance Research Caveats

1. Subject Variables

Some of the more likely candidates to serve as moderating variables include the level of prior physical training of the subjects. Well-conditioned athletes exhibit different physiological responses to exercise protocols than do their less fit counterparts.[5] Athletes in particular sports are known to possess differing muscle fiber type ratios and caffeine has been demonstrated to have varying effects related to muscle fiber type.[39] Another experimental subject variable is nutritional status, especially whether subjects have been maintaining a high carbohydrate diet, since research has indicated that carbohydrate loading may negate caffeine's ergogenic effects.[53]

An extremely important subject variable is whether subjects are habituated to caffeine and to what extent, if any, they may be caffeine tolerant. To test the influence of caffeine habituation on exercise performance, Fisher et al.[64] recruited six habituated (>600 mg/d) caffeine users for a 1-h treadmill running protocol in both caffeine and placebo trials. In one set of trials, caffeine tolerant subjects continued their normal caffeine ingestion, while in another set they were tested after a 4-d withdrawal from caffeine. A caffeine dosage of 5 mg/kg of body weight was administered 1 h prior to the experimental trials. The researchers failed to detect significant differences between placebo and caffeine trials before the 4-d withdrawal from caffeine suggesting that the subjects had developed a tolerance to the ergogenic effects of caffeine. After the 4-d abstinence, however, significant improvements were noted including a near doubling of pre-exercise plasma FFA levels.

Finally, there is virtually no mention of the fact that the majority of test subjects in the caffeine research literature are reported to be males, so that hormonal differences in respect to caffeine's ergogenic effects may be a topic that requires further examination.

2. Dosing Variables

Another category of potential confounding variables includes dosing issues. Caffeine researchers have administered a wide variety of experimental dosages, an issue related obviously to physiological effects but also of interest to those concerned with caffeine doping. The timing of the administration of the caffeine may also be an important factor.[53] The majority of the studies administer caffeine 60 min before testing, ostensibly because plasma caffeine levels peak 30 to 60 min after administration, yet research also indicates that plasma FFA levels peak 3 to 4 h after the consumption of caffeine.[1]

Problems may also be associated with the difficulty of separating caffeine's potential ergogenic effects from its psychostimulant effects. Many studies suggest caffeine decreases subjects' rate of perceived exertion (RPE),[61,63,65-67] providing a psychological advantage facilitating greater effort during exercise. Closely related is the notion that in placebo controlled studies, it is virtually impossible to blind subjects to the experimental treatment, since caffeine produces an easily detectable psychostimulant effect.[65]

3. *Exercise Regimen Variables*

A final category of potential confounders includes the variety of exercise regimens and environments utilized in the research, everything from laboratory cycle ergometers (most common) to cross-country skiing at high altitude in adverse weather conditions.

Even this brief survey suggests the complexity of attempting to determine the efficacy of caffeine as an ergogenic aid for endurance activity in view of so many serious potential limitations to the research. With this in mind, the next section reviews some of the more significant research findings.

Since the focus of this chapter is on caffeine as an ergogenic aid for humans, the major emphasis will be on human studies but it should be noted that most of the animal research has produced no effects or, in some cases, negative results associated with endurance performance.[9] It has been suggested that variability in muscle glycogen storage capabilities between rodents and humans may be a significant variable for explaining why caffeine seems ineffective at improving metabolic performance or endurance in rodents.[9] These findings may have some bearing on the notion that caffeine produces some of its ergogenic effects in humans and not in animals as a result of its psychostimulant properties, since attitude and motivation may be of lesser importance in less cerebral animal species.

4. *Research Producing Positive Findings*

Perhaps the most influential and most cited work on the topic of caffeine and endurance is the original study by Costill et al.[61] in which nine competitive cyclists (including two women) exercised to exhaustion on a bicycle ergometer. In the experiemental protocol, subjects received 330 mg caffeine 1-h prior to exercise. Results unequivocably demonstated that caffeine allowed subjects to cycle significantly longer, to perceive their efforts as significantly easier, and to exhibit significantly higher rates of fat oxidation.

The next major study, in this series, was conducted by Ivy and colleagues[62] and it apparently employed many of the same nine cyclists from the first study. This experiment measured work production during 2 h on a cycle ergometer. One hour prior to testing, subjects received half of a 500-mg dose of caffeine, the rest of which was administered periodically throughout the session. Again the results were clear cut. RPEs were the same for experimental and placebo trials but significantly more work was accomplished during the caffeine trials.

The last in this series of studies was lead by Essig[63] and it investigated the glycogen sparing effects of caffeine on seven male subjects using leg ergometer cycling, after the administration of 5 ml/kg body weight of caffeine, 1 h prior to testing. Again the results were unequivocal and showed a 42% decrease in use of muscle glycogen during the caffeine trials.

A decade later, in a published interview, Costill reflected on the diversity of subsequent research findings following this intial spate of positive results and he speculated that they may be related to subject selection variables. He felt that some people may be positive responders to caffeine, since in the first two studies his group conducted, several of the same subjects were employed.[39]

Many other studies have subsequently produced positive results. Berglund and Hemmingsson[65] examined the effects of 6 mg/kg caffeine on 14 competitive cross-country skiers in a 20-km ski run at both high (2900 m) and low (300 m) altitude. Subjects were administered caffeine 1 h prior to testing. There were significant decreases in time needed to complete the run at low altitude and even greater improvements at high altitude. It should be noted that dramatic differences in weather conditions during the different trials may have contaminated results. Also of interest, the authors observed that when the double blind code was broken, approximately 80% of the subjects had been able to distinguish between placebo and caffeine.

Cadarette et al.[68] found significant improvement associated with the administration of 2 to 9 mg/kg caffeine 60 min prior to conducting a treadmill endurance protocol. Sasaki and co-workers[69] also reported similar results. Sasaki used five male distance runners and in both of these last two studies, caffeine was administered 1 h prior to testing. Interestingly, Sasaki's group also examined the effects of sucrose and sucrose with caffeine and found that all three treatments yielded significant improvement in endurance running but fat utilization was highest in the caffeine trials.

McNaughton[70] used a bicycle ergometer to examine caffeine's effects on high intensity, short duration (approximately 7 min) activity using relatively caffeine naive subjects who received a high dose (10 to 15 mg/kg) of caffeine one hour before testing. This study showed significant enhancement of work performance and increases in FFA associated with caffeine use by caffeine naive subjects.

Flinn et al.[66] conducted an interesting study using nine recreational athletes who were caffeine naive. A 10 mg/kg dose was administered 3 h prior to testing on a cycle ergometer. These researchers attributed their positive results to (1) the use of caffeine naive subjects, (2) high doses of caffeine, (3) the timing of the dose, 3 h prior to exercise allowing FFA levels to peak, and (4) the use of recreational rather than elite athletes.

In another well-designed study, Graham and Spriet[71] used seven competitive runners, who were tested both in cycling and running to exhaustion protocols using 9 mg/kg doses of caffeine administered 1 h prior to testing. Their results, dramatic increases in endurance times following administration of caffeine, provided some useful insights. Mode of exercise (running vs. cycling) did not seem to affect the outcomes; well-trained athletes on high carbohydrate diets clearly derived ergogenic effects in contradiction to previous research results. This study also demonstrated that there was no effect related to subjects' history of caffeine use.

In another study, Spriet et al.[72] examined the glycogen sparing effects of caffeine on eight recreational cyclists following the administration of 9 mg/kg of caffeine 1 h prior to testing. This research also showed a significant glycogen sparing effect.

In an interesting twist, Fulco et al.[73] examined caffeine's effects on endurance both at sea level and at altitude (4300 m). Eight healthy, male soldiers, who were not elite athletes but who were regular joggers, were instructed to cycle to exhaustion. Caffeine (4 mg/kg) was administered 1 h prior to testing. Results were surprising in that no ergogenic effects were detected at sea level but a 54% improvement in time to exhaustion was observed at altitude. Decreased RPE was noted for the caffeine trials but the researchers attributed the ergogenic effects to either a caffeine-induced increase in tidal volume or diminished altitude-induced impairment in muscular force production during exercise.

In yet another interesting protocol, Passman and colleagues[74] focused on dose-response effects. Nine well-trained cyclists received either 0, 5, 9, or 13 mg/kg caffeine 1 h prior to cycling to exhaustion. All subjects were habituated to caffeine (minimum use 100 mg/d). Significant increases in both endurance and FFA production were associated with caffeine but no significant dose-response effects were noted.

Similar results were obtained by Graham and Spriet[75] using eight well trained, male endurance athletes who received either 0, 3, 6, or 9 mg/kg caffeine 1 h before testing. Subjects ran to exhaustion and showed significant improvements in endurance for the 3- and 6-mg doses but not for the 9-mg dose. The authors suggested the lack of significant results at the higher dose may have been related to the large number of caffeine naive subjects in the study.

Cole and co-workers[67] examined perceived exertion and work output using a cycle ergometer with 10 healthy males, 8 of whom were classified as caffeine naive. In the experimental trials, subjects consumed 6 mg/kg caffeine 1 h before testing. Caffeine significantly improved work performance, even though the perception of effort was held constant for each trial. Subjects did more work on caffeine even while they were instructed to work at a predetermined RPE during both experimental and placebo trials.

VI. RESEARCH INDICATING NO EFFECTS ON ENDURANCE

Despite the impressive number of studies suggesting an ergogenic effect related to caffeine use prior to engagement in endurance activities, there are also many studies that have failed to demonstrate significant effects. Powers et al.[30] examined time to exhaustion on a cycle ergometer for seven trained, male runners who were also recreational cyclists. Subjects received 5 mg/kg caffeine 1 h prior to testing. No significant effects were noted in time to exhaustion despite significant increases in FFA.

Butts and Crowell,[58] in an attempt to replicate the early work of Costill, recruited 28 untrained subjects (15 males) to participate in a cycle ergometer test. Subjects were administered 300-mg caffeine 1 h prior to testing. No significant effects were detected in time to exhaustion but a wide variation in subject response to caffeine was observed by the researchers.

Bond et al.,[76] using a similar protocol, administered 5 mg/kg caffeine 1 h prior to testing to six healthy, male volunteers. No significant improvements in performance on a cycle ergometer were noted. Sasaki and colleagues[77] also failed to demonstrate any ergogenic effects for treadmill running among seven male subjects who ingested 800-mg caffeine over 2 h of running.

Falk et al.[54] examined time to exhaustion on a cycle ergometer following a 40-km march. Subjects consisted of 23 caffeine naive males who were administered 5-mg/kg caffeine. Despite significant decreases in RPE for the experimental group, there were no significant differences in time to exhaustion between experimental and control groups.

Tarnopolsky and colleagues[78] studied six trained, male runners using a 90-min treadmill run. Subjects, who were habituated to caffeine (200 mg/day) were administerd 6-mg/kg caffeine 1 h prior to testing. No significant differences in metabolic or neuromuscular effects were detected, although plasma FFA was significantly elevated following administration of caffeine.

Dodd et al.[48] tested 17 moderately trained males for VO_2 max and time to exhaustion on a bicycle ergometer. Experimental trials involved the administration of 3- or 5-mg/kg caffeine 1 h prior to testing. Caffeine had no effect on exercise performance. Since nearly half of the subjects were caffeine naive (<25 mg/d), while the other half were caffeine tolerant (>310 mg/d), the researchers were able to conclude that even though caffeine had no significant effects on performance, it did produce a variety of physiologically significant effects (heart rate and expired ventilation volume) in the caffeine naive group.

Fulco et al.,[73] in a study described earlier, noted significant caffeine moderated effects on endurance at altitude but failed to detect significant effects in the same untrained subjects when cycling at sea level.

VII. SUMMARY OF CAFFEINE'S EFFECTS AS AN ERGOGENIC AID

A. Muscular Strength

In vitro and *in situ* laboratory results have consistently indicated that caffeine may be useful for improving the production of muscular force.[34-37] Human studies, though producing mixed results, have consistently been suggestive of no significant effects of caffeine on anaerobic power.[29,31,37,44-52] A variety of explanations have been proposed to reconcile the differences between laboratory and human studies including the possibilities that larger, potentially toxic doses used in the laboratory may elicit different physiological responses than those available to living human subjects using much lower and safer doses.[5, 19,21,23] Of greater concern are the handful of studies that used human subjects and also produced positive results, such as increased swimming velocity,[40] increased maximal anaerobic power,[41] improved leg strength,[43] and faster running times.[42] Most of the positive results in strength tests have involved trained subjects.

Such results suggest a need for further research comparing trained with untrained subjects, along with an examination of muscle fiber type ratios of experimental subjects. Also, the question of subjects' habituation to caffeine needs to be explored more fully. For the present, the reported ergogenic effects of caffeine on muscular strength must be viewed with skepticism and perhaps be attributed to the psychostimulant properties of caffeine.

B. Endurance Activities

In the case of caffeine's ergogenic effects on endurance during extended exercise of submaximal intensity (70 to 85% VO_2 max), animal studies do not offer much support.[9] A large number of human studies, however, are clearly suggestive of significant ergogenic effects on endurance.

Since there are also a large number of studies indicating no effects, it is apparent that caffeine's ergogenic properties are mediated by one or more intervening variables that have not been fully elucidated. There are a number of intriguing candidates to serve as mediating variables. Some researchers believe that untrained persons are better candidates to respond positively to caffeine as an endurance enhancing agent but lack of training may simply be a marker for dietary differences. Some research has suggested that a high carbohydrate diet negates caffeine's ergogenic effects and trained athletes often include a high carbohydrate diet as part of their training program.[53] Unfortunately for this line of thought, not all studies have shown that a high carbohydrate diet negates caffeine's ergogenicity.[71]

Type of exercise has been suggested as an intervening variable but at least one well-designed study has contradicted this hypothesis.[71] Caffeine dose would seem like a logical candidate as a moderating variable, yet research suggests that relatively low doses equivalent to one or two cups of coffee may be sufficient to elicit an ergogenic response in some subjects and that high doses may not elicit such a response.[2] A major consideration concerns the subjects' prior use of caffeine and, in the case of aerobic activity, there is strong evidence that caffeine naive subjects are more responsive to its ergogenic effects.[66] Caffeine tolerant individuals would benefit from a 4-d withdrawal period prior to competition.

Perhaps the most intriguing perspective is that caffeine's major effects have little to do with muscles and fat metabolism but result from its psychostimulant effects, enhancing mood, improving attitude towards exercise, and thus motivating athletes to work harder and longer. This would account for its purported inability to alter strength, which may be a less psychologically malleable variable, while endurance performance is sometimes believed to be more amenable to force of will.

VIII. ETHICAL CONSIDERATIONS

Athletes have been trying to get an edge on their competitors probably even before the ancient Greek Olympians and Macedonian athletes were purported to have eaten ground donkey hooves to improve their running abilities. Today, a variety of ergogenically effective anabolic steroids are used by internationally renowned athletes. A few years ago, a successful Olympic track star confided to this writer that he did not want to use anabolic steroids but he was forced to do so because all of his competitors used them and he needed the extra edge just to stay even.

Caffeine occupies a special place among ergogenic aids. First, it is a widely used and readily available legal drug. It is safer than most other ergogenic agents. The research in this chapter leaves little doubt as to its effectiveness in endurance activities. Historically, caffeine has been employed by athletes at least since the 1920s but its popularity has peaked in recent decades following more convincing research as to its ergogenicity.[2]

The idea of regulating caffeine use in connection with athletic competition is not new but it has gained an impetus from the recent widespread abuse by athletes at all levels of competition. Currently, the IOC bans the use of high doses of caffeine, equivalent to approximately eight cups of coffee,[5] an amount that would not be reached by a casual coffee drinker.

Graham et al.[79] noted that more than a quarter of Canadian youth surveyed reported use of caffeine during the last year to improve their athletic performance. The current allowable levels of caffeine permitted by the IOC are well above the minimum dose needed to elicit an ergogenic effect. If the IOC and other regulatory bodies are serious about controlling the use of performance enhancing drugs, then it may be necessary to ban caffeine entirely from competition.

REFERENCES

1. Clarkson, P. M., Nutritional ergogenic aids: Caffeine, *International Journal of Sport Nutrition*, 3, 103, 1993.
2. Jacobson, B. H. and Kulling, F. A., Health and ergogenic effects of caffeine, *British Journal of Sports Medicine*, 23, 34, 1989.
3. Wilcox, J. A., Caffeine and endurance performance, *Sports Science Exchange*, 3, 1990.
4. Grossman, E., Some methodological issues in the conduct of caffeine research, *Food and Chemical Toxicology*, 22, 245, 1984.
5. Nehlig, A. and Debry, G., Caffeine and sport activity: A review, *Journal of Sports Medicine*, 15, 215, 1994.
6. Daly, J. W., Mechanism of action of caffeine, in *Coffee, Caffeine, and Health*, Garattini, S., Ed., Ravens Press, New York, 1993, chap. 4.
7. Nehlig, A., Daval, J. L., and Debry, G., Caffeine and the central nervous system: Mechanisms of action, biochemical, metabolic, and psychostimulant effects, *Brain Research Reviews*, 17, 139, 1992.
8. Snyder, S. H., Adenosine as a mediator of the behavioral effects of xanthines, in *Caffeine: Perspective from Recent Research*, Dews, P. B., Ed., Springer Verlag, Berlin, 1984, chap. 3.
9. Dodd, S. L., Herb, R. A., and Power, S. K., Caffeine and exercise performance, *Sports Medicine*, 15, 14, 1993.
10. Bianchi, C. P., The effect of caffeine on radiocalcium movement in frog sartorius, *Journal of General Physiology*, 44, 845, 1961.
11. Blinks, J. R., Olson, C. B., Jewell, B. R., and Braveny, P., Influence of caffeine and other methyxanthines on mechanical properties of isolated mammalian heart muscle, *Circ Research*, 30, 367, 1972.

12. Isaacson, A., Hinks, M. J., and Taylor, S. R., Contracture and twitch potentiation of fast and slow muscles at 20° and 37° C. *American Journal of Physiology*, 218, 33, 1970.
13. Endo, M., Calcium release from the sarcoplasmic reticulum, *Physiology Review*, 57, 71, 1977.
14. Endo, M., Tanaka, M., and Ogawa, Y., Calcium induced release of calcium from sarcoplasmic reticulum of skinned skeletal muscle fibers, *Nature*, 228, 34, 1970.
15. Fabiato, A. and Fabiato, F., Calcium release from sarcoplasmic reticulum, *Circ Research*, 40, 119, 1977.
16. Stephenson, E. W., Activation of fast skeletal muscle: Contribution of studies on skinned fibers, *American Journal of Physiology*, 240, C1, 1981.
17. Gulati, J. and Babu, A., Contraction kinetics of intact and skinned frog fibers and degree of activation, *Journal of General Physiology*, 86, 479, 1985.
18. Wendt, I. and Stephenson, D., Effects of caffeine on calcium-activated force production in skinned cardiac and skeletal muscle fibers of the rat, *European Journal of Physiology*, 398, 210, 1983.
19. Beavo, J. A., Rogers, N. L., Crofford, O. B., Hardman, J. G., Sutherland, E. W., and Newman, E. V., Effects of xanthine derivatives on lipolysis and on adenosine 3′,5′-monophosphate phosphodiesterase activity, *Molecular Pharmacology*, 6, 597, 1970.
20. Butcher, R. W. and Sutherland, E. W., Adenosine 3′,5′,-monophosphate in biological materials, *Journal of Biological Chemistry*, 237, 1244, 1962.
21. Knapik, J. J., Jones, B. H., Toner, M. M., Daniels, W. L., and Evans, W. J., Influence of caffeine on serum substrate changes during running in trained and untrained individuals, *Biochem Exercise*, 13, 514, 1983.
22. Rall, T. W., Evolution of the mechanism of action of methylxanthines: From calcium mobilizers to antagonists of adenosine receptors, *Pharmacologist*, 24, 277, 1982.
23. Weiss, B. and Hart, W. N., Selective cyclic nucleotide phosphodiesterase inhibitors as potential therapeutic agents, *Annual Review of Pharmacol Toxicol*, 17, 441, 1977.
24. Hollins, C. and Stone, T. W., Adenosine inhibition of aminobutyric release from slices of rat cerebral cortex, *British Journal of Pharmocology*, 69, 107, 1980.
25. Kostopoulos, G. K. and Phillis, J. W., Purinergic depression of neurons in different areas of the rat brain, *Exp Neurol*, 55, 719, 1977.
26. Okada, Y. and Kuroda, Y., Inhibitory action of adenosine and adenosine analogs on neurotransmission in the olfactory cortex slice of guinea pig: Structure-activity relationships, *European Journal of Pharmacology*, 61, 137, 1980.
27. Phillis, J. W. and Wu, J. H., The role of adenosine and its nucleotides in central synaptic transmission, *Prog Neurobiol*, 16, 187, 1983.
28. Zhang, Y. and Wells, J., The effects of chronic caffeine administration on peripheral adenosine receptors, *Journal of Pharmacology and Experimental Therapeutics*, 254, 757, 1990.
29. Bond, V., Gresham, K., McRae, J., and Tearney, R., Caffeine ingestion and isokinetic strength, *British Journal of Sports Medicine*, 20, 135, 1986.
30. Powers, S., Byrd, R., Tulley, R., and Callendar, T., Effects of caffeine ingestion on metabolism and performance during graded exercise, *European Journal of Applied Physiology*, 50, 301, 1983.
31. Williams, J., Signorile, J., Barnes, W., and Henrich, T., Caffeine, maximal power output and fatigue, *British Journal of Sports Medicine*, 22, 132, 1988.
32. Fredholm, B., Effects of methylxanthines on skeletal muscle and on respiration, in *The Methylxanthine Beverages and Foods*, Spiller, G., Ed., Alan R. Liss, New York, 1984, chap. 15.

33. Foltz, E., Ivy, A., and Barborka, C., The use of double work periods in the study of fatigue and the influence of caffeine on recovery, *American Journal of Physiology*, 136, 79, 1942.
34. Waldeck, B., Sensitization by caffeine of central catecholamine receptors, *Journal of Neural Transmission*, 34, 61, 1973.
35. MacIntosh, B. R., Barbee, R. W., and Stainsby, W. N., Contractile response to caffeine of rested and fatigued skeletal muscle, *Medicine and Science in Sports and Exercise*, 13, 95, 1981.
36. Varagic, V. M. and Zugic, M., Interactions of xanthine derivatives, catecholamines, and glucose-6-phosphate on the isolated phrenic nerve diaphragm preparation of the rat, *Pharmacology*, 5, 275, 1971.
37. Yamaguchi, T., Caffeine-induced potentiation of twitches in frog single muscle fiber, *Japanese Journal of Physiology*, 25, 693, 1975.
38. Lopes, J. M., Aubier, M., Jardin, J., Aranda, J. V., and Macklem, P. T., Effects of caffeine on skeletal muscle function before and after fatigue, *Journal of Applied Physiology*, 54, 1303, 1983.
39. Conlee, R. K., Amphetamine, caffeine, and cocaine, in *Ergogenics-Enhancement of Performance in Exercise and Sport*, Lamb, D. R. and Williams, M. H., Eds., Brown & Benchmark, Dubuque, IA, 1991, chap. 8.
40. Collomp, K., Ahmaidi, S., Chatard, J. C., Audran, M., and Prefaut, C., Benefits of caffeine ingestion on sprint performance in trained and untrained swimmers, *International Journal of Applied Physiology*, 64, 377, 1992.
41. Anselme, F., Collomp, K., Mercier, B., Ahmaidi, S., and Prefaut, C., Caffeine increases maximal anaerobic power and blood lactate concentration, *European Journal of Applied Physiology*, 65, 188, 1992.
42. Wiles, J. D., Bird, S. R., Hopkins, J., and Riley, M., Effects of caffeinated coffee on running speed, respiratory factors, blood lactate, and perceived exertion during 1500-m treadmill running, *British Journal of Sports Medicine*, 26 , 116, 1992.
43. Jacobson, B. H., Weber, M. D., Claypool, L., and Hunt, L. E., Effects of caffeine on maximal strength and power in elite male athletes, *British Journal of Sports Medicine*, 26, 276, 1992.
44. Blyth, C. S., Allen, E. M., and Lovingood, B. W., Effects of amphetamine (dexedrine) and caffeine on subjects exposed to heat and exercise stress, *Research Quarterly*, 31, 553, 1960.
45. Bugyi, G. J., The effects of moderate doses of caffeine on fatigue parameters of the forearm flexor muscles, *American Corrective Therapy Journal*, 34, 49, 1980.
46. Jacobson, B. H. and Edwards, S. W., Influence of two levels of caffeine on maximal torque at selected velocities, *Journal of Sports Medicine and Physical Fitness*, 31, 147, 1991.
47. Powers, S. K. and Dodd, S., Caffeine and endurance performance, *Sports Medicine*, 2, 165, 1985.
48. Dodd, S. L., Brooks, E., Powers, S. K., and Tulley, R., The effects of caffeine on graded exercise performance in caffeine naive versus caffeine habituated subjects, *European Journal of Applied Physiology*, 62, 424, 1991.
49. Ganslen, R. V., Balke, B., Nagle, F. J., and Phillips, E. E., Effects of some tranquilizing analeptic and vasodilatory drugs on physical work capacity and orthostatic tolerance, *Aerospace Medicine*, 35, 630, 1974.
50. Perkins, R. and Williams, M. H., Effects of caffeine upon maximal muscular endurance of females, *Medical Science and Sports*, 7, 221, 1975.
51. Williams, J. H., Barnes, W. S., and Gadberry, W. L., Influence of caffeine on force and EMG in rested and fatigued muscle, *American J Phys Med*, 66, 169, 1987.
52. Collomp, K., Ahmaidi, S., Audran, M., Chanal, J. L., and Prefaut, C., Effects of caffeine ingestion on performance and anaerobic metabolism during the Wingate Test, *International Journal of Sports Medicine*, 12, 439, 1991.

53. Weir, J., Noakes, T.D., Myburgh, K., and Adams, B., A high carbohydrate diet negates the metabolic effects of caffeine during exercise, *Medicine and Science in Sports and Exercise*, 19, 100, 1987.
54. Falk, B., Burstein, R., Ashkenazi, I., Spillberg, O., Alter, J., Zylber-Katz, E., Rubinstein, A., Bashan, N., and Shapiro, Y., The effect of caffeine on physical performance after prolonged exercise, *European Journal of Applied Physiology*, 59, 168, 1989.
55. Deuster, P. A., Bockman, E. L., amd Muldoon, S. M., In vitro responses of cat skeletal muscle to halothane and caffeine, *Journal of Applied Physiology*, 58, 521, 1985.
56. Huerta, M. and Stefani, E., Potassium and caffeine contractures in fast and slow muscles of the chicken, *Journal of Physiology*, 318, 181, 1981.
57. Mitsumoto, H., Deboer, G. E., Bunge, G., Andrish, J. T., Tetzlaff, J. E., and Cruse, R. P., Fiber-type specific caffeine sensitivities in normal human skinned muscle fiber, *Anesthesiology*, 72, 50, 1990.
58. Butts, N. and Crowell, O., Effects of caffeine ingestion on cardiorespiratory endurance in men and women, *Research Quarterly in Exercise and Sports*, 56, 301, 1985.
59. Robertson, D., Frolich, J., Carr, R., Watson, J., Hollifield, J., Shand, D., and Oates, J., Effects of caffeine on plasma renin activity, catecholamines, and blood pressure, *New England Journal of Medicine*, 298, 181, 1978.
60. Williams, J. H., Caffeine, neuromuscular function and high-intensity exercise performance, *Journal of Sports Medicine and Physical Fitness*, 31, 481, 1991.
61. Costill, D. L., Dalsky, G. P., and Fink, W. J., Effects of caffeine ingestion on metabolism and exercise performance, *Medicine and Science in Sports*, 10, 155, 1978.
62. Ivy, J. L., Costill, D. L., Fink, W. J., and Lower, R. W., Influences of caffeine and carbohydrate feedings on endurance performance, *Medicine and Science in Sports*, 11, 6, 1979.
63. Essig, D., Costill, D. L., and Van Handel, P. J., Effects of caffeine ingestion on utilization of muscle glycogen and lipid during leg ergometer cycling, *International Journal of Sports Medicine*, 1, 86, 1980.
64. Fisher, S. M., McMurray, R. G., Berry, M., Mar, M. H., and Forsythe, W. A., Influence of caffeine on exercise performance in habitual caffeine users, *International Journal of Sports Medicine*, 7, 276, 1986.
65. Berglund, B. and Hemmingsson, P., Effects of caffeine ingestion on exercise performance at low and high altitudes in cross-country skiers, *International Journal of Sports Medicine*, 3, 234, 1982.
66. Flinn, S., Gregory, J., McNaughton, L. R. Tristan, S., and Davies, R., Caffeine ingestion prior to incremental cycling to exhaustion in recreational cyclists, *International Journal of Sports Medicine*, 11, 188, 1990.
67. Cole, K. J., Costill, D. L., Starling, R. D., Goodpaster, B. H., Trappe, S. W., and Fink, W. J., Effects of caffeine ingestion on perception of effort and subsequent work production, *International Journal of Sport Nutrition*, 6, 14, 1996.
68. Cadarette, B., Levine, L., Berube, C., Posner, B., and Evans, W., Effects of varied doses of caffeine on endurance exercise to fatigue, *Biochemistry of Exercise*, 13, 871, 1983.
69. Sasaki, H., Maeda, J., Usui, S, and Ishiko, T., Effect of sucrose and caffeine ingestion on performance of prolonged strenuous running, *International Journal of Sports Medicine*, 8, 261, 1987.
70. McNaughton, L., Two levels of caffeine ingestion on blood lactate and free fatty acid responses during incremental exercise, *Research Quarterly*, 58, 255, 1987.

71. Graham, T. E. and Spriet, L. L., Performance and metabolic responses to a high caffeine dose during prolonged exercise, *Journal of Applied Physiology*, 71, 2292, 1991.
72. Spriet, L. L., MacLean, D. A., Dyck, D. J., Hultman, E., Cederblad, G., and Graham, T. E., Caffeine ingestion and muscle metabolism during prolonged exercise in humans, *American Journal of Applied Physiology*, 262, E891, 1992.
73. Fulco, C. S., Rock, P. B., Trad, L. A., Rose, M. S., Forte, V. A., Young, P. M., and Cymerman, A., Effects of caffeine on submaximal exercise performance at altitude, *Aviation, Space, and Environmental Medicine*, 65, 539, 1994.
74. Passman, W. J., van Baak, M. A., Jeukendrup, A. E., and de Haan, A., The effect of different dosages of caffeine on endurance performance, *International Journal of Sports Medicine*, 16, 225, 1995.
75. Graham, T. E. and Spriet, L. L., Metabolic, catecholamine, and exercise performance response to various doses of caffeine, *Journal of Applied Physiology*, 78, 867, 1995.
76. Bond, V., Adams, R., Balkissoon, B., McRae, J., Knight, E., Robbins, S., and Banks, M., Effects of caffeine on cardiorespiratory function and glucose metabolism during rest and graded exercise, *International Journal of Sports Medicine*, 27, 47, 1987.
77. Sasaki, H., Takaoka, I, and Ishiko, T., Effects of sucrose or caffeine ingestion on running performance and biochemical responses to endurance running, *International Journal of Sports Medicine*, 8, 203, 1987.
78. Tarnopolsky, M. A., Atkinson, S. A., Macdougall, J. D., Sale, D. G., and Sutton, J. R., Physiological responses to caffeine during endurance running in habitual caffeine users, *Medicine and Science in Sports and Exercise*, 21, 418, 1989.
79. Graham, T. E., Rush, J. W. E., and van Soeren, M. H., Caffeine and exercise: Metabolism and performance, *Canadian Journal of Applied Physiology*, 19, 111, 1994.

Chapter 12

CAFFEINE: EFFECTS ON PSYCHOLOGICAL FUNCTIONING AND PERFORMANCE

Barry D. Smith and Kenneth Tola

CONTENTS

0-8493-2647-8/98/$0.00+$.50

I. INTRODUCTION

Caffeine is undoubtedly the most widely consumed of all psychotropic drugs.[1-4] Its popularity is typically attributed to its stimulant effects,[4] though its role in slowing and smoothing habituation[5,6] and in enhancing and sustaining attentional focus[7,8] may also be factors. The focus of this paper is on psychological functioning and performance. As we address the effects of caffeine in these areas, we will necessarily also review literature concerned with underlying physiological effects and attempt to integrate current knowledge under a biobehavioral model.

The increasing scientific attention devoted to caffeine in recent years[9] reflects not only its popularity and widespread use, but also concern that it may have detrimental physiological effects and interest in its impact on psychological functioning and behavior. Health concerns have focused primarily on cardiovascular function.[4,10] Early studies suggested that caffeine consumption may increase the risk of some cardiovascular problems.[11,12] However, more recent studies provide little support for this concern, with the possible exception of blood pressure.[13] Lipid profiles appear to be unaffected by habitual caffeine consumption.[14-17] Moreover, there is little or no elevated risk of myocardial infarction,[18] ischemic heart disease,[19] arrhythmia,[20,21] or other disorders.[22] As to coronary heart disease (CHD), which was a primary concern following earlier studies, mounting evidence clearly suggests no increased risk.[15,23] Most recently, a major prospective cohort study followed 85,747 women aged 34 to 59 for 10 years. After adjustment for other risk factors, there was no positive association of coffee consumption with CHD.[24] However, there is still a possibility that when coffee is boiled, there may be adverse effects on lipid profiles and elevated cardiovascular risk,[25] so caution is still in order.[26]

The effects of caffeine on mental performance and emotional functioning have only begun to receive scientific attention in recent years,[27] despite the fact that its popularity presumably stems primarily from these effects. Moreover, some of these consequences have very likely been noted by users for centuries. In an interesting history of caffeine consumption, Roberts and Barone[28] note that the recorded history of tea consumption dates at least to the Tang Dynasty in China (AD 618–907), where it was widely consumed. The Chinese, perhaps observing the alerting and other psychological effects of the drug, were convinced that tea improved health and prolonged life. Coffee, by far the most common source of caffeine[1] first appeared in written records in the tenth century A.D., but had probably been in use in Ethiopia since the sixth century. By the 12th century, coffeehouses were common in the Middle East, and by the 17th century they had spread throughout Germany, France, Holland, Austria, and England. Histories of these centuries clearly suggest that the reason for the widespread use of this popular drink was its effect on mental states. One early writer summed it up well:

> Coffee is the common man's gold, and like gold, it brings to every man the feeling of luxury and nobility.
>
> Abd-al-Kadir, *In Praise of Coffee*, 1587

Many since the 16th century have also experienced that "feeling of luxury and nobility", but we knew little more than did Abd-al-Kadir about the exact nature of or basis for the psychological effects of caffeine until a relatively few years ago — nearly the end of the 20th century.

A. Caffeine: Consumption And Major Sources

Caffeine is so pervasive that about 80% of U.S. adults drink coffee or tea daily, in addition to consuming other caffeinated foods. The average adult in the U.S. and Canada consumes 4 mg/kg/day,[29] and many exceed 15 mg/kg.[1,30] While coffee is the most popular drink in the U.S., most drinkers in Asian countries prefer tea. Coffee (5 oz) averages 85 mg for ground roasted and 60 mg for instant, while leaf tea (5 oz) averages 30 mg and instant tea averages 20.[29]

In addition to coffee and tea, the psychological effects of caffeine can be obtained from a number of other food sources. Chocolate is a popular and widely consumed source, but the drug is also found in considerable quantities in a number of medications, both prescription and over-the-counter (OTC). Caffeine tablets (e.g., No-Doz) are sold for those who use the drug to study, drive, or engage in other activities. Less obvious is the caffeine content in analgesics, cold preparations, and anorectants.

The multi-source availability of caffeine means that investigators studying total consumption must be exceptionally careful to query subjects concerning all possible sources in their dietary and drug intakes. It also means that in experimental studies where the desire is to dose caffeine relative to the subject's typical intake or to population averages, those consumption levels should be calculated taking all common sources into account. In some kinds of studies, where the concern is not only with caffeine per se but with arousal drugs more generally, other pharmacological sources of arousal must also be assessed. Ginseng, for example, has been widely advertised in recent years. It is available OTC and does act to increase arousal. Similarly, theobromine (2,7-dimethylxanthine) is found in cocoa and some other foods and may affect arousal.[31] And theophylline (1,3-dimethylxanthine) is found in some medications, in small amounts in tea, and in trace quantities in cocoa and coffee.[31]

II. HUMAN FUNCTIONING: A BIOBEHAVIORAL MODEL

To approach an integrative understanding of the psychological, behavioral, and underlying physiological consequences of caffeine consumption, a theoretical model is essential. The biobehavioral theory of arousal proposed by the present author[9,32] provides one such model. It is contained within a broader dual-interaction model of psychological, behavioral, and physiological functioning (Figure 1). The advantage of this approach for understanding caffeine is that it predicts the effects of the drug in the broader context of a theory that recognizes it as one of a number of arousal agents.

A. The Dual-Interaction Model

Briefly, the dual-interaction approach postulates that two interactions — that between biology and environment and that between person and situation — work together to determine behavior. The Person and the Situational context interact to determine behavior in the short term. The Person, in turn, is a product of developmental factors that are both Biologi-

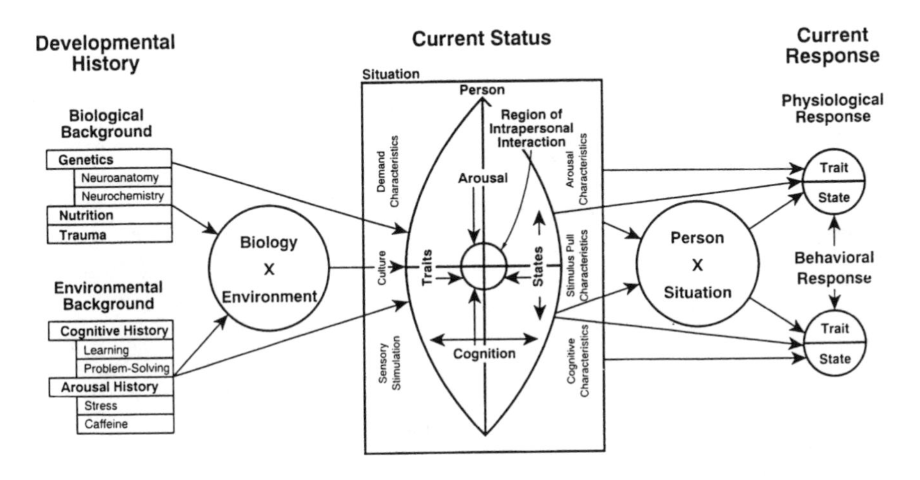

FIGURE 1
Human functioning: the dual-interaction model. (From Smith, B.D., Effects of acute and habitual caffeine ingestion in physiology and behavior: Tests of a biobehavioral arousal theory. Special issue: Caffeine Research, *Pharmacopsychoecologia*, 7(2), 151-167, 1994. With permission.)

cal (e.g., genetic) and Environmental (e.g., learning, long-term caffeine exposure), and the interaction of the two forms a separate source of variance. The Person comprises both long-term (trait) and short-term (state) dimensions and has two important functional components termed arousal and cognition.

Arousal and cognition cross with the state-trait distinction in the Region-of-Intrapersonal Interaction to permit both state and trait forms of both arousal and cognition. The model places the Person in a Situational context, and both the Person and the Situation contribute separately and interactively to both physiological functioning and behavior.

B. The Arousal Model

The arousal component of the dual-interaction model, which governs the effects of caffeine, can be split out and amplified to provide a multi-dimensional model of arousal (Figure 2). Biological and Environmental background factors contribute separately and interactively to both chronic and acute arousal. The individual can be exposed either chronically or acutely or both to such environmental arousal agents as caffeine and stress. Chronic exposure contributes to arousal traits and thereby affects arousal states, while acute exposure contributes directly to the current arousal state. The multi-dimensional nature of both traits and states can be seen in Figure 2. The trait arousal dimensions are intensity, type (emotional or general), and individual differences. The latter include extraver-

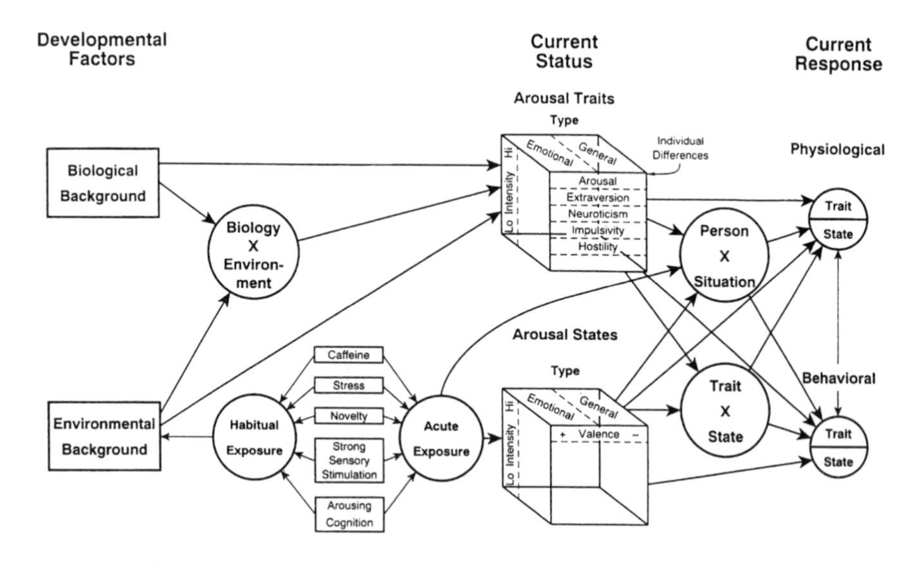

FIGURE 2
Arousal: a biobehavioral model. (From Smith, B.D., Effects of acute and habitual caffeine ingestion in physiology and behavior: Tests of a biobehavioral arousal theory. Special issue: Caffeine Research, *Pharmacopsychoecologia,* 7(2), 151-167, 1994. With permission.)

sion, impulsivity, neuroticism, sensation-seeking, hostility, and potentially others. Intensity and type are also dimensions of state arousal, and the third dimension is valence (positive or negative). There are both separate and interactive contributions of both arousal traits and arousal states to current physiological functioning and behavior.

C. Principles Applied To Caffeine

Four general theoretical principles derived from the arousal model are especially relevant to the effects of caffeine.

1. Moderate levels of chronic use of caffeine and other arousal agents tend to reduce the effects of acute exposure. However, higher chronic levels can exacerbate the impact of acute exposure.
2. Arousal output is an inverted U-shaped function of arousal input (Figure 3). That is, the effect of arousal input on mental performance and such physiological indicators as electrodermal activity (EDA) initially rises. With further arousal input from trait and state sources, it asymptotes, then decreases as arousal input increases.
3. Individual differences in arousal or arousability (susceptibility) interact with strength of exposure to affect mental performance, psychological functioning, and physiology.

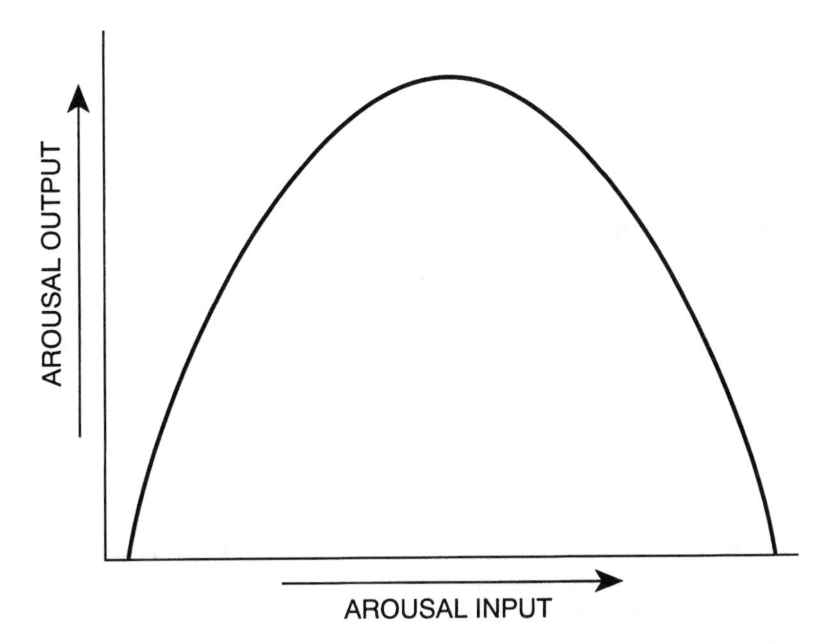

FIGURE 3
Arousal input and arousal output: the invert-U function.

4. The arousal effects of multiple agents are additive: Exposure to several agents produces higher overall arousal and stronger effects than exposure to any one. It is for this reason that the possibility of several agents must be taken into account in experimental work. The arousal level resulting from multiple agents is subject to the inverted-U principle.

D. Hypotheses Relating to Caffeine

Given the general principles of the arousal model, we can derive several more specific hypotheses that are particularly relevant to caffeine effects. These hypotheses have been tested to varying degrees in the caffeine literature.

1. The individual's average habitual exposure to caffeine moderates the effect of acute exposure on both physiological and psychological functioning.
2. Only those areas of functioning that are directly relevant to arousal are affected by caffeine. Included would be certain aspects of emotion, performance affected by focused attention, and behavior relating to certain personality dimensions.
3. Acute exposure to caffeine raises arousal levels, subject to the inverted-U principle.

4. Acute exposure to caffeine reduces the rate of habituation of physiological responses, subject to the inverted-U principle.
5. Acute exposure smooths and stabilizes the habituation function.

III. EFFECTS OF CAFFEINE ON COGNITIVE PERFORMANCE

Beginning with Wilhelm Wundt's research on vigilance, the effects of caffeine on cognitive functioning and related mental performance have been studied fairly extensively. Researchers have investigated cognitive-motor performance,[34] memory functions in both adults[27] and children,[35] reaction times,[36] and decision making,[37] among other areas.

A. Information Processing

Information-processing theory[38] has served, at least loosely, as the basis for a number of studies of the effects of caffeine on cognitive functioning. Several studies have shown beneficial effects of the drug in rapid information processing (RIP) tasks.[39-41] Other work demonstrates that caffeine enhances problem-solving[42] and improves logical reasoning,[43,44] as well as increasing performance on mental arithmetic tasks.[45,46] Some studies have even shown that caffeine counteracts sleep deprivation effects in spatial capacity tasks[47] and partially reverses age-related deficits in cognitive functioning.[48]

Using a rapid information-processing task, Hasenfratz and Battig[49] had a subject look for a 3-digit odd or even target on a computer screen that also presented other, non-target digits. When the subject saw the target number, he or she was to press a response key as quickly as possible. The investigators found that a low dose (150 mg) of caffeine improved performance on the RIP task, while a higher dose (600 mg) impaired performance.

Other studies have also shown that high doses of caffeine can interfere with performance on complex tasks,[50] including the processing of ambiguous information.[51] They can also negatively affect scores on such cognitive tasks as spatial abilities in refreshed subjects.[47] In other work, however, caffeine has not affected the search/detection domain of information processing[52] or reading comprehension.[53]

One factor in the differential cognitive results may be baseline or prestimulation arousal level. When baseline arousal is already elevated, highly arousing tasks, such as those that are complex or involve intense stimuli, can result in overstimulation. As Hasenfratz and Battig[49] note, it may be such excessive levels of stimulation that account for the commission errors seen in the RIP paradigm. Baseline arousal levels therefore need to be taken into account in estimating or calculating overall levels of stimulation and resultant activation.

One influence on prestimulation arousal level appears to be gender. When gender differences in arousal or activation have been specifically examined, female subjects have been quite consistently shown to exhibit higher levels of arousal or greater arousability than males. Physiologically, this arousal differential has been reported for both EEG[54-56] and EDA[57,58] measures. In studies involving mixed-gender groups with no analysis of the gender factor, it is possible that caffeine-induced increases in information processing in males would be counteracted by decrements in females. Depending on the gender balances of the groups, results could be considerably distorted. Stimulation that is highly arousing for males could lead to overarousal in females, whose responses would be dampened as suggested by the inverted U-shaped principle.

Interestingly enough, most of the studies reporting positive effects of caffeine in information-processing tasks have used primarily or exclusively male subjects.[39,42,43,45,46,59] In fact the only study that found positive cognitive effects of caffeine on females employed fatigued females, whose baseline arousal levels may have been lower.[41]

Conversely, most studies that have shown either detrimental effects[47,50] or no effects[52,53] of caffeine on information processing have used both males and females in the same study. In fact, the only study with this result that used exclusively male subjects also used moderate (250 mg) doses of caffeine with a difficult (visual Stroop) task. The combined effect of the drug and the task probably produced a degree of arousal high enough to interfere with cognitive performance. Caffeine, in this case, therefore contributed to an overall detrimental effect of arousal.[51] A different type of study showing detrimental effects used the same caffeine dose on both tired and refreshed subjects.[47] The tired subjects were aroused to the point of showing beneficial effects from the drugs. Therefore, the same dose should be expected to overarouse the refreshed subjects and decrease their information processing abilities, as was the case.

In addition to gender, task difficulty or complexity appears to be a substantial factor in arousal. Information processing tasks, particularly complex ones, have been shown to increase arousal levels in otherwise unstimulated subjects.[60] The more complex the task, the higher the arousal level and the greater the chance that a given caffeine dosage would contribute to overstimulation. The additive nature of arousal sources — in this case caffeine and complexity — means that arousal is high when caffeine is present and complexity or difficulty level is substantial. The result is that caffeine impairs performance on complex tasks,[50,51] particularly in female subjects.

B. Memory

A major focus of cognitive psychology, memory has been studied intensively, and a number of investigations have addressed the effects of caffeine. Unfortunately, results in this important area of mental performance are quite mixed. A number of studies have found that caffeine enhances memory performance in several paradigms. It has been shown to improve delayed recall,[42] recognition memory,[61,62] semantic memory,[63] and verbal memory in general.[64] Other studies have shown significant increases in memory performance on both easy[65] and difficult[66] memory tasks. And females (but not males) in one study showed positive effects of caffeine on word list retention, though only when the words were presented at a slow rate.[67]

Some studies have gotten opposite or equivocal results for memory tasks. Caffeine can actually decrease immediate word list recall, at least under some circumstances.[68,69] It has even been shown to amplify the detrimental effects of alcohol on memory.[70] Complicating the picture further, other studies have shown that caffeine has no effect on recall.[7,53,71]

Both short- and long-term verbal memory have been assessed. There is no effect on short-term memory with 64 mg of caffeine[72] or with 100,[73] and no effect on long-term memory with 64 or 128 mg.[72] Verbal learning and memory were also unaffected by doses of 125 to 500 mg.[74] In addition, no effect was seen on implicit or incidental memory,[75] as was also true for delayed recall with 3 and 6 mg/kg[76] or with 200, 400, or 600 mg.[69] This latter result is somewhat offset by a study in which delayed recall was improved by caffeine, even though immediate recall was not.[42] Finally, Linde[77] tested both fatigued and non-fatigued subjects on an auditory attention task requiring immediate recall. She found no effects of 150 or 200 mg doses of caffeine.

Given the mixed results in the literature, it is difficult to know just how caffeine does affect memory. To some extent, the differential effects may depend on the memory assessment method (recall or recognition) and the time frame (immediate or delayed). Gender differences may also cloud the picture, as discussed above. Even when these differences are taken into account, however, unexplained discrepancies remain. One partial explanation may be that the differential effects of caffeine are a function of the subject's memory load. For example, Anderson[65] found that caffeine enhanced low load memory tasks but was detrimental in high load tasks. This could be due to the increased arousal induced by the high load task, which, in the presence of caffeine, could produce overarousal. The drop in arousal output as the subject crossed the peak of the inverted U-shaped function could cause the memory deficits observed in some studies.

Since many studies do not control for memory load,[78] it is difficult to determine the impact of this factor. If load is important, investigators might find no caffeine effects when the memory load is too low to elicit differentials. At the same time, a very difficult task that carries a high memory load may push arousal near the peak of the inverted-U. Caffeine could then produce overarousal, leading to a decrement in memory performance. Further work is clearly needed to determine the extent to which the memory load factor has affected results to date.

An alternative or additional explanation for the mixed results may lie in the differentially arousing effects of other factors present in the experimental situation. One study in our laboratories involved a backward recall task. Each subject received three blocks of four recall trials each. In a repetitive condition, each block involved one particular stimulus type (letters, digits, or color names). In a novel condition, each block contained one trial of each of the three stimulus types. Using a double-blind procedure, each subject was randomly assigned to receive either 300 mg caffeine or a placebo prior to performing the memory task. Half of each drug group was randomly assigned to a noise condition, involving a constant 80-dB white noise stimulus and half to a no noise control condition.

Results showed that both novelty and white noise improved recall performance under placebo and decreased it under caffeine.[6] It appears that the additional arousal generated by novelty and white noise served to push caffeine subjects over the top of the inverted-U curve and hence decrease their recall performance. Thus, it may be that caffeine does improve memory performance under conditions that otherwise produce low arousal. However, any condition causing overarousal, whether or not it is a part of the memory task itself, can yield performance decrements.

C. Vigilance Performance

One aspect of cognitive performance in which there is considerable consistency in the literature as to the effects of caffeine is vigilance. One example is a study conducted by Lieberman and his colleagues,[79] who used the Wilkenson Vigilance Test.[80] Above a white noise background, subjects were presented with a 400-ms tone every 2 s for 1 h. Targets were 70-ms tones that were randomly interspersed among the longer tones, and subjects responded by pressing a key on a keyboard. Hits, misses, and false alarms were recorded. They found that low (32 mg) to moderate (256 mg) doses of caffeine increased the number of correct hits without affecting the error rate.

A number of other studies have also shown that caffeine improves vigilance performance[47,81] on both auditory[77,82-84] and visual[84,85] tasks. Conversely, decrements in performance have been attributed to low levels of arousal,[86] while higher levels improve performance on sustained attention tasks.[7,8,87,88] Although some earlier work suggested negative effects on cognitive functioning in children, a recent meta-analysis found no supportive evidence.[89] In fact, children exhibit improved functioning on both auditory vigilance[90] and sustained attention[91] tasks when caffeine is given. In addition, moderate doses (200 mg) decrease self-reported feelings of boredom, possibly providing a partial explanation for the positive effect of caffeine in vigilance and sustained attention tasks.[66] More generally, a recent review showed that caffeine improved vigilance performance in 14 of 17 studies.[92]

Despite the apparent overall positive effect of caffeine on vigilance, there is evidence to suggest that there may be a limitation on the size of the arousal increment (induced by caffeine, intense stimulation, or both) that will produce improvement in vigilance studies. If that limit is exceeded, performance may asymptote or deteriorate. Frewer and Laden[93] found that low doses of caffeine improved vigilance performance, while high doses initially impaired it. After 2 h, however, these high doses also improved vigilance.

In another study, the senior author and colleagues preselected subjects high and low in habitual caffeine ingestion. Using double-blind controls, they were given either caffeine (4.0 mg/kg) or a placebo and exposed to 93-dB background white noise or no noise. A visual vigilance task consisted of three blocks of ten 1-min trials with targets appearing on trials 1, 3, 4, 7, and 10 of each block. Stimuli were angled lines appearing on a computer screen; targets were vertical lines. Results showed that caffeine decreased target response times (improved performance) when there was no white noise, but increased response times when the 93-dB noise was present.[94] In addition, subjects with histories of habitually high levels of caffeine use exhibited relative decrements in vigilance performance.

The results of these two studies and others provide further support for the theoretical inverted U-shaped arousal function. In the first case,[93] high doses of caffeine pushed subjects over the top of the curve and hence impaired vigilance performance. As time passed and the subject became more accustomed to the experimental situation, arousal returned to more optimal levels and performance improved. In the second study,[94] caffeine combined with moderately high intensity situational stimulation (white noise) to drive arousal up beyond the point of transmarginal inhibition and, again, decrease performance.

D. Distraction

Caffeine affects not only information processing, memory, and vigilance performance, but also other aspects of cognitive functioning. One of those is distractibility and, therefore, the effects of situational distractors on differential functioning during cognitive tasks.[95] The TUIT (Task Unrelated Image and Thought) questionnaire assesses distractibility by determining the extent to which the subject tends to respond to distractors and hence to deviate attention from the focal task at hand. It appears to provide a measure of cognitive arousal or arousability. In one study, for example, normal control subjects had moderate TUIT scores. Depressive (less aroused) patients had lower TUIT scores and anxiety (more aroused) patients higher TUIT scores than did these controls.[96] In effect, higher levels of arousal were associated with higher distractibility scores on the TUIT. Accordingly, we might predict that caffeine, by raising arousal, would also increase distractibility and raise TUIT scores. In a test of that hypothesis, Giambra and colleagues[97] gave subjects caffeine and used the TUIT to determine its effect on distractibility. Results showed that TUIT scores increased with caffeine, supporting the theory that caffeine increases cognitive arousal.

E. Complex Cognitive Functioning

Real-life settings, including work settings, often require more complex and varied cognitive functioning than is the case for many laboratory tasks. One case in point is decision-making, in which multiple types and sources of information are logically combined to yield an informed decision.[98] What effect does caffeine have on such complex reasoning processes as those involved in arriving at decisions? While little work has been done in this area, it thus far appears that the drug has a positive effect, at least in reducing the amount of time required to arrive at a decision.[37,99]

Research on the effects of caffeine in the work place is also rather sparse. However, there have been some studies. The use of caffeine at work, primarily through coffee consumption in the U.S., Canada, and some other countries and through tea consumption in some Asian countries, has a long history. Indeed, much of the substantial daily intake of the average adult, whether of coffee or tea, occurs in job settings. Moreover, it does appear to have positive effects on mental performance. In one study, for example, managerial effectiveness was reduced when employees abstained from caffeine.[100] Whether the withdrawal from caffeine or the lack of the drug caused this outcome is not entirely clear, but the job-enhancing effect of the drug is.

It is commonly assumed that the ubiquitous office coffee pot is heavily used by workers in order to increase their levels of wakefulness, alertness, and, more generally, arousal.[4] There may, however, be a number of additional perceived or actual benefits of work-related caffeine intake. Headaches, for example, are often reported in work settings, and one study showed that workers sometimes consume caffeine primarily to relieve them.[101] This finding is consistent with the widespread medical use of caffeine to treat headache.[102,103]

A more common and salient, though more subtle, basis for on-the-job consumption may be boredom. For some people, work is perceived as boring, and boredom is, in part, a function of habituation. The habituation process takes place when there are multiple repetitions of the same stimulus complex or a continuation of that complex over time.[104] Habituation is basically a process of physiological and psychological adaptation to stimuli that cease to yield new information.[105] While it is an adaptive mechanism in that it moves noninformative stimuli into the background and permits active attention to focus on new information, it can also have negative effects. In particular, subjects who become highly habituated or overhabituated experience psychological discomfort, fatigue, and boredom.[5] Caffeine can partially offset these detrimental effects of repeated stimulation (e.g., in the work place) by slowing the rate at which habituation occurs and smoothing the process.[6] Thus, workers may consume the drug not only to increase alertness, but also to slow and smooth habituation.

There are also documented negative effects of the amounts of caffeine often consumed at work.[106] Most of these revolve around the stresses commonly perceived to be present in job settings. Caffeine has been shown to exacerbate the effects of stress on neuroendocrine responses[107] and cardiovascular functioning, particularly blood pressure[45, 108-110] It is no surprise, then, that it has these same effects in work settings, predisposing the individual toward strong physiological and psychological responses to work stressors.[111] The blood-pressure response to work stress appears to be particularly prone to caffeine enhancement.[20, 112] In addition, a study of telemarketers showed that employees became more psychologically sensitive to job stressors after consuming caffeine.[113]

F. Cognitive Aspects of Psychomotor Functioning

From a cognitive perspective,[38,114] psychomotor performance follows from or is influenced by the cognitive processing of both incoming sensory-perceptual information and available memory stores. The role of memory as a cognitive process in psychomotor performance has been increasingly studied in recent years as work on procedural or nondeclarative memory has progressed.[114] From this cognitive perspective, whenever motor performance occurs, it is potentially influenced by related prior practice and skill development, which have been stored in memory. Reflex activity is, of course, often involved, but it can be readily modified by procedural memory for motor skills. Thus, even such basic responses as reaction time to a simple stimulus are, in part, a function of cognitive processes. In effect, a physical response is secondary to mental (cognitive) performance.

Some studies of the influence of cognition on motor performance in adults have found that acute doses of caffeine improve psychomotor performance[34, 115] in such areas as simple visual selection[116] and fine motor control.[117] However, others show no effect of the drug on performance[118] or an impact only on initial learning and not on later performance,[119] especially at low dosage levels.[79] Studies of children and adolescents are even more inconsistent. Some report caffeine-related improvement on manual dexterity tasks[91] and even a dose-response relationship in some cases.[120] One study, for example, found that both 2.5 and 5.0 mg/kg of caffeine improved the manual dexterity of the dominant hand in 8- to 12-year-olds.[91] Other work shows decrements in overall psychomotor accuracy, speed, or both.[121–123] For example, one investigation showed that 200 mg of caffeine decreased performance on a recently learned tactile discrimination task in 10-year-olds.[123] A third group of studies suggests that caffeine has no effect at all, at least on gross motor performance.[35,121]

The inconsistent effects of caffeine in cognitively mediated performance tasks may result from differences in age groups, dosage levels, and environmental factors.[124,125] The latter have been shown to substantially affect arousal[126,127] in both adults[128,129] and children.[130,131] Office noise is effective in increasing self-reported arousal,[132] as are white noise in the laboratory,[94] exercise,[133] and stress.[134] Such environmental factors are sources of arousal and can interact with stimulants like caffeine.[135]

External conditions can also cause a decrease in arousal that may also affect cognitive/psychomotor performance. An interesting stimulation study conducted by Suedfield and Eich[136] showed how arousal can be reduced. They used Restricted Environmental Stimulation Technique (REST), in which a subject floats in a dense solution of skin temperature water and Epsom salts. This technique was shown to decrease subjective reports of arousal. Similar reports come from studies of meditation[137,138] and systematic relaxation.[139]

Experimental demonstrations of the increments and decrements in arousal that can be produced by environmental conditions suggest a need to carefully examine this aspect of the literature concerned with the effects of caffeine on psychomotor performance. Variability in the environmental conditions and extraneous stimuli that differentiate experiments may have contributed substantially to the mixed results in that literature. Considerably more research, systematically varying environmental factors, and caffeine dosage levels will be needed before firm conclusions can be drawn in this area.

G. Cognitive Aspects of Reaction-Time Performance

One of the most fundamental measurements of cognitive activity and efficiency is reaction time (RT).[36] Rapid response to a stimulus is based on the cognitive processing of sensory information to yield motor output. Although what we observe is a motor response, the underlying process is clearly cognitive. Studies show that caffeine can either speed or slow reaction times, depending on drug dosage and task complexity. On relatively simple tasks, such as rapid information processing[40] and the numeric Stroop,[59,140] caffeine typically decreases reaction times,[116,117,135] though not all studies are consistent.[141] This effect may be even more pronounced in elderly people, who show greater RT improvement than younger subjects under the influence of the drug.[142]

To some degree, the association between caffeine and RT forms a dose-response relationship, higher acute doses producing faster reaction times than lower doses.[64,81] The drug has also been shown to counteract the negative effects of alcohol[70] and sleep deprivation on reaction time.[140] These findings apply to both high and low habitual users. Both groups show the positive effect of caffeine on simple RT.[53]

There does, however, appear to be a ceiling on the acute dosage of caffeine that will enhance reaction time. At relatively low doses given prior to simple tasks or highly practiced complex tasks, the drug does enhance RT.[41,104,117,143,144] However, these results may not apply to more complex tasks that have not been extensively practiced. For example, Lieberman[79] found that 64 mg of caffeine decreased RT on a simple visual task in which the subject had to identify an object. However, the same dose of caffeine had no effect on RT when the subject had to choose objects in a more complex task. In fact, caffeine has been found to have detrimental effects on reaction times in some complex tasks.[51,104,145] Again, there appears to be an inverted-U relationship between overall arousal — induced by the combination of caffeine and other arousal factors — and performance on reaction time tasks.

IV. CAFFEINE AND EMOTIONAL FUNCTIONING

The other side of the psychological coin from cognition is emotion, and caffeine has also been shown to have important effects on this aspect of functioning as well. Depending on dosage level and concurrent factors, caffeine can result in either positive or negative mood changes.

A. Mood State Effects

Several studies have shown that caffeine can improve mood states, increasing the frequency of positive mood self-reports[7,63,115,147] in both regular caffeine users and non-users.[148] In fact, some evidence suggests that long-term use of the drug may improve overall mood.[149] Caffeine has also been shown to improve the negative moods often seen early in the morning[146] and after lunch[159] and can even counteract the mood deficits found after up to 48 h of sleep deprivation.[151] In fact, the increases seen in cognitive tasks have been attributed to the positive mood effects of caffeine.[8] In drug interaction studies, caffeine has been shown to amplify the positive mood changes induced by other stimulants. In one study, for example, the drug enhanced positive mood states induced by nicotine.[152] In another, relatively low doses of caffeine enhanced mood states and increased the desire for cocaine in drug abusers.[153] At higher doses, it had a slight negative effect on mood.

While caffeine consumption has resulted in improved mood, abstinence has resulted in negative moods.[147] Both acute withdrawal[154] and overnight abstinence[148] appear to cause dysphoric mood states.

The mood effects of caffeine appear to be dose dependent.[81] Although some work does show a positive, linear dose–response relationship,[155] most studies show mood decrements at high doses. Low doses seem to improve mood, while higher doses have negative mood effects.[49] Caffeine doses of 100 mg have been shown to increase vigor[156] and feelings of well-being.[157] Even doses as high as 300 mg have been shown to create positive mood states of "mental sedation" in some studies.[73] However, doses over 300 mg tend to increase tension and anxiety.[66] High caffeine doses, for example, caused inmates in one study to experience anxiety, frustration, and irritability,[158] and the drug has been shown to increase tenseness and nervousness as well.[66] Complicating matters further, there are individual differences in sensitivity to the mood state effects of varied doses of caffeine.[159] As with cognitive performance, the inverted-U function may best explain the mood effect of the drug.

Another factor that influences the effects of caffeine on mood is the expectation of the person consuming it. In one study, for example, subjects showed no mood effects until they reached caffeine dosage levels that they could detect.[160] Similarly, Evans and Griffiths[161] found that people who knew they were consuming caffeine reported positive mood effects. On the other hand, if they unknowingly consumed the same amount of caffeine, they reported negative mood changes. Totten and France[162] found that caffeine combines with anticipatory anxiety to increase self-reports of anxiety. A final study showed that subjects who chose to take caffeine felt no increase in anxiety, while those who had no choice did self-report increased anxiety with the same levels of caffeine.[163]

B. Anxiety

Anxiety is related to higher physiological and behavioral arousal levels,[96,164] especially levels of affective arousal.[165,166] Similarly, caffeine has long been shown to increase arousal.[58, 109, 167, 168] This parallel may suggest both underlying causal relationships and interactions.

A number of studies document an increase in anxiety with caffeine ingestion,[76, 169, 170] a phenomenon seen in both users and non-users.[135] In addition, caffeine has been found to increase anxiety levels in smokers,[50] alcoholics,[172] and ECT patients.[173] Elevations of anxiety have also been observed in children as young as 8 years old,[91] and males appear to be more sensitive to this anxiety-producing effect of caffeine.[81,135] Taking this finding a step further, some investigators have reported a dose-response relationship: higher doses of caffeine produce greater elevations in anxiety.[49,174] Doses of 400 mg increase anxiety more than doses of 200 mg,[66,175] and 600 mg increases anxiety more than 400 mg.[69] It is not clear, however, whether or not this relationship is linear. Although some work does suggest linearity,[69] other studies have shown that any dose over 300 mg may push anxiety to asymptotic levels, with no further increase at higher doses.[27,174,176]

To the extent that caffeine increases anxiety and tracks its effects, it is worth considering the possibility of some underlying physiological relationship between the drug and the emotion. Some work suggests that feelings of anxiety and anxiety symptoms such as sweating, palpitations, nausea, irritability, loss of appetite, tension, and lack of concentration,[175] may be associated with adenosine receptors in the brain.[177] Caffeine acts as an antagonist for these same adenosine receptors,[178] possibly suggesting a neural association between the emotion and the drug.

It may also be no coincidence that both habitual levels of anxiety and the preference for and consumption of caffeine have been shown to be subject to genetic predispositions. Increasing evidence in recent years suggests the presence of a substantial genetic factor in anxiety.[179] This predisposition may be expressed in the serotonin system of the brain[180-182] and possibly also the norepinephrine system.[183] Evidence indicates that levels of habitual caffeine consumption and the intensity of responses to single doses may also be subject to a hereditary predisposition.[184,185] It appears to involve the bimodally distributed ability to acetylate molecules possessing an amino functional group. The genetic predisposition very likely has a direct effect on the extent to which caffeine acts as an adenosine receptor antagonist in a given individual and may also influence caffeine-relevant taste preferences. Depending on the percentage of variance accounted for by the genetic predisposition, early exposure to and experience with caffeinated substances interacts with heredity to shape both the preference for caffeine and the reaction to ingestion. The potential for a genetically based neurophysiological relationship between anxiety and caffeine is clear, but a considerable amount of research will be required to further confirm it.

Despite the well-documented association of caffeine with anxiety and the possibility that there is a neural association between the two, the literature has not been entirely consistent. In fact, a survey of over 9,000 people in England found no relationship between caffeine and anxiety.[186] In addition, even though panic disorder patients are hypersensitive to anxiety-producing stimuli and situations,[187-189] doses of caffeine under 100 mg do not increase their anxiety levels.[188]

C. Stress

One of the major contributing factors in anxiety and anxiety disorders is stress, and it is reasonable to hypothesize that this is an area of psychological functioning in which caffeine may be implicated.[9] Ongoing research has clearly demonstrated the destructive psychological and physiological effects of stress. One of the most serious reactions is post-traumatic stress disorder (PTSD), which was reported at least as far back as 1755 when a peasant family was trapped by an avalanche in the Italian Alps.[190] It has been widely studied in Vietnam veterans[191,192] and in veterans of World War II and the Korean War.[193] In civilians, PTSD is seen in 38% of burn victims[194] and 46% of those involved in motor vehicle accidents.[195] More generally, a study of college students revealed that any of a wide variety of prior traumatic experiences could produce the symptoms of PTSD.[196] There is now some evidence that caffeine may be a contributing factor in this disorder.[197]

Other psychological consequences of stress include its role in reducing college performance[198] and in suicide, which takes 30,000 lives in the U.S. each year — about one every 18 minutes.[199] Interestingly enough, however, caffeine consumption appears to have precisely the opposite effect in this regard. In a large-scale 10-year follow-up study of women, caffeine consumption was inversely related to suicide.[149] It is likely that this effect is due to the mood-enhancing properties of moderate amounts of the drug.[149]

Stress also has destructive physiological effects. Stressors significantly modify the number of NK cells and the number of T-cells, thereby reducing the immune response and becoming a contributing factor in infectious and other disorders.[200,201] Stress is also a factor in cardiovascular disorders, where it contributes to the gradual development of coronary artery disease and hypertension[202] and is a precipitating factor in heart attacks.[203] In addition, stress contributes to the development of a number of other physical disease processes, such as asthma[204] and rheumatoid arthritis.[205]

The role of caffeine in stress and stress reactions has been well documented.[206] It affects the neuroendocrine[107] and heart rate[207,208] responses to stress, as well as the skin conductance response to stressful anagram tasks.[94] Best documented, however, are the additive effects of stress and caffeine on blood pressure and related cardiovascular indicators.[45,108] In one investigation, subjects were exposed to stressful mental arithmetic, cold pressor, and static exercise tasks after taking caffeine (250 mg) or a placebo. The drug enhanced the impact of the stressors, yielding an additive effect on blood pressure.[109] Confirming studies show interactive effects of caffeine and stress on both resting pressures[46] and the blood pressure response.[209,210] For example, as little as 250 mg of caffeine exacerbates the cold pressor stress response.[49,109] The interaction is seen not only in adults, but also in teenagers[109] and even prepubertal boys.[211]

One widely employed experimental paradigm is the Rapid Information Processing (RIP) task. In a recent RIP study, Lovallo and colleagues[212] had subjects respond to random light presentations of 3 ms duration. They pressed a response key with each light onset and were given 50 cents for "very rapid" responses. Using 3.3 mg/kg of caffeine (an average of 264 mg per subject), they found that the drug produced a significantly greater increase in the blood pressure response than did a placebo. Many other studies confirm the exacerbating effect of caffeine on the blood pressure response to stress.[43,107,213-216]

D. Anger, Aggression and Violence

Caffeine may also be a factor in anger and its expression in aggressive behavior. One of the most rampant problems in U.S. society today is violence, an extreme form of aggressive behavior often precipitated by anger. Between 1960 and 1991, mortality from all causes decreased, but deaths from murder more than doubled from 7.7 to 16.6 per 100,000 population.[217] A 4-year longitudinal study of violent injury and death in the urban African-American population of western Philadelphia, totaling 68,000 people, confirmed the high levels of aggression in society. Of the men in the sample between ages 20 and 29, 94% visited the emergency department of an area hospital at least once during the four years. Overall, violence-induced injuries accounted for 31% of all hospital admissions and 42% of deaths, both representing substantial increases from earlier years.[218]

Violence has also expanded into the public schools to a degree never before observed. Metropolitan areas are seeing almost daily reports of students bringing knives and guns into the schools. In fact, a recent survey showed that 11% of teachers and 23% of students nationwide have been victims of violence in school.[219] In addition to the suffering and loss of life, the monetary cost to society of every murder is calculated at $2.4 million.[220]

Is caffeine a contributing factor in anger and violence? Preliminary indications are that it may well be. It has been clearly demonstrated that elevations in affective arousal are associated with increases in aggression.[221-224] Higher arousal states are also seen with anger[225] and with aggression in children as young as 8 years of age.[226] Since caffeine contributes to affective arousal,[96,165] it may also contribute to anger and aggression. In fact, however, very few studies have addressed this issue directly. Increases in caffeine have been shown to increase aggression in both normal subjects[158,227,228] and psychiatric patients.[229] In addition, studies show that caffeine increases hostility[174] and that abstinence from the drug decreases it.[230] However, these effects have not been entirely consistent, with some studies finding no effects of caffeine on aggression.[231] Considerably more research in this important area will be required.

These inconsistencies can perhaps best be explained by examining the perception of arousal. Both physiological arousal and cognitive assessment of that arousal are necessary to produce aggression.[223,224] In one study, individuated people reacted more aggressively when they were informed that their heightened arousal came from the previously unknown consumption of caffeine. De-individuated people showed decreases in aggression levels when they were told that they consumed caffeine.[232] The individuated person would theoretically attribute arousal to some internal factor before knowing about the caffeine. With the emergence of an external object, attention is focused on the deception, and aggression therefore increases. The de-individuated person, on the other hand, would already assume that the experimenters had caused the arousal, and specific knowledge of caffeine consumption would only confirm that suspicion.

Attribution of the arousal source more generally has been shown to influence the level of resultant aggressiveness in a subject.[233] In addition, when subjects think they have no control over their stimulation, they become more aggressive,[234] and that effect may also be exacerbated by caffeine.

E. Happiness

On the more positive side, caffeine has been shown not only to have positive mood effects under some circumstances, as discussed above, but more specifically to increase self-reported happiness and feelings of pleasure. This hedonic effect may, however, occur only at relatively low doses.[42] More generally, any dose under 300 mg may, depending on other conditions contributing to arousal, promote happiness[27] and can even cause euphoria-like symptoms in animals.[235] As the dosage increases above 300 mg, levels of contentedness decrease.[175]

Confirming the pleasurable effects of arousal, Russell[236] used the Affect Grid to assess happiness. It was found that reports of pleasure increased with increasing arousal up to a point. Beyond this point, further arousal led to decreases in pleasure. This finding, like many others, supports the theoretical inverted U-shaped function. What remains in this area is to further assess the effects of caffeine and its interaction with other arousal and perceptual factors to better understand the optimal arousal function.

V. THE CAFFEINE RESPONSE: INDIVIDUAL DIFFERENCES

The biobehavioral arousal model[9] holds that arousal is multidimensional and hence affected by a number of interacting factors. Caffeine is thus clearly not the only agent that influences psychological and physiological functioning through its impact on arousal, and it is important to determine just how the drug interacts with other elements to affect arousal and its psychological sequelae. Other situational factors, such as stimulus intensity and multiple arousal sources, as well as individual difference dimensions, are among the important considerations.[237] Individual differences in the response to caffeine, and to arousal and arousability more generally, must, in particular, be taken into account. Some subjects have strong reactions to arousal agents, others considerably weaker responses. While this general arousal-responsiveness dimension may cut across a number of arousal agents, there may also be arousability differences in reactions to specific agents, such as caffeine.

We have already noted evidence for genetic factors that underlie the preference for and response to caffeine. These factors create a biologically based set of individual difference dimensions that may be modified by experience with the drug. In addition, there is evidence for a number of broader individual difference dimensions that appear to be relevant. These bipolar continua differentiate between subjects who are habitually high in arousal or arousability and those who are habitually low. The factors in question are personality dimensions that theoretically reflect underlying biological continua of arousal or arousability.[238] Included among these dimensions are extraversion,[58] impulsivity,[239,240] and sensation-seeking.[94,241,242] We will take up the first two of these.

A. Extraversion

Eysenck hypothesizes that extraversion reflects an underlying continuum of activation or arousal.[243-245] Many studies have been conducted to test this assumption, and caffeine is sometimes employed in order to determine how its effects vary as a function of the individual differences in arousability reflected by the Eysenck dimension. Interactions involving EEG,[246,247] EDA,[248,249] mood,[148] and task performance[148,247] have been examined.

The validity of Eysenck's arousal hypothesis and the differential effects of caffeine on introverts and extraverts are generally well documented, primarily in studies involving various EDA measures. Investigations of the arousal hypothesis quite consistently confirm that introverts are more aroused or arousable than extraverts.[9,56,250] As compared with extraverts, introverts show larger phasic skin conductance responses,[238,241,248] higher skin conductance levels,[241] slower electrodermal habituation,[248] higher heart rate reactivity,[251] and shorter Wave V latencies.[247] Since EDA has been shown to be a reliable measure of arousal,[6,94,249.252] these results support Eysenck's hypothesis. They also support the present arousal theory, which postulates the existence of individual difference dimensions reflecting an underlying arousal continuum.

Studies of the interaction of extraversion and caffeine test the hypothesis that the effects of caffeine on psychological and physiological functioning are subject to variability as a function of individual difference dimensions. An earlier series of double-blinded, placebo-controlled studies in our laboratories addressed this issue. In each study, a large group of subjects completed the Eysenck Personality Inventory (EPI)[253] as a measure of extraversion. Scores were used to establish extreme groups of introverts and extraverts, and subjects in each of these groups were randomly assigned to receive one of several doses of caffeine or a placebo. Subjects were then exposed to a series of auditory stimuli of varied intensity.

Results showed a clear interaction between extraversion and caffeine. Introverts, who have been shown to exhibit higher baseline arousal levels and greater arousability,[104] exhibited larger phasic electrodermal responses under placebo and low caffeine doses than did extraverts. However, the reverse was true under high doses of caffeine.[105,238] In addition, when a preparatory signal preceded intense auditory stimulation, it reversed dosage-related response patterns in introverts, but had little effect on extraverts.[254]

These group reversals clearly show that the arousal effects of caffeine are mediated by individual differences. The generally expected linear increment in response amplitude exhibited by extraverts under increasing levels of caffeine-induced arousal was sharply contrasted with the decrement exhibited by introverts. The best explanation for this differential effect of caffeine is the presence of an inverted U-shaped arousal function: the augmentation of arousal input as caffeine dosage increases produces a corresponding elevation of arousal output up to a point. Further input increments then produce a decrease in output in introverts, who are more highly aroused at baseline. The introverts are essentially pushed over the top of the inverted-U by the caffeine.

The finding of an inverted-U function is consistent with the biobehavioral theory, which predicts this biologically protective effect of multiple sources of arousal.[9,255] Two alternative, though compatible, theoretical explanations are Pavlov's concept of transmarginal inhibition[256,257] and Wilder's law of initial values.[258] Pavlov suggested that there is a protective physiological mechanism designed to avert damage to the cortex due to excessive stimulation and resultant arousal. This transmarginal inhibitory mechanism goes into action when arousal from multiple sources — such as caffeine and personality predispositions — summates to push overall arousal to dangerously high levels. The result, as with the inverted-U function of the biobehavioral theory, is a decrement in arousal output as measured psychophysiologically and a corresponding decrease in psychologically perceived arousal.

Wilder[258] hypothesized that there are protective biological limits on a variety of organs and systems, such that the extent to which caffeine or any other agent will increase measured arousal is dependent on the starting or baseline value of the physiological parameter. For example, a high intensity auditory stimulus may raise heart rate by 60 bpm to a total of 125 bpm if the prestimulation HR is only 65 bpm. However, if the resting baseline is 130 bpm, the same stimulus may raise it only 40 bpm to 170 bpm. In effect, Wilder is proposing the same inverted-U function, though it is less clear whether there will be an arousal output decrement when the margin is crossed or whether the function will simply reach a stable asymptote.

B. Impulsivity

Further confirmation of the inverted U-shaped arousal function relating caffeine to personality is seen in studies of impulsivity. Impulsives typically exhibit lower levels of arousal than nonimpulsives under baseline experimental conditions.[259,260] However, caffeine can modify[44] and even reverse the relative positions of the two groups. In one study, impulsives and nonimpulsives were tested on easy (letter cancellation) and difficult (verbal ability) tasks under each of five different caffeine dosages. Increasing drug doses improved the performance of both groups on the easy (less arousing) task. However, on the difficult task only the impulsives showed the positive dose-response relationship. Nonimpulsives improved with increasing caffeine dose up to a point, then deteriorated, supporting the inverted-U theory.[261]

Other research has typically confirmed the interactive effect of caffeine and impulsivity on mental task performance. The more highly aroused nonimpulsive group performs better than the impulsive group under placebo conditions. However, impulsives show greater improvement when given caffeine.[44] This same interaction is seen in studies of recognition memory[61] and visual search.[65] Exceptions to this common finding are seen in studies of recall memory for supraspan word lists, where no caffeine-impulsivity interaction has been observed.[67,71]

IV. CAFFEINE AND PSYCHOPATHOLOGY: ADDICTION AND CAFFEINISM

The DSM IV notes the potential for caffeine to be abused and includes Caffeine Intoxication under the category of Substance Abuse Disorders.[262] Despite this official classification, there continues to be controversy as to whether or not caffeine is actually a drug of abuse. Some researchers maintain that caffeine has very low, if any, potential for abuse,[235] while others believe that it can be addictive and has characteristics similar to those of other addictive drugs.[263]

A. The Potential For Abuse

In 1988, the Surgeon General established three criteria for addiction liability.[264] These general areas are Psychoactivity, Compulsive Use (Substance Dependence), and Drug-Reinforced Behavior (Reinforcing Effects).

1. Psychoactivity

As we have seen, low doses of caffeine (75 to 300 mg) have been shown to increase positive mood states,[153] with higher doses leading to more and more positive mood states, at least up to a point.[155,265] At the very high levels of consumption (greater than 500 mg) seen in heavy caffeine users,[157] the drug can elevate anxiety and depress affect.[34] Our more general review of the mood state literature above leaves little doubt that caffeine is a psychoactive drug.

2. Substance Dependence

A formal diagnosis of substance dependence requires a maladaptive pattern of abuse that leads to clinically significant impairment or distress. More detailed criteria revolve around the development of tolerance, the experience of withdrawal when abstinence is required, the inability to stop using the drug, and continued use over a protracted period of time. The question is whether or not these criteria, clearly applicable to cocaine, heroin, and other drugs, are met by caffeine.

Some research suggests that there is a group of coffee drinkers who are dependent on caffeine,[4] and liking for coffee has been shown to increase as dependency increases.[266] Moreover, in one study, regular caffeine consumers preferred drinks with 100 mg of caffeine over placebo drinks, while non-users had an opposite preference.[267] Dependency on caffeine results from repeated exposure to the drug[155] in either acute high doses or repetitive lower doses[235] and can produce considerable behavioral disruption.[268] Using DSM-IV criteria, one team of investigators found, in fact, that 16 out of 27 self-assessed caffeine-dependent people fulfilled clinical requirements for dependency.[269] Animal studies have also confirmed the dependence potential of caffeine.[235] For example, self-administration trials in rats provide an animal model for the development of dependence on the drug.[270]

Consistent with these observations, there is some evidence that caffeine may act, in part, on dopaminergic fibers that project into the medial forebrain bundle. Other psychostimulants also appear to act on this system, which may be at least one of the neural mechanisms involved in the development of dependence.[271] Further work has suggested a parallel between caffeine and another highly addictive drug, alcohol. Many of the same factors that enter into the development of alcoholism may also influence the development of dependence on caffeine.[272]

3. Tolerance

Tolerance is generally taken as one of the hallmarks of addiction liability. Moreover, to the extent that tolerance develops in a habitual caffeine consumer, any positive effects on mental performance may be eradicated. Addressing the tolerance literature in their earlier review, Gilliland and Bullock[34] concluded that there was little evidence for tolerance at that time. Since then, there have been several other tolerance studies, some confirming that earlier conclusion.[25,107] One study, for example, showed that relatively low doses (250 mg) of caffeine have similar effects on cerebral blood flow in non-users and heavy users,[273] evidence against substantial tolerance in heavy users. Moreover, habitual caffeine use does not eliminate its acute effects[274] or its enhancement of the stress response[214] in some studies.

There are, however, opposing findings suggesting that tolerance to caffeine does develop,[155,167,275,276] perhaps in as little as five days.[277] One team of investigators examined adults who consumed caffeine on a regular daily schedule and found evidence for significant tolerance.[277] Similarly, Evans and Griffiths[161] demonstrated the development of tolerance with a high dose of caffeine. In addition, the reticular formation in male rats has been shown to develop complete tolerance to caffeine within 2 weeks.[279]

A variety of factors differentiating tolerance studies could have contributed to the observed discrepancy. Lower doses are less likely to lead to tolerance than higher doses or will do so less rapidly. The habitual coffee drinkers in some studies may have had different levels or durations of consumption. In the cases of acute dosing, caffeine consumed by subjects outside the laboratory on the day of the experiment may have varied. This is particularly true when some investigators request in advance that subjects abstain from caffeine prior to the experiment, while others do not. Differences in age, gender, and arousal-relevant personality dimensions, such as extraversion and impulsivity, may have affected results. Finally, in the population at large, underlying genetic factors may make some people more susceptible to the development of caffeine tolerance. Unfortunately, there is no clear pattern in the studies to date that would specifically target one or more of these explanations. As a result, the tolerance issue remains unresolved.

4. Withdrawal

Guellot[280] first reported caffeine withdrawal symptoms that included insomnia and psychomotor impairment. Other studies confirm the psychomotor impairment,[281] and the list of withdrawal symptoms has grown to include headaches,[282-284] tension,[283] and fatigue.[285] There is also decreased attention,[281] increased anxiety,[263] irritability, disturbed concentration,[286] nausea/vomiting,[235] depression,[160] dysphoric mood,[148] and symptoms of stress,[147] such as increased heart rates.[287] These symptoms, similar to nicotine withdrawal effects,[288] can substantially impair the functioning of the individual during the withdrawal period.[289,290] However, it appears that very low doses of caffeine do not lead to withdrawal symptoms when stopped,[115] and some investigators have found that withdrawal symptoms occur only with total abstinence.[291] Fatigue is usually the first symptom to appear, followed by headaches,[292] which constitute 35 to 49% of all withdrawal complaints.[293] Withdrawal symptoms usually appear 12 to 24 h after abstinence and peak 8 to 16 h later.[4,290,294,295] The headaches disappear after a few days,[31] and the other symptoms also weaken over time.[148]

Confirming that the observed withdrawal is physiological are studies in which a placebo is substituted for caffeine in dependent users. Withdrawal symptoms appear even under these conditions.[269] In addition, the placebo substitution results in higher scores on depression scales.[160,296]

5. Reinforcing Effects

Psychological aspects of caffeine dependency, to the extent that they occur, may be due to the reinforcing effects of the drug.[235,297] In fact, doses as low as 25 mg have been shown to have reinforcing properties.[284] Although caffeine may not be as reinforcing as other psychostimulants,[163] animal studies have shown that it does have the properties of a positive reinforcer.[298]

These reinforcing effects are especially prevalent in coffee drinking, where the two major reasons for consumption appear to be the stimulation and relief given by the caffeine.[299] One study showed that, while nondependent heavy coffee drinkers consumed the same amount of coffee regardless of the presence of caffeine, those who were caffeine dependent consumed significantly more coffee when it was caffeinated.[290] In addition, recent caffeine use has been shown to cause people to choose caffeinated over decaffeinated coffee[290] even though de-caffeinated coffee and caffeinated coffee have been shown to taste the same.[300]

6. Caffeine Addiction in Perspective

Is caffeine an addictive drug? It is clearly psychoactive, and both withdrawal and reinforcement data document its addiction liability. Tolerance data are much less consistent, and this phenomenon will require further investigation. Although there is support for its addictive properties, caffeine obviously cannot be equated in this regard with such powerfully addictive substances as nicotine, cocaine, alcohol, or the narcotics. Caffeine withdrawal symptoms are nowhere nearly as severe as those for these other drugs, and the drug itself is much less psychologically, physiologically, or socially destructive.

B. Caffeinism

The first published report of caffeinism appeared in 1967 and described the case of a woman thought to have an anxiety disorder until it was determined that she was consuming 15 to 18 cups of brewed coffee per day. She showed rapid improvement when her caffeine intake was drastically reduced.[301] In 1974, John Greden[302] alerted clinicians to this newly identified disorder, which can produce symptoms indistinguishable from those of the anxiety disorders. He highlighted the diagnostic dilemma this situation can present and noted the need for care in making a differential diagnosis. Most of the research on caffeinism followed his article and was conducted primarily in the 1970s and 1980s. While there has been little recent research, the problem remains a potentially important one that may require further empirical attention.

Wilfrid Pilette[303] defined caffeinism as "...a pharmacological state of acute or chronic toxicity that results from the ingestion of high doses of caffeine...". As Greden[302] had suggested, the symptoms are highly correlated with those of the anxiety disorders. Commonly included among observed psychological manifestations are excessive anxiety, sleep disturbances,[303] irritability, and agitation.[304] Accompanying physical symptoms can include tremulousness, muscle twitches, diuresis, arrhythmias, flushing, tachypnea, palpitations, gastrointestinal disturbances,[302] psychophysiological complaints, sensory disturbances,[304] tachycardia,[305] and respiratory distress.[306] At extreme doses, the drug can be severely toxic or even fatal. In one case, a 27-year-old male patient experienced epileptoid convulsions, shallow respiration, and unconsciousness, as well as hyperpyrexia, tachycardia, and hypertension. He had ingested 500 g of ground coffee to obtain a "high".[307] In another case, a 20-year-old bulimic woman consumed 20 g of caffeine in a suicide attempt. In addition to severe manifestations of the more common symptoms of caffeine intoxication, she suffered a subendocardial infarction.[308]

The existence of caffeinism and its major symptom patterns were repeatedly confirmed in the early studies,[306] and it may be fairly common. Behar,[309] for example, diagnosed it in 16% of veterans referred to an outpatient clinic for PTSD. However, the more general prevalence of the disorder is unknown, definitive differential diagnostic signs have not been identified, and contributing causal factors are not well understood. Since many people who consume large amounts of caffeine apparently do not develop caffeinism,[1,30] while others manifest the symptoms on lower (though substantial) doses,[303] there are clearly factors other than dosage.

Gender and tobacco use both appear to be among the factors that contribute to caffeinism liability. Women and non-smokers are at higher risk.[185] Body weight, pattern of consumption, and exposure to other psychostimulants are other obvious possibilities. Somewhat more subtle is the likelihood that a predisposing factor may be present, and the genetic factor discussed above may provide this missing link. It may affect the adenosine receptor antagonism potency of caffeine[185] and may involve the serotonin[180] or norepinephrine[183] system or both.

Supporting this possibility is an interesting study in which patients with generalized anxiety disorder (GAD) were given 250 or 500 mg of caffeine prior to the recording of psychophysiological measures. They showed greater increases in EEG, skin conductance level, and blood pressure indicators of arousal than did normal controls.[175] The authors concluded that GAD patients appear to be abnormally sensitive to caffeine, an observation that both supports the likelihood of a genetic factor and helps to further understand the relationship between caffeine and GAD. Supportive studies show a similar caffeine hypersensitivity in patients with panic disorder.[75,310,311]

VII. CAFFEINE, AROUSAL, AND PSYCHOLOGICAL FUNCTIONING

Two decades ago we had very little scientific evidence concerning the effects of caffeine on psychological functioning. However, both scientific and public interest in the effects of this widely used psychostimulant increased dramatically when the Framingham heart study[312] and other early reports[11,12] pointed to its cardiopathogenic potential. With reports of caffeinism also entering the literature,[301,302] interest in studying the psychological, as well as physical, effects of the drug grew. The resulting pursuit of scientific research on caffeine has addressed a wide variety of areas of psychological functioning and performance. Among these, we have reviewed here literature on cognitive performance, emotional functioning, and psychopathological potential. We turn now to an attempt at achieving a further theoretical understanding of the factors that interact with and enter into the impact of caffeine.

A. The Biobehavioral Model Revisited

While conflicting results and unresolved issues remain, there are also increasing consistencies concerning the impact of caffeine on psychological and underlying physiological functioning. These consistencies become more apparent in the context of the biobehavioral model and the inverted-U arousal function that it includes. This model holds that arousal level is only one of several elements entering into the dual-interaction model that determines behavior and that caffeine is only one of a number of common contributors to arousal. Its effects in any given individual or situation thus depend on other relevant factors. Among these are arousal traits and arousal states. Biological and environmental backgrounds contribute to current traits, and both habitual and acute exposure to caffeine and other arousal agents contribute to current states. We have also postulated for some time a genetic factor that differentially predisposes individuals to have stronger or weaker physiological, and therefore psychological, reactions to caffeine. As we have seen, there is now evidence for such a factor and additional evidence that caffeine sensitivity and anxiety proneness may be genetically related. The several factors in the arousal model and their interactions combine to determine current physiological and psychological responses.

To reach a full understanding of caffeine effects, the biobehavioral model clearly suggests that we must learn how this psychostimulant interacts with other arousal-relevant factors. While not all studies are consistent, it now appears that the inverted U-shaped function provides the best available integration of both arousal-performance and arousal-arousal (arousal input-arousal output) data. The cognitive literature shows that this curvilinear relationship applies to information-processing, memory, vigilance, reaction time, and other cognitive-psychomotor data, among others.

Most findings for emotional functioning are also consistent with this theory. Mood states become more positive until arousal, including the caffeine component, crosses threshold, then deteriorate with further arousal increments. Happiness similarly increases, then decreases as arousal rises. Data on such arousal-relevant personality dimensions as extraversion and impulsivity clearly support the inverted-U hypothesis. What this suggests, then, is that many of the effects of caffeine are mediated by its effect on arousal and its interaction with other arousal agents. Such a finding supports most aspects of the biobehavioral model and also requires that we achieve the fullest possible understanding of the arousal properties of caffeine.

B. Effects On Arousal And Alertness

In the context of the biobehavioral theory, the relationship between caffeine and psychological functioning appears to be quite straightforward. It revolves around the well-documented impact of the drug on arousal and alertness. The vast literature in this area is quite consistent in demonstrating that caffeine increases both physiological arousal[9,313] and self-reported wakefulness and alertness.[148,202,314,315] Most of the effects on physiological arousal that serve to modify psychological performance are straightforward. Caffeine elevates skin conductance level (SCL), a reliable measure of tonic arousal[6,105,254,316] and also slows and stabilizes its habituation.[6] Skin conductance response (SCR) amplitude is also increased by caffeine,[58] and again habituation rate is reduced and the rate function smoothed by the drug.[5,317]

Electroencephalographic (EEG) changes following acute caffeine administration also support the observed effects of the drug on arousal level, though the exact nature of the changes depends on the subject population and the experimental situation. Studies have documented relative EEG activation[318] and decreased alpha activity,[116,168] with a demonstrable dose-response relationship,[49] under caffeine. In fact, the arousing effect of caffeine is so substantial that a 200-mg dose taken in the morning affects sleep EEG during the subsequent night.[319] The drug also produces changes in auditory evoked potentials recorded during a visual vigilance task, including a significant decrease in P2-N2 amplitude.[320] Other work has shown decreases in beta[59,310] and delta[50] amplitudes.

Cardiovascular studies show typically small but quite consistent increases in blood pressure.[108,153,167,212,321] In fact, normal dietary amounts of the drug elevate both systolic and diastolic pressures,[212,322,323] and there is some evidence that it may be a contributing factor in hypertension.[324] Studies using nuclear ventriculography and impedance cardiography suggest that this elevation may be based on increased systemic vascular resistance.[325] The blood-pressure elevation effect may be subject to tolerance with regular consumption,[167,267] though it may not be complete.[326] In addition, expectancy regarding the effect of caffeine on blood pressure may play a role.[327] Heart rate effects are much less consistent. Some studies show a decrease,[153,328-332] others an increase,[207,274,326,333] and still others no change.[167,209,334-337]

Overall, there is strong support for the hypothesis that caffeine elevates physiological arousal. It may be of particular behavioral significance that it also slows and smooths the process of habituation.[9] However, the mixed results for some measures, particularly heart rate, suggest the need to examine other mechanisms and effects.[9]

Self-report measures confirm the arousing effects of caffeine. It quite consistently produces an increase in alertness,[8,63,338] and this remains true even when nightly sleep has been restricted to five hours in subjects who normally sleep eight.[140] In fact, caffeine increases sleep latency[82,140] and, when given at night, elevates alertness to daytime levels.[314] It is no wonder, then, that the benefits of sleep on performance are reduced when caffeine is consumed prior to sleeping.[339] Even caffeine consumed during the morning hours disturbs the quality of sleep that night.[319] Other studies show that the drug substantially counteracts even 48 hours of sleep deprivation[151] and that the substitution of decaffeinated coffee in regular coffee drinkers decreases wakefulness.[287]

Further indication of the powerful effects of caffeine on psychological functioning comes from studies comparing the effects of the drug with other methods of elevating mental alertness. One such method is the prophylactic nap, which has been shown to maintain or increase alertness.[340] One recent investigation accordingly compared the effects of caffeine with those of prophylactic naps. Subjects were assigned to one of four nap conditions (0, 2, 4, or 8 h) and to one of four caffeine dosage groups (a single 400 mg dose, repeated doses of 150 or 300 mg every 6 h, or placebo). All then underwent two nights and days of sleep loss, during which they completed mood scales and performance tests. Results showed a dose-response elevation of alertness for both caffeine and prophylactic sleep. The authors concluded that the alertness increment produced by 150 to 300 mg of caffeine was approximately equivalent to that seen after 2 to 4 h of prophylactic nap time.[341]

A second study compared morning caffeine with eating breakfast. Interestingly enough — and contrary to popular advice — morning caffeine was more effective in increasing alertness, as well as performance on certain tasks, than was breakfast.[7] These self-report and observational measures of alertness are consistent with the bulk of the physiological literature in confirming the activating effects of caffeine.

C. Conclusion

As we noted earlier, caffeine affects not only arousal, but also other behavioral influences such as attentional focus. However, it now appears that these other effects may be secondary to the impact of the drug on arousal and that a multi-factorial model incorporating the inverted-U function may best describe that relationship. Most results in the literature to date are supportive of the biobehavioral model proposed here. However, research on the psychological effects of acute and habitual caffeine consumption is still in its infancy — or at best early childhood — and it is hoped that the biobehavioral model will help to guide further research in this important area.

REFERENCES

1. Gilbert, R. M., Caffeine as a drug of abuse, in *Research advances in alcohol and drug problems*. Edited by Gibbins, R. J., Israel, Y., and Kalant, H., Eds., John Wiley and Sons, New York, 1976.
2. Gilbert, R., Caffeine consumption, in *The Methlaxine Beverages and Foods: Chemistry, Consumptions and Health Effects*; New York: Liss, 1984.
3. Murray, J., Physiological aspects of coaffeine consumption. *Psychological Reports*; 62, 575-587, 1988.
4. Benowitz, N. L., Clinical pharmacology of caffeine. *Annual Review of Medicine*; 41, 277-288, 1990.
5. Davidson, R. and Smith, B., Arousal and habituation: Differential effects of caffeine, sensation seeking and task difficulty. *Personality and Individual Differences*; 10(1), 111-119, 1989.
6. Davidson, R. and Smith, B., Caffeine and novelty: Effects on electrodermal activity and performance. *Physiol Behav; 49*, 1169-1175, 1991.
7. Smith, A., Caffeine, performance, mood and states of reduced alertness. Special Issue: Caffeine research. *Pharmacopsychoecologia*; 7(2), 75-86, 1994.
8. Rusted, J., Caffeine and cognitive performance: Effects on mood or mental processing? Special Issue: Caffeine research. *Pharmacopsychoecologia*; 7(2), 49-54, 1994.
9. Smith, B. Effects of acute and habitual caffeine ingestion in physiology and behavior: Tests of a biobehvioral arousal theory. Special Issue: Caffeine Research. *Pharmacopsychoecologia*, 7(2), 151-167, 1994.
10. La Vecchia, C., Gentile, A., Negri, E., Parezzini, F. and Franceschi, S., Coffee consumption and myocardial infarction in women. *American Journal of Epidemology*; 130, 481-485, 1989.
11. Darragh, A., Kenny, M., Lambe, R. and O'Kelly, D., Adeverse effects of caffeine. *Irish Journal of Medical Science*; 150, 47-53, 1981.
12. Dobmeyer, D., Stino, R., Leier, C., Greenberg, R. and Schaal, S., The arrythmogenic effects of caffeine in human beings. *New Engalnd Journal of Medicine*; 308, 814-816, 1983.
13. Pincomb, G., Lovallo, W., McKey, B., Sung, B., Passey, R., Everson, S. and Wilson, M., Acute blood pressure elevations with caffeine in men with borderline systemic hypertension. *Am J Cardiol*; 77(4), 270-274, 1996.
14. Bak, A. and Grobbee, D., Caffeine, blood pressure and serum lipids. *Am J Clin Nutr*; 53(4), 971-975, 1991.
15. Battig, K., Cardiovascular effects of everyday coffee consumption. *Schweizerische Medizimische*; 122, 1536-1543, 1992.
16. Lewis, C. and Caan, B., Funkhouser, E., Hilner, J., Bragg, C., Dyer, A., Reczynski, J., Savage, P., Armstrong, M. and Friedman, G., Inconsistent associations of caffeine-containing beverages with blood pressure and with lipoproteins. The CARDIA study: Coronary artery risk developemnt in young adults. *American Journal of Epidemiology*; 138, 502-507, 1993.

17. Superko, H., Bortz, W., Williams, P., Albers, J. and Wood, P. , Caffeinated and decaffeinated coffee effects on plasma lipoprotein cholestrol, apolipoprotiens and lipase activity: A controlled, randomized trial. *American Journal of Clinical Nutrition*; 54, 599-605, 1991.
18. Etherton, G. and Kochar, M., Coffee: Facts and contreversy. *Archives of Family Medicine*; 293, 317-322, 1993.
19. Lynn, L. and Kissinger, J., Coronary precautions: Should caffeine be restricted to patientsafter myocardial invarction? *Heart and Lung*; 21, 365-371, 1992.
20. Myers, M. G. and Reeves, R. A., The effect of caffeine on daytime ambulatory blood pressure. *American Journal of Hypertension*; 4, 427-431, 1991.
21. Chou, T., Wake up and smell the coffee: Caffeine, coffee and the medical consequences. *Western Journal of Medicine*; 157, 544-553, 1992.
22. Suter, P. and Vetter, W., Coffee and caffeine: Various selceted reports for everyday practive. *Schweiz Runssch Med Prax*; 82, 1122-1128, 1993.
23. Gartside, P. and Glueck, C., Relationship of dietary intake to hospital admission for coronary heart and vascular disease: The NHANES II national probability study. *Journal of the American College of Nutrition*; 12, 676-684, 1993.
24. Willett, W., Stampfer, M., Manson, J., Colditz, G., Rosner, B. and Hennekens, C., Coffee consumption and coronary heart disease. *JAMA*; 285(6), 458-462, 1996.
25. Pirich, C., O-Grady, J. and Sininger, H., Coffee, lipoprotiens and cardiovascular disease. *Wien Klinical Wochenschr*; 104, 3-6, 1993.
26. Stavric, B., An update on research with coffee caffeine. *Food Chemistry and Toxicology*; 30, 533-555, 1992.
27. Lieberman, H., Wurtman, R., Emde, C. and Coviella, I., The effects of caffeine and aspirin on mood and performance. *J Clin Psychopharm*; *7*, 315-320, 1987.
27. Lieberman, H., Caffeine, in *Handbook of Human Performance (Vol. 2)*. Academic Press Ltd., 1992.
28. Roberts, H. and Barone, J., Biological effects of caffeine: History and use. *Food and Tehcnology*; 37, 32-39, 1983.
29. Barone, J. and Roberts, H., Caffeine consumption. *Food Chem Toxicol*; 34(1), 119-129, 1996.
30. Wells, S. J., Caffeine: Implications of recent research for clinical practice. *American Journal of Orthopsychiatry*; 54(3), 375-389, 1984.
31. Hirsh, K., *Central nervous system pharmacology of the dietary methylxanthines. In The Methylxanthine Beverages and Foods: Chemistry, Consumption, and Health Effects*, Edited by Spiller, G.A., New York: Allan R. Liss, Inc., 1984.
32. Smith, B., Rafferty, J., Lindgren, K., Smtih, D. and Nespor, A. Effects of habitual caffeine use and acute ingestion: Testing a biobehavioral model. *Physiology and Behavior*; 51, 131-137, 1992.
33. Koelega, H. Extraversion and vigilance performance: 30 yeaors of inconsistencies. *Psychological Bulliten*; 112(2), 239-258, 1992.
34. Gilliland, K., Bullock, W., Caffeine: A potential drug of abuse. *Advances in Alcohol and Substance Abuse*; 3(1-2), 53-73, 1984.
35. Baer, R., Effects of caffeine on classroom behavior, sustained attention, and a memory task in preschool childern. *Journal of Applied Behavior Analysis*; *20*(3), 225-234, 1987.
36. King, D. and Henry, G., The effect of neuroleptics on cognitive and psychomotor function: A preliminary study of helath volunteers. *British Journal of Psychiatry*; 160, 647-653., 1992.
37. Lubit, R., Russett,-Bruce The effects of drugs on decision-making. *Journal of Conflict Resolution*; Mar Vol 28(1), 85-102, 1984.
38. Stratta, P., Mancini, F., Mattei, P. and Casacchia, M., Information processing strategy to remediate Wisconson Cart Sorting test performance in schizophrenia: A pilot study. *American Journal of Psychiatry*; 151(6), 915-918, 1994.

39. Hasenfratz, M., Jaquet, F., Aeschbach, D., and Battig, K., Interactions of smoking and lunch with the effects of caffeine on cardiovascular functions and information processing. *Human Psychopharmacology Clinical and Experimental*; 6(4), 277-284, 1991.
40. Hasenfratz, M., Bunge, A., Dal-Pra, G., Battig, K., Antagonistic effects of caffeine and alcohol on mental performance parameters. *Pharmacology, Biochemistry and Behavior*; 46(2), 463-465, 1993.
41. Battig, K., and Buzzi, R., Effect of coffee on the speed of subject paced information processing. *Neuropsychobiology*; 16, 12, 1986.
42. Warburton, D. M., Effects of caffeine on cognition and mood without caffeine abstinence. *Psychopharmacology*; 119(1), 66-70, 1995.
43. Bonnet, M. and Arand, D., The use of prophylactic naps and caffeine to maintain performance during a continuous operation. *Ergonomics*; *37*(6), 1009-1020, 1994.
44. Smith, A. P., Rusted, J. M., Savory, M., and Eaton-Williams, P., The effects of caffeine, impulsivity and time of day on performance, mood and cardiovascular function. *Journal of Psychopharmacology*; 5(2), 120-128, 1991.
44. Massaro, D. and Ferguson, E., Cognitive style and perception: The relationship between category width and speech perception, categorization and discrimination. *The American Journal of Psychology*, 106(1), 25-50,1993.
45. France, C., Ditto, B., Caffeine effects on several indices of cardiovascular activity at rest and during stress. *Journal of Behavioral Medicine*; 11(5), 473-482, 1988.
46. Lane, J. D., and Williams, R. B., Caffeine affects cardiovascular responses to stress. *Psychophysiology*; 22(6), 648-655, 1985.
47. Linde, L., An auditory attention task: A note on the processing of verbal information. *Perceptual and Motor Skills*; 78(2), 563-570, 1994.
48. Riedel, W. and Jolles, J., Cognition enhancers in age related cognitive decline. *Drugs Aging*, 8(4), 245-474, 1996.
49. Hasenfratz, M., Battig, K., Acute dose-effect relationships of caffeine and mental performance, EEG, cardiovascular and subjective parameters. *Psychopharmacology*; 114(2), 281-287, 1994.
50. Pritchard, W. S., Robinson, J. H., deBethizy, J. D., Davis, R. A., et-al., Caffeine and smoking: Subjective, performance, and psychophysiological effects. *Psychophysiology*; 32(1), 19-27, 1995.
51. Foreman, N., Barraclough, S., Morre, C., Mehta, A., and Madon, M., High doses of caffeine impair performance of a numerical version of the Stroop task in men. *Pharmacology, Biochemistry, and Behavior*; 32, 399-403, 1989.
52. Loke, W. H., The effects of caffeine and automaticity on a visual information processing task. *Human- Psychopharmacology- Clinical-and-Experimental*; 7(6), 379-388, 1992.
53. Landrum, R., Meliska, C. and Loke, W., Effects of caffeine and task experience on task performance. *Psychologia: Int J Psych Orient*; *37*, 801-812, 1988.
54. Ketterer, M., Lateralized representation of affect, affect cognizance and the coronary prone personality. *Biol Psych*; *15*, 509-516, 1982.
55. Smith, B., Meyers, M. and Kline, R., Hemispheric assymetry and emotion: Lateralized parietal processing of affect and cognition. *Biol Psych*; *29*, 11-26. 1987.
56. Smith, B., Kline, R., Lindgren, K., Ferro, M., Smith, D. and Nespor, A., The laterlaized processing of affect in emotional liable extraverts and introverts: central and autonomic effects. *Biol Psych*; *39*, 143-157, 1995.
57. Roman, F., Garcia-Sanchez, F., Martinez-Selva, J., Gomez-Amor, J. and Carrillo, E., Sex differences and bilateral electrodermal activity. *Pavl J Biol Science*; *24*, 150-155, 1989.
58. Smith, B. D., Davidson, R. A., Green, R. L. Effects of caffeine and gender on physiology and performance: Further tests of a biobehavioral model. *Physiology and Behavior*; 54, 415-522, 1993.

59. Hasenfratz, M., and Battig, K., Action profiles of smoking and caffeine: Stroop effect, EEG, and peripheral physiology. *Pharmacology, -Biochemistry-and-Behavior;* 42(1), 155-161, 1992.
60. de-Brabander, B., Effect of short lateralized signals on arousal versus activation on tasks requiring visuospatial or elementary semantic visual processing. *Perceptual and Motor Skills; 67*(3), 783-788, 1988.
61. Bowyer, P., Humphreys, M. and Revelle, W., Arosual and recognition memory: The effects of impulsivity, caffeine and time on a task. *Personality and Individual Differences;* 4(1), 41-49, 1983.
62. Bowyer, P., Humphreys, M. and Reville, W., Arousal and recognition memory. The effects of impulsivity, caffeine and time on task. *Person Individ Diff; 4,* 41-49, 1985.
63. Smith, A. P., Kendrick, A. M., Maben, A. L., Effects of breakfast and caffeine on performance and mood in the late morning and after lunch. *Neuropsychobiology;* 26, 198-204, 1992.
64. Jarvis, M., Does caffeine intake enhance absolute levels of cognitive performance? *Psychopharmacology; 110,* 45-52, 1993.
65. Anderson, K. and Revelle, W., The interactive effects of caffeine, impulsivity and task demands on visual search task. *Personality and Individual Differences;* 4(2), 127-134, 1983.
66. Loke, W. H., Effects of caffeine on mood and memory. *Physiology-and-Behavior;* Vol 44(3), 367-372, 1988.
67. Erikson, G. The effects of caffeine on memory for word lists. *Physiology and Behavior; 35*(1), 47-51, 1985.
68. Terry, W. and Phifer, B., Caffeine and memory performance on the AVLT. *Journal of Clinical Psychology;* 42(6), 860-863, 1986.
69. Roache, J. and Griffiths, R., Interaction of diazepam and caffeie: Behavioral and subjective dose effects in humans. *Pharmacology, Biochemistry and Behavior;* 26(4), 801-812, 1987.
70. Oborne, D. J., Rogers, Y., Interactions of alcohol and caffeine on human reaction time. *Aviation, -Space,-and -Environmental- Medicine;* 54(6), 528-534, 1983.
71. Arnold, M., Petros, T., Beckwith, B., Coons, G. and Gorman, N., The effects of cafeine, impulsivity and sex on memory for word lists. *Physiol Behav, 41,* 25-30, 1987.
72. Lieberman, H. R., Beneficial effects of caffeine. *In Twelfth International Scientific Colloquium on Coffee;* Paris: ASIC. 1988.
73. Clubley, M., Bye, C. E., Henson, T. A., Peck, A. W. and Riddington, C. J., Effects of caffeine and cyclizine alone and in combination on human performance, subjective effects and EEG activity. *British Journal of Clinical Pharmacology;* 7: 157-63, 1979.
74. File, S., Bond, A. and Lister, R., Interaction between effects of caffeine and lorazepam in performance and self ratings. *Journal of Clinical Psychopharmacology;* 2, 102-106, 1982.
75. Turner, J., Incidental information processing: Effects of mood, sex and caffeine. *International-Journal-of-Neuroscience;* 72(1-2), 1-14, 1993.
76. Loke, W. H., Hinrichs, J. V., and Ghoneim, M. M., Caffeine and diazepam: Separate and combined effects on mood, memory, and psychomotor performance. *Psychopharmacology;* 87, 344-350, 1985.
77. Linde, L., Mental effects of caffeine in fatigued and non-fatigued female and male subjects. *Ergonomics;* 38(5), 864-885, 1995.
78. Revelle, W., Loftus, D. A., Individual differences and arousal: Implications for the study of mood and memory. Special Issue: Development of relationships between emotion and cognition. *Cognition-and-Emotion;* 4(3), 209-237, 1990.

79. Lieberman, H. R., Wurtman, R. J., Emde, G. G., Roberts, C., and Coviella, I. L. G., The effects of low doses of caffeine on human performance and mood. *Psychopharmacology*; 92, 308-312, 1987a.
80. Wilkinson, R., Methods for research on sleep deprivation and sleep function. In, *Sleep and Dreaming*. (Hartmann,E., ed.). Boston: Little and Brown, 1970.
81. Loke, W. and Meliska, C., Effects of caffeine use and ingestion on a protracted vigilance test. *Psychopharmacology; 87*, 344-350, 1984.
82. Zwyghuizen-Doorenbos, A., Roehrs, T., Lipshutz, L., Timms, V. and Roth, T., Effects of caffeine on alertness. *Psychopharmacology; 100*, 36-39, 1990.
83. Pons, L., Trenque, T., Bielcki, M. and Moulin, M., Attentional deficits of caffeine in man: Comparison with drugs acting on performance. *Psychiatry Research*; 23(3), 329-333, 1988.
84. Fagan, D., Swift, C. G., and Tiplady, B., Effects of caffeine on vigilance and other performance tests in normal subjects. *Journal of Psychopharmacology*; 2, 19-25, 1988.
85. Fine, B. J., Kobrick, J. L., Lieberman, H. R., Marlowe, B., et-al., Effects of caffeine or diphenhydramine on visual vigilance. *Psychopharmacology*; 114(2), 233-238, 1994.
86. Belyavin, A., and Wright, N. A., Changes in electrical activity of the brain with vigilance. *Electroencephalography and Clinical Neurophysiology*; 66(2), 137-144, 1987.
87. Lorist, M., Snel, J., Kok, A. and Madler, G., Acute effects of selective attention and visual search processes. *Psychophysiology*; 3(4), 354-361, 1996.
88. Munte, T. F., Heinze, H. J., Kunkel, H., and Scholz, M., Personality traits influence the effects of diazepam and caffeine on CNV magnitude. *Neuropsychobiology*;12(1), 60-67, 1984.
89. Stein, M., Krasowski, M. Leventhal, B., Phillips, W. and Bender, B., Behavioral and cognitive effects of methylxanthines: A meta-analysis of theophyliine and caffeine. *Arch Pediatr Adolesc Med*; 150(3), 284-288, 1996.
90. Kupietz, S. and Winsberg, B., Caffeie and inattentiveness in reading-disabled childern. *Perceptual and Motor Skills*; 44 (3, pt. 2), 1238, 1977.
91. Bernstein, G. A., Carroll, M. E., Crosby, R. D., Perwein, A. R., et-al., An investigation of personality and caffeine use. *Journal of the American Academy of Child and Adolescent Psychiatry*; 33(3), 407-415, 1994.
92. Koelega, H. S., Stimulant drugs and vigilance performance: A review. *Psychopharmacology*; 111(1), 1-16, 1993.
93. Frewer, L. and Lader, M., The effetcs of caffeine on two computerized tests of attention and vigilance. *Human Psychopharmacology Clinical and Experimental*; 6(2), 119-128, 1991.
94. Smith, B., Rafferty, J., Lindgren, K., Smith, D. and Nespor, A., Chronic and acute effects of caffeine: Testing a biobehavorial model. *Physiol Behav, 51*, 131-137, 1991.
95. Wegner, D. M., Shortt, J. W., Blake, A. W., Page, M. S., The suppression of exciting thoughts. *Journal of Personality and Social Psychology*; 58(3), 409-418, 1990.
96. Giambra, L. M., Grodsky, A., Belongie, C., and Rosenberg, E. H., Depression and thought intrusions, relating thought frequency to activation and arousal. *Imagination, Cognition and Personality*; 14(1), 19-29, 1995.
97. Giambra, L. M., Wise, K., Rosenberg, E. H., Jung, R. E., The influence of caffeine arousal on the frequency of task-unrelated image and thought intrusions. *Imagination Cognition and Personality*; 13(3), 215-223, 1994.
98. Johnson, M., Thinking about strategies during, before and after making a decision. *Psychology and Aging*; 8(2), 231-241, 1993.
99. Smith, D., Tong, J. and Leigh, G., Combined effects of caffeine and tobacco on the components of choice reaction time, heart rate and hand steadiness. Perc and Motor Skills; *45*(2), 635-639, 1977.

100. Struefert, S., Pogash, R., Miler, J. and Gingrich, D., Efects of caffeine deprivation on complex human fuctioning. *Psychopharmacology; 118*(4), 377-384, 1995.
101. Sargent, J., and Solbach, P., Stress and headache in the workplace: The role of caffeine. *Medical Psychotherapy An International Journal;* 1, 83-86, 1988.
102. Choi, A., Laurito, C. and Cummingham, F., Pharmacologic managment of postdural puncture headache. *Ann Pharmacother;* 30(7-8), 831-839, 1996.
103. Ramadan, N., Headache caused by intracranial pressure and intracranial hypotension. *Curr Opin Neurol;* 9(3), 214-218., 1996.
104. Smith, B., Concannon, M., Campbell, S. and Bozman, A., Regression and criterion measures of habituation: A comparitive analysis in extraverts and introverts. *Journal of Research in Personality;* 24(2), 123-132, 1990.
105. Smith, B., Rypma, C. and Wilson, R., Dishabiuation and spontaneous recovery of the electrodermal orienting response: Effects of extraversion, impulsivity, sociabiltiy and caffeine. *Journal of Research in Personality;* 15, 475-487, 1981.
106. Dekker, D., Paley, M. Popken, S. and Tepas, D., Locomotive engineers and their spouses: Coffee consumption, mood and sleep disorders. *Ergonomics; 36*(1-3), 233-238, 1993.
107. Lane, J. D., Adcock, A., Williams, R. B., and Kuhn, C. M. , Caffeine effects on cardiovascular and neuroendocrine responses to acute psychosocial stress and their relationship to level of habitual caffeine consumption. *Psychosomatic Medicine;* 52, 320-336, 1990.
108. Greenberg, W., and Shapiro, D., The effects of caffeine and stress on blood pressure in individuals with and without a family history of hypertension. *Psychophysiology;* 24(2), 151-156, 1987.
109. France, C., and Ditto, B., Cardiovascular responses to the combination of caffeine and mental arithmetic, cold pressor, and static exercise stressors. *Psychophysiology;* 29, 272-282, 1992.
110. Shapiro, D and Oakley, M., Methodological issues in the evaluation of drug behavioral interactions in the treatment of hypertension. *Psychosomatic Medicine;* 51(3), 269-276, 1989.
111. Lane, J., Neuroendocrine responses to caffeine in the work environment. *Psychosomatic Medicine; 56*(3), 267-270, 1994.
112. Jeong, D. U., and Dimsdale, J. E., The effects of caffeine on blood pressure in the work environment. *American Journal of Hypertension;* 3, 749-753, 1990.
113. France, C., and Ditto, B., Cardiovascular responses to occupational stress and caffeine in telemarketing employees. *Psychosomatic Medicine;*51(2), 145-151, 1989.
114. Tulving, E., What is episodic memory? *Current Directions in Psychological Science;* 2(3), 67-70, 1993.
115. Rogers, P., Richardson, N. and Dernoncourt, C., Caffeine use: Is there a net benifit for mood and psychomotor performance? *Neuropyshobiology; 31*(4), 195-199, 1995.
116. Kenemans, J. L., and Lorist, M. M., Caffeine and selective visual processing. *Pharmacology, Biochemistry and Behavior;* 52(3), 461-471, 1995.
118. Kuznicki, J. and Turner, L., The effects of caffeine on users and non-users. *Physiol Behav; 37*, 397-408, 1986.
119. Miller, L. and Miller, S., Caffeine enhances initial but not extended learning of a proprioceptive-based discrimination taskin non smoking moderate users. *Percept Mot Skills;* 82(3), 891-898, 1996.
120. Rapoport, J., Jensvold, M. and Elkins, R., Behavioral and autonomic effects of caffeine in normal boys. *Dev Pharmacol Ther; 3*, 74-82, 1981.
121. Barr, H. M., Streissguth, A. P., Darby, B. L., Sampson, P. D., Prenatal exposure to alcohol, caffeine, tobacco, and aspirin: Effects on fine and gross motor performance in 4-year-old children. *Developmental-Psychology;* 26(3), 339-348, 1990.

122. Elkins, R., Rapoport, J. and Zahn, T., Acute effects of caffeine in prepubertal boys. *Am J Psychiatry; 138,* 178-183, 1981.
123. Powers, H., Caffeine, behavior and the LD child. *Academic Therapy; 11*(1), 5-19, 1975.
124. Robertson, D., Wade, D., Workman, R., Woosley, R. L., and Oates, J.A., Tolerance to the humoral and hemodynamic effects of caffeine in man. *J. Clin. Invest;* 67: 1111-17, 1981.
125. Goldstein, A., Kaizer, S., Whitby, O., Psychotropic effects of caffeine in man. IV. Quantitative and qualitative differences associated with habituation to coffee. *Clin. Pharmacol. Ther;* 10: 489-497, 1969.
126. Donovan, R., Rossiter, J., Marcoolyn, G. and Nesdale, A., Store atmosphere and purchasing behavior. *Journal of Retailing; 70*(3), 283-294, 1994.
127. Mehrabian, A., Effects of affective and informational characteristics of work environments on worker satisfaction. *Imagination, Cognition and Personality;* 9(4), 293-301, 1990.
128. Sinclair, R., Hoffman, C., Mark, M. and Martin, L., Construct accessibility and the misattribution of arousal: Schachter and Singer Revisited. *Psychological Science; 5*(1), 15-19, 1994.
129. Baker, J., Levy, M. and Grewal, D. An experimental approach to making retail store environmental decisions. *Journal of Retailing;* 68(4), 445-460, 1992.
130. Guess, D. and Carr, E., Rejoinder to Lovass and Smith, Mulick and Meinhold and Baumeister. *American Journal on Retardation; 96*(3), 335-344, 1991.
131. Kaplan-Estrin, M., Jacobson, S. and Jacobson, J., Alternaitve approaches to clustering and scoring the Bayley Infant Behavior Record. *Infant Behavior and Development; 17*(2), 149-157, 1994.
132. Loewen, L. and Suedfeld, P., Cognitive and arousal effects of masking office noise. *Environment and Behavior; 24*(3), 381-395, 1992.
133. Achee, J., Tesser, A., and Pilkington, C., Social perception: A test of the role of arousal in self-evaluation maintenance processes. Special Issue: Affect in social judgments and cognition. *European Journal of Social Psychology;* 24(1), 147-159, 1994.
134. Prins, D., Hubbard, C. and Krause, M., Syllabic stress and the occurence of stuttering. *Journal of Speech and Hearing Research;* 34(5), 1011-1016, 1991.
135. James, J. E., The influence of user status and anxious disposition on the hypertensive effects of caffeine. *International Journal of Psychophysiology;*10(2), 171-179, 1991.
136. Suedfeld, P. and Eich, E., Autobiographical memory and affect conditions of reduced environmental stimulation. *Journal of Environmental Psychology;* 15(4), 321-326, 1995.
137. Alexander, C., Robinson, P., Orme-Johnson, D. and Schneider,R., The effects of transcendental meditation compared to other methods of relaxation and meditation in reducing risk factors, morbidity and mortality. *Homeostasis in Health and Disease;* 35(4-5), 243-263, 1994.
138. Taub, E., Steiner, S., Weingarten, E., and Walton, K. , Effectiveness of broad spectrum approaches to relapse prevention in severe alcohlism: A long term, randomized, controlled trial of Transcendental Meditation, EMG biofeedback and electronic eurotherapy. Special Issue: Self-recovery: Treating addictions using transcendental meditation and Maharishi Ayur-Veda. *Alcoholism Treatment Quarterly;* 11 (1-2), 187-220, 1994.
139. Benson, H., Kornhaber, A., Kornhaber, C. and LeChanu, M. , Increases in positive psychological characteristics with a new relaxation response curriculum in high school students. *Journal of Research and Development in Education;* 27(4), 226, 1994.

140. Rosenthal, L., Roehrs, T., Zwyghuizen-Doorenbos, A., Plath, D., et-al., Alerting effects of caffeine after normal and restricted sleep. *Neuropsychopharmacology;* 4(2), 103-108, 1991.
141. Edwards, S., Brice, L., Craig, C. and Perri-Jones, R., Effects of caffeine, practice and mode of presentation on Stroop task performance. *Pharmacol Biochem Behav;* 54(2), 309-315, 1996.
142. Swift, C. and Tiplady, B., The effect of age on the response to caffeine. *Psychopharmacology;* 67, 73-80, 1988.
143. Azcona, O., Barbanoj, M. J., Torrent, J., and Jane, F. , Evaluation of the effects of alcohol-caffeine interaction on the central nervous system. *Journal of Psychopharmacology;* 6, 136, 1992.
144. Jacobsen, B. H., and Edgley B. M., Effects of caffeine on simple reaction time and movement time. *Aviation, Space, and Environmental Medicine;* 58, 1153-1156, 1987.
145. Anderson, K. J., Revelle, W., and Lynch, M. J., Caffeine, impulsivity, and memory scanning: A comparison of two explanations for the Yerkes-Dodson effect. *Motivation and Emotion;* 13, 1-20, 1989.
146. Johnson, L. C., Spinweber, C. L., and Gomez, S. A., Benzodiazepines and caffeine: Effect on daytime sleepiness, performance, and mood. *Psychopharmacology;*101, 160-167, 1990.
147. Ratliff-Crain, J., O'Keeffe, M. K., and Baum, A., Cardiovascular reactivity, mood, and task performance in deprived and nondeprived coffee drinkers. *Health-Psychology;* 8(4), 427-447, 1989.
148. Richardson, N. J., Rogers, P. J., and Elliman, N. A., Effects of comprehensive relaxation training (CRT) on mood: A preliminary report on relaxation training plus caffeine cessation. *Pharmacology, Biochemistry and Behavior;* 52(2), 313-320, 1995.
149. Kawachi, I., Willett, W., Colditz, G., Stampfer, M. and Speizer, F., A prospective study of coffee drinking and suicide in women. *Arch Intern Med;* 156(5), 521-525, 1996.
150. Richardson, N., Rogers, P. and Elliman, N., Conditioned flavor preferences reinforced by caffeine consumed after lunch. *Physiol Behav;* 60(1), 257-263, 1996.
151. Penetar, D., McCann, U., Thorne, D. and Kamimori, G., Caffeine reversal of sleep deprivation effects on alertness and mood. *Psychopharmacology;* 112(2-3), 359-365, 1993.
152. Perkins, K. A., Sexton, J. E., Stiller, R. L., Fonte, C., et-al., Subjective and cardiovascular responses to nicotine combined with caffeine during rest and casual activity. *Psychopharmacology;* 113(3-4), 438-444, 1994.
153. Rush, C., Sullivan, J. and Griffiths, R., Intravenous caffeine in stimulant drug abusers: Subjective reports and physiological effects. *Journal of Pharmacology and Experimental Therapeutics;* 273(1), 351-358, 1995.
154. Cohen, C., Pickworth, W. B., Bunker, E. B., and Henningfield, J. E., Caffeine antagonizes EEG effects of tobacco withdrawal. *Pharmacology, Biochemistry and Behavior;* 47(4), 919-926, 1994.
155. Heishman, S. J., Henningfield, J. E., Is caffeine a drug of dependence? Criteria and comparisons. Special Issue: Caffeine research. *Pharmacopsychoecologia;* 7(2),127-135, 1994.
156. Leathwood, P. and Pollet, P., Diet-induced mood changes in normal populations. *Journal of Psychiatric Research;* 17: 147-54, 1982.
157. Griffiths, R. R., Evans, S. M., Heisman, S. J., Preston, K. L., Sannerud, C. A., Wolf, B. and Woodson, P. P., Low-dose caffeine discrimination in humans. *Journal of Pharmacology and Experimental Therapeutics;* 252: 970-8, 1990.
158. Hughes, G. V., and Boland, F. J., The effects of caffeine and nicotine consumption on mood and somatic variables in a penitentiary inmate population. *Addictive Behaviors;*17(5), 447-457, 1992.

159. Loke, W.H., Effects of repeated caffeine administration on cognition and mood. *Human Psychopharmacology Clinical and Experimental*; 5(4), 339-348, 1990.
160. Silverman, K., Evans, S. M., Strain, E. C., Griffiths, R. R., Withdrawal syndrome after the double-blind cessation of caffeine consumption. *N. Engl. J. Med.*; 327: 1109-1114, 1992.
161. Evans, S. M., and Griffiths, R. R., Caffeine tolerance and choice in humans. *Psychopharmacology*; 108(1-2), 51-59, 1992.
162. Totten, G. L., and France, C. R., Physiological and subjective anxiety responses to caffeine and stress in nonclinical panic. *Journal of Anxiety Disorders*; Vol 9(6), 473-488, 1995.
163. Stern, K. N., Chait, L. D., and Johanson, C. E., Reinforcing and subjective effects of caffeine in normal human volunteers. *Psychopharmacology*; 98, 81-88, 1989.
164. Kenardy, J., Oei, T.P., Weir, D., and Evans, L., Phobic anxiety in panic disorder: Cognition, heart rate, and subjective anxiety. *Journal of Anxiety Disorders*; 7(4), 359-371, 1993.
165. Mauri, M., Sarno, N., Rossi, V. M., Armani, A., et al., Personality disorders associated with generalized anxiety, panic, and recurrent depressive disorders. *Journal of Personality Disorders* 6(2), 162-167, 1992.
166. Fonagy, P. and Calloway, S., The effect of emotional arousal on spontaneous swallowing rates. *Journal of Psychosomatic Research*; 30(2), 183-188, 1986.
167. Casiglia, E., Paleari, C. D., Petucco, S., Bongiovi, S., Colangeli, G., Baccilieri, M. S., Pavan, L., Pernice, M., and Pessina, A. C., Haemodynamic effects of coffee and purified caffeine in normal volunteers: A placebo-controlled clinical study. *Journal of Human Hypertension*; 6, 95-99, 1992.
168. Dimpfel, W., Schober, F., and Spuler, M., The influence of caffeine on human EEG under resting conditions and during mental loads. *Clinical Inverstigations*; 71, 197-207, 1993.
169. Hughes, J. R., Higgins, S. T., and Hatsukami, D., Effects of abstinence from tobacco: A critical review. In Kozlowski, L. T., Annis, H. M., Cappell, H. D., Glaser, F. B., Goodstadt, M. S., Israel, Y., Kalant, H., Sellers, E. M., and Vingilis, E. R., (Eds.) *Research advances in alcohol and drug problems*. (Vol. 10, pp. 317-398). New York: Plenum Press, 1990.
170. Sachs, D., and Benowitz, N. *The nicotine withdrawal syndrome: Nicotine absence or caffeine excess?* Proceedings of the Fiftieth Annual Meeting of the Committee on Problems of Drug Dependence: NIDA Research Monograph. 90, p. 38. Washington, DC: U.S. Government Printing Office, 1988.
171. Chait, L. D., and Griffiths, R. R., Effects of caffeine administration on human cigarette smoking. *Clinical Pharmacology and Therapeutics*; 34, 612-622, 1982.
172. Zeiner, A. R., Stanitis, T., Spurgeon, M., Nichols, N., Treatment of alcoholism and concomitant drugs of abuse. *Alcohol*; 2(3), 555-559, 1985.
173. Coffey, C. E., Weiner, R. D., Hinkle, P. E., Cress, M., et al., Adverse reaction to use of caffeine in ECT. *Biological Psychiatry*; 22(5), 637-649, 1987.
174. Veleber, D. M., Templer, D. I., Effects of caffeine on anxiety and depression. *Journal of Abnormal Psychology*; 93(1), 120-122, 1984.
175. Bruce, M., Scott, N., Shine, P., and Lader, M., Anxiogenic effects of caffeine in patients with anxiety disorders. *Archives of General Psychiatry*; 49(11), 867-869, 1992.
176. Shanahan, M. P., and Hughes, R. N., Potentiation of performance-induced anxiety by caffeine in coffee. *Psychological Reports*; 59, 83-86, 1986.
177. Dubovsky, S. L., Generalized anxiety disorder: New concepts and psychopharmacologic therapies. 142nd Annual Meeting of the American Psychiatric Association (1989, San Francisco, California). *Journal of Clinical Psychiatry*; 51(Suppl) 3-10, 1990.

178. Fredholm, B. B., On the mechanism of action of theophylline and caffeine. *Acta Med. Scand*; 217: 149-53, 1985.
179. Kendler, K., Neale, M., Kessler, R. and Heath, A., Generalized Anxiety disorder in women: A population based twin study. *Archives of General Psychiatry*; 49(4), 267-272, 1992.
180. Rauch, S. and Jenike, M., Neurobiological models of obsessive-compulsive disorder. *Psychosomatics*; 34(1), 20-32, 1993.
181. Otto, M., Normal and abnormal information processing: A neuropsychological perspective on obsessive compulsive disorder. *Psychiatric Clinics of North America*; 15(4), 825-848, 1992.
182. Scarone, S., Colombo, C., Livian, S. and Abbruzzese, M. , Increased right caudate nucleus size in obsessive compulsive disorder: Detection with magnetic resosnance imaging. *Psychiatry Research Neuroimaging*; 45(2), 115-121, 1992.
183. Nutt, D., Glue, P. and Lawson, C., The neurochemistry of anxiety: An update. *Progress in Neuropsychopharmacology and Biological Psychiatry*; 14(5), 737, 1990.
184. Hildebrand, M. and Seifert, W., Determination of acetylator phenotype in caucasians with caffeine. *Journal of Clinical Pharmacology*; 37, 525-526, 1981.
185. Carrillo, J. and Benitez, J., Caffeine metabolism in a healthy spanish population: N-Acetylator phenotype and oxidation pathways. *Clinical Pharmacological Therapeutics*; 55, 293-304, 1994.
186. Warburton, D. M., Thompson, D. H., An evaluation of the effects of caffeine in terms of anxiety, depression and headache in the general population. Special Issue: Caffeine research. *Pharmacopsychoecologia*; 7(2), 55-61, 1994.
187. Smith, G. A., Caffeine reduction as an adjunct to anxiety management. *British Journal of Clinical Psychology*; 27(3), 265-266, 1988.
188. Charney, D. S., Heninger, G. R., and Jatlow, P. I., Increased anxiogenic effects of caffeine in panic disorders. *Archives of General Psychiatry*; 42(3), 233-243, 1985.
189. Lee, M. A., Flegel, P., Greden, J. F., andCameron, O. G., Anxiogenic effects of caffeine on panic and depressed patients. 41st Annual Meeting of the Society of Biological Psychiatry (1986, Washington, DC). *American Journal of Psychiatry*; 145(5), 632-635, 1988.
190. Parry-Jones, B. and Parry-Jones, W., Post-traumatic stress disorder: Supportive evidence from an eighteenth century natural disaster. *Psychological Medicine*; 24(1), 15-27, 1994.
191. Kramer, T., Lindy, J., Green, B., Grace, M. and Leonard, A., The lombordity of post traumatic stress disorder and suicidality in vietnam veterans. *Suicide and Life Threatening Behaviors*; 24(1), 58, 1994.
192. Long, N., Chamberlain, K. and Vincent, C., Effect of the Gulf War on reactivation of adverse combat-related memories in Vietnam veterans. *Journal of Clinical Psychology*; 50(2), 138-144, 1994.
193. Spiro, A., Schnurr, P. and Aldwin, C., Combat related post traumatic stress disorder symptoms in older men. *Psychology and Aging*; 9(1), 17-26, 1994.
194. Powers, P., Cruse, C., Daniels, S. and Stevens, B., Posttraumatic stress disorder in patients with burns. *J Burn Care Rehabil*; 15(2), 147-153, 1994.
195. Blanchard, E., Hickling, E., Taylor, A. and Loos, W., The psychophysiology of motor vechicle accident related posttraumatic stress disorder. *Behavior Therapy*; 25(3), 453-467, 1994.
196. Vrana, S. and Lauterbuch, D., Prevelance of traumatic events and post traumatic symptoms in college students. *Journal of Traumatic Stress*; 7(2), 289-302, 1994.
197. Iancu, I., Dolberg, O. and Zohar, J., Is caffeine involved i nthe pathgenesis of scombat stress reaction. *Mil Med*; 161(4), 230-232, 1996.
198. Schreiber, E. and Schreiber, K., Using relaxation techniques and positive self esteem to improve academic acheivement of college students. *Psychological Reports*; 76(3), 929-930., 1995.

199. National Center for Health Statistics. *Health USA: 1994*. Hyattsville,MD.: Public Health Service, 1995.
200. Herbert, T. and Cohen, S., Stress and Immunology in humans: a meta analysis review. *Psychosomatic Medicine*; 55(4), 364-379, 1993.
201. Sgoutas-Emch, S., Cacioppo, J., Uchino, B. and Malarkey, W., The effects of an acute psychological stressor on cardiovascular, endocrine, and cellular immune response: A prospective study of individuals high and low in heart rate reactivity. *Psychophysiology*; 31(3), 264-271, 1994.
202. Miller, S. and Sita, A., Parental history of hypertension, menstrual cycle phase and cardiovascular response to stress. *Psychosomatic Medicine*; 56(1), 61-69, 1994.
203. Petch, M., Triggering a heart attack. *BMJ*, 312(7029), 459, 1996.
204. Klinnert, M., Mrazek, P. and Mrazek, D., Early asthma onset: The interaction between family stressors and adaptive parenting. *Psychiatry Interpersonal and Biological Processes*; 57(1), 51-61, 1994.
205. Stewart, S. and Pihl, R., Effects of alcohol administration on psychophysiological and subjective-emotional responses to aversive stimulation in anxiety sensitive women. *Psychology of Addictive Behaviors*; 8(1), 29-42, 1994.
206. James, J. *Caffeine and Health*. London: Academic Press, 1991.
207. MacDougall, J. M., Musante, L., Castillo, S., and Acevedo, M.C., Smoking, caffeine, and stress: Effects on blood pressure and heart rate in male and female college students. *Health Psychology*; 7, 461-478, 1988.
208. Goldstein, I. B., and Shapiro, D., The effects of stress and caffeine on hypertensives. *Psychosomatic Medicine*; 49(3), 26-235, 1987.
209. Myers, H. F., Shapiro, D., McClure, F., Daims, R., Impact of caffeine and psychological stress on blood pressure in Black and White men. Special Issue: Race, reactivity, and blood pressure regulation. *Health Psychology*; 8(5), 597-612, 1989.
210. Lovallo, W. R., Pincomb, G. A., Sung, B. H., Everson, S. A., Passey, R. B., and Wilson, M. F., Hypertension risk and caffeine's effect on cardiovascular activity during mental stress in young men. *Health Psychology*; 10, 236-243, 1991.
211. Zahn, T. and Rapoport, J., Autonomic nervous system effects of acute doses of caffeine in caffeine users and abstainers. *Int J Psychophsiol*; 5, 33-41, 1987.
212. Lovallo, W. R., al'Absi, M., Pincomb, G. A., Everson, S. A., et al., Caffeine and behavioral stress effects on blood pressure in borderline hypertensive Caucasian men. *Health Psychology*; 15(1), 11-17, 1996.
213. James, J. E., The influence of user status and anxious disposition on hypertensive effects of caffeine. *International Journal of Psychophysiology*; 10, 171-179, 1990.
214. Lane, J. D., and Williams, R.B., Cardiovascular effects of caffeine and stress in regular coffee drinkers. *Psychophysiology*; 24(2), 157-164, 1987.
215. Lovallo, W. R., Pincomb, G. A., Sung, B. H., Passey, R. B., Sausen, K. P., and Wilson, M. F., Caffeine may potentiate adrenocortical stress responses in hypertension-prone men. *Hypertension*; 14, 170-176, 1989.
216. Pincomb, G. A., Lovallo, W. R., Passey, R. B., Wilson M. F., Effect of behavior state of caffeine's ability to alter blood pressure. *American Journal of Cardiology*; 61: 798-802, 1988.
217. Seltzer, A., Multiple personality: A psychiatric misadventure. *Canadian Journal of Psychiatry*; 39(7), 442-445, 1994.
218. Schwarz, D., Grisso, J., Miles, C., Holmes, J., Wishner, A. and Sutton,R., A logitudinal study of injury morbidity in an African American population. *JAMA*. 271(10), 755-760, 1994.
219. Mushinski, M., Violence in America's public schools. *Stat Bull Metrop Insur Co*; 75(2), 2-9, 1994.
220. Miller, T., Cohen, M. and Rossman, S., Victim costs of violent crime and resulting injuries. *Health Aff Millwood*; 12(4), 186-197, 1993.

221. Zeichner, A., Allen, J. D., Giancola, P. R., Lating, J. M., Alcohol and aggression: Effects of personal threat on human aggression and affective arousal. *Alcoholism Clinical and experimental Research*; 18(3), 657-663, 1994.
222. Bond, A. J., Pharmacological manipulation of aggressiveness and impulsiveness in healthy volunteers. *Progress in Neuro Psychopharmacology and Biological Psychiatry*; 16(1), 1-7, 1992.
223. Augsburger, D., An existential approach to anger management training. *Journal of Psychology and Christianity*; 1986 Win Vol 5(4), 25-29, 1986.
224. Anderson, C. A., Deuser, W. E., and DeNeve, K. M., Hot temperatures, hostile affect, hostile cognition, and arousal: Tests of a general model of affective aggression. *Personality and Social Psychology Bulletin*; 21(5), 434-448, 1995.
225. Shields, S. A., Reports of bodily change in anxiety, sadness, and anger. *Motivation and Emotion*;8(1), 1-21, 1984.
226. Klaczynski, P. A., Cummings, E. M., Responding to anger in aggressive and nonaggressive boys: A research note. *Journal of Child Psychology and Psychiatry and Allied Disciplines*; Mar Vol 30(2), 309-314, 1989.
227. Ketterer, M. W., and Maercklein, G. H., Caffeinated beverage use among Type A male patients suspected of CAD/CHD: A mechanism for increased risk? *Stress Medicine*; 7(2), 119-124, 1991.
228. Branscombe, N. R., Wann, D. L., Role of identification with a group, arousal, categorization processes, and self-esteem in sports spectator aggression. *Human Relations*; 45(10), 1013-1033, 1992.
229. Zaslav, M., Psychology or comorbid posttraumatic stress disorder and substance abuse: lessons for combat veterans. *J Psychoactive Drugs*; 26(4), 393-400, 1994.
230. de-Freitas, B., and Schwartz, G., Effects of caffeine in chronic psychiatric patients. *American Journal of Psychiatry*; 136(10), 1337-1338, 1979.
231. Carmel, H., Caffeine and aggression. *Hospital and Community Psychiatry*; 42(6), 637-639, 1991.
232. Taylor, S. L., O'Neal, E. C., Langley, T., Butcher, A. H., Anger arousal, deindividuation, and aggression. *Aggressive Behavior*; 17(4), 193-206, 1991.
233. Gustafson, R., Alcohol and aggression. *Journal of Offender Rehabilitation*; 21(3-4), 41-80, 1994.
234. Geen, R. G., McCown, E. J., Effects of noise and attack on aggression and physiological arousal. *Motivation and Emotion*; 8(3), 231-241, 1984.
235. Griffiths, R.R. and Woodson, P.P., Caffeine physical dependence: a review of human and laboratory animal studies. *Psychopharmacology*; 94: 437-51, 1988.
236. Russell, J. A., Weiss, A., Mendelsohn, G. A, Affect Grid: A single-item scale of pleasure and arousal. *Journal of Personality and Social Psychology*;57(3), 493-502, 1989.
237. Walsh, J. J., Wilding, J. M., Eysenck, M. W., Stress responsivity: The role of individual differences. *Personality and Individual Differences*; 16(3), 385-394, 1994.
238. Smith, B., Wilson, R. and Jones, B., Extraversion and multiple levels of caffeine induced arousal: Effects of overhabituation and dishabituation. *Psychophysiology*; 20(1), 29-34, 1983.
239. Gupta, U., Differential effects of caffeine on free recall ofter semantic and ryhme tasks in high and low impulsives, *Psychopharmacology*; 105, 137-140, 1991.
240. Gupta, U., Effects of caffine in recognition. *Pharmacolgy, Biochemistry and Behavior*; 44, 393-396, 1993.
241. Smith, B. D., Rockwell-Tischer, S., Davidson, R. , Extraversion and arousal: Effects of attentional conditions on electrodermal activity. *Personality and Individual Differences*; 7, 293-303, 1986.

242. Smith, B., Davidosn, R., Smith, D., Goldstein, H. and Perlstein, W., Sensation seeking and arousal: Effects of strong stimulation on electrodermal activation and memory task performance. *Personality and Individual Differences*; 6, 671-679, 1989.
243. Eysenck, H., *The Biological Basis of Personality*. Springfield,IL: Charles C. Thomas, 1967.
244. Eysenck, H., A reply to Costa and MaCrea: P or A and C - the role of theory. *Personality and Individual Differences*; 13, 867-868, 1992.
245. Broke, B., and Battmann, W., The arousal-activation theory of extraversion and neuroticism: A systematic analysis and principal conclusions. *Advances in Behaviour Research and Therapy*; 14(4), 211-246, 1992.
246. Berenbaum, H., andWilliams, M., Extraversion, hemispatial bias, and eyeblink rates. *Personality and Individual Differences*;17(6), 849-852, 1994.
247. Bullock, W. A., and Gilliland, K., Eysenck's arousal theory of introversion-extraversion: A converging measures investigation. *Journal of Personality and Social Psychology*; 64(1), 113-123, 1993.
248. Smith, B. D., Kline, R., and Meyers, M., The differential hemispheric processing of emotion: A comparative analysis in strongly lateralized sinistrals and dextrals. *International Journal of Neuroscience*; 50, 59-71, 1990.
249. Davidson, R., Fedio, P., Smith, B., Aurielle, E. and Martin, A., Lateralized mediation of arousal and habiuation: Diffeential bilateral electrodermal activity in unilateral temporal lobectomy patients. *Neuropschologia; 30*, 1053-1063, 1992.
250. Stelmack, R. M., Biological bases of extraversion: Psychophysiological evidence. Special Issue: Biological foundations of personality: Evolution, behavioral genetics, and psychophysiology. *Journal of Personality*; 58(1), 293-311, 1990.
251. Pearson, G. L., and Freeman, F. G., Effects of extraversion and mental arithmetic on heart-rate reactivity. *Perceptual and Motor Skills*, 72, 1239-1248, 1991.
252. Davidson, R., Smith, B., Tamny, T. and Fedio, P., Emotional arousal in temporal lobectomy: autonomic and performance effects of success and failure feedback. *Journal of Clinical and Experimental Neuropsychology*; 1995.
253. Eysenck, H. and Eysenck, S., *Manual for the Eysenck Personality Inventory*, San Diego: Educational and Testing Service, 1968.
254. Smith, B., Wilson, R. and Davidson, R., Electrodermal activity and extraversion: Caffeine, preparatory signal and stimulus intensity effects. *Personality and Individual Differences*; 5, 59-65, 1984.
255. Smith, B. D., Extraversion and electrodermal activity: Arousability and the inverted-U. *Personality and Individual Differences*, 4, 411-419, 1983.
256. Smith, B., Wilson, R. and Davidson, R., Electrodermanl activity and extraversion. *Personality and Individual Differences*; 5, 59-65, 1984.
257. Nebylitsyn, V., Current problems in differential psychophysiology. *Soviet Psychology*; 11(3), 47-70, 1973.
258. Wilder, D. and Shapiro. P., Effects of anxiety on impressin formation in a group of context: An anxiety-assimilation hypothesis. *Journal of Experimental and Social Psychology*; 25, 481-499, 1988.
259. Ellis, L., Relationships of criminality and psychopathy with eight other apparent behavioral manifestations of sub-optimal arousal. *Personality and Individual Differences*; 8(6), 905-925, 1987.
260. Stenberg, G., Personality and the EEG: Arousal and emotional arousability. *Personality and Individual Differences*; 13(10), 1097-1113, 1992.
261. Anderson, K., Impulsivity, caffeine, and task difficulty: A within-subjects test of the Yerkes-Dodson law. *Personality and Idividual Differences*, *16*(6), 813-829, 1994.

262. American Psychiatric Association. *Diagnostic and Statistical Manual of Mental Disorders. (4th ed).* Washington,D.C: American Psychiatric Association, 1994.
263. Holtzman, S. G., Caffeine as a model drug of abuse. *Trends in Pharmacological Sciences II*; (9); 355-6, 1990.
264. US Dept. Health and Human Services. *The Health Consequences of Smoking: Nicotine Addiction.* A Report of the Surgeon General. DHSS Publ. No. (CDC) 88-8406. Washington, DC: Govt. Print. Off., 1988.
265. Kruger, A., Chronic psychiatric patients' use of caffeine: pharmacological effects and mechanisms. *Psychol Rep*; 78(3), 915-923, 1996.
266. Clines, B. M., Rozin, P., Some aspects of the liking for hot coffee and coffee flavor. *Appetite*; 3(1), 23-34, 1982.
267. Carrillo, J., Dahl, M., Svensson, J., Alm, C., Rodriguez, I. and Bertilsson, L., Disposition of fluvoxamine in humans is determined by the polymorphic CYP2D6 and also by the CYP1A2 activity. *Clin Pharmacol Ther*; 60(2), 183-190, 1996.
268. Carroll, M. E., Hagen, E. W., Asencio, M., Brauer, L. H., Behavioral dependence on caffeine and phencyclidine in rhesus monkeys: Interactive effects. *Pharmacology, Biochemistry and Behavior*; 31(4), 927-932, 1988.
269. Strain, E. C., Mumford, G., Silverman, K.,; Griffiths, R. R., et-al., Caffeine dependence syndrome: Evidence from case histories and experimental evaluations. American College of Neuropsychopharmacology (1993, Honolulu, Hawaii). JAMA *Journal of the American Medical Association*; 272(13), 1043-1048, 1994.
270. Falk, J. L., Zhang, J., Chen, R., and Lau, C. E., A schedule induction probe technique for evaluating abuse potential: Comparison of ethanol, nicotine and caffeine, and caffeine-midazolam interaction. Special Issue: Behavioural pharmacology of alcohol. *Behavioural Pharmacology*; 5(4-5), 513-520, 1994.
271. Wise, R. A., and Bozarth, M. A., A psychomotor stimulant theory of addiction. *Psychological Review*; 1987 Oct Vol 94(4), 469-492, 1987.
272. Kozlowski, L. T., Henningfield, J. E., Keenan, R. M., Lei, H., et al., Patterns of alcohol, cigarette, and caffeine and other drug use in two drug abusing populations. Special Issue: Towards a broader view of recovery: Integrating nicotine addiction and chemical dependency treatments. *Journal of Substance Abuse Treatment*, 1993 Mar-Apr Vol 10(2), 171-179, 1993.
273. Mathew, R. J., and Wilson, W. H., Substance abuse and cerebral blood flow. *American Journal of Psychiatry*; 148(3), 292-305, 1991.
274. Van-Dusseldorf, M., Smits, P., Lenders, J. W., Temme, L., et al., Effects of coffee on cardiovascular responses to stress: A 14-week controlled trial. *Psychosomatic Medicine*;54(3), 344-353, 1992.
275. Bolton, S., and Null, G., Caffeine: Psychological effects, use and abuse. *Journal of Orthomolecular Psychiatry*; 10(3), 202-211, 1981.
276. Myers, M. G., and Reeves, R. A., The effect of caffeine on daytime ambulatory blood pressure. *American Journal of Hypertension*; 4, 427-431, 1993.
277. Denaro, C. P., Brown, C. R., Jacob, P., Benowitz, N. L. , Effects of caffeine with repeated dosing. *European Journal of Clinical Pharmacology*, 40, 273-278, 1991.
278. Robertson, C., Gatchel, R. and Fowler, C., Effectiveness of a videotaped behavioral intervention in reducing anxiety in emrgency oral surgery patients. *Behavioral Medicine*; 17(2), 77-85, 1991.
279. Chou, D. T., Khan, S., Forde, J., and Hirsh, K. R., Caffeine tolerance: Behavioral, electrophysiological and neurochemical evidence. *Life Sciences*; 36(24), 2347-2358, 1985.
280. Guelliot, O., *Du cafeisme chronique*. Union Med. Sci. Nordest 9: 181-194, 1885a.
281. Rizzo, A. A., Stamps, L. E., Fehr, L. A., Effects of caffeine withdrawal on motor performance and heart rate changes. *International Journal of Psychophysiology*;6(1), 9-14, 1988.

282. Hughes, J. R., Higgins, S. T., Bickel, W. K., Hunt, W. K., Fenwick, J. W., Gulliver, S. B., and Mireault, G. C., Caffeine self-administration, withdrawal, and adverse effects among coffee drinkers. *Arch. Gen. Psychiatry*; 48: 611-617, 1991.
283. Hughes, J. R., Oliveto, A. H., Helzer, J. E., Higgins, S. T., et al., Should caffeine abuse, dependence, or withdrawal be added to DSM-IV and ICD-10? *American Journal of Psychiatry*; 149(1), 33-40, 1992.
284. Hughes, J., Oliveto, A., Bickel, W. and Higgins, S., The ability of low doses of caffeine to serve as reinforcers in humans: A replication. *Experimental and Clinical Psychopharmacology*; 3(4), 358-363, 1995.
285. Evans, S. M., and Griffiths, R. R., Dose-related caffeine discrimination in normal volunteers: Individual differences in subjective effects and self-reported cues. *Behavioral Pharmacology*; 2, 345-356, 1991.
286. Cacciatore, R., Helbing, A., Jost, C., and Bess, B., Episodic headache, diminished performance and depressive mood. *Schweiz Rundsch Med Prax*, 85(22), 727-729, 1996.
287. Hofer, I., and Battig, K., Cardiovascular, behavioral, and subjective effects of caffeine under field conditions. *Pharmacology, Biochemistry and Behavior*; 48(4), 899-908, 1994.
288. Swanson, J. A., Lee, J. W., Hopp, J. W., Caffeine and nicotine: A review of their joint use and possible interactive effects in tobacco withdrawal. *Addictive Behaviors*; 19(3), 229-256, 1994.
289. Rainey, J. T., Headache related to chronic caffeine addiction. *Tex. Dent. J*; 102: 29-30, 1985.
290. Griffiths, R. R., Bigelow, G. E., and Liebson, I. A., Human coffee drinking: reinforcing and physical dependence producing effects of caffeine. *J. Pharmacol. Exp. Ther*; 239: 416-425, 1986a.
291. Mitchell, S. H., de-Wit, H., Zacny, J. P., Caffeine withdrawal symptoms and self-administration following caffeine deprivation. *Pharmacology, Biochemistry and Behavior*; 51(4), 941-945, 1995.
292. Bruce, M., Scott, N., Shine, P., Lader, M., Caffeine withdrawal: A contrast of withdrawal symptoms in normal subjects who have abstained from caffeine for 24 hours and for 7 days. *Journal of Psychopharmacology*; Vol 5(2), 129-134, 1991.
293. Hughes, J. R., Oliveto, A. H., Bickel, W. K., Higgins, S. T., et al., Caffeine self-administration and withdrawal. *Drug and Alcohol Dependence*; 32(3), 239-246, 1993.
294. Mathew, R. J., and Wilson, W. H., Caffeine consumption, withdrawal and cerebral blood flow. *Headache*; 25: 305-309, 1985.
295. Wilkin, J. K., The caffeine withdrawal flush: Report of a case of †weekend flushing. *Milit. Med*; 151: 123-124, 1986.
296. Oliveto, A. H., Hughes, J. R., Terry, S., Bickel, W. K., Higgins, S. T., Pepper, S. L., and Fenwick, J. W., Effects of caffeine on tobacco withdrawal. *Clinical Pharmacology and Therapeutics*; 50, 157-164, 1991.
297. Griffiths, R. R., and Woodson, P. P., Reinforcing properties of caffeine: studies in humans and laboratory animals. *Pharmacol. Biochem. Behav.* 1987.
298. Foltin, R. W., The importance of drug self-administration studies in the analysis of abuse liability: An analysis of caffeine, nicotine, anabolic steroids, and designer drugs. Annual Meeting of the American Academy of Psychiatrists in Alcoholism and Addictions (1990, Santa Monica, California). *American Journal on Addictions*; Spr Vol 1(2), 139-149, 1992.
299. Graham, K., Reasons for consumption and heavy caffeine use: Generalization of a model based on alcohol research. *Addictive Behaviors*; 13(2), 209-214, 1988.
300. Brauer, L. H., Buican, B., de-Wit, H., Effects of caffeine deprivation on taste and mood. *Behavioural Pharmacology*; 5(2), 111-118, 1994.

301. Reimann, H. Caffeinism: A cause of long-continued, low-grade fever. *JAMA*, 202, 131-132, 1967.
302. Greden, J. F., Anxiety or caffeinism: A diagnostic dilemma. *American Journal of Psychiatry*; 131, 1089-1096, 1974.
303. Pilette, W. L., Caffeine: Psychiatric grounds for concern. *Journal of Psychosocial Nursing and Mental Health Services*; 21(8), 19-24, 1983.
304. James, J. and Stirling, K., Caffeine: A survey of some of the known and suspected deleterious effects of habitual use. *British Journal of Addiction*; 78(3), 251-258.
305. Victor, B. S., Lubetsky, M., andGreden, J. F., Somatic manifestations of caffeinism. *Journal of Clinical Psychiatry*; 42(5), 185-188, 1981.
306. Kits van Waveren, L., Cafeinisme (Caffeinism). *Tijdschrift voor Psychiatrie*; 30(6), 403-407, 1988.
307. Wurl,P., Life threatening caffeine poisoning by using coffee as a psychoactive drug. *Wien Klin Wochenschr*; 106(11), 359-361, 1994.
308. Forman, J., Aizer, A. and Young, C. Myocardial infarction resulting from caffeine overdose in an anorectic woman, *Ann Emerg Med*; 29(1), 178-180, 1997.
309. Behar, D., Flashbacks and posttraumatic stress symptoms in combat veterans. *Comprehansive Psychiatry*, 28(6), 459-466, 1987.
310. Newman, F. X., Stein, M. B., Trettau, J. R., Coppola, R., et al., Quantitative electroencephalographic effects of caffeine in panic disorder. *Psychiatry Research Neuroimaging*; 45(2), 105-113, 1992.
311. Beck, J. G., Berisford, M. A., The effects of caffeine on panic patients: Response components of anxiety. *Behavior Therapy*; 23(3), 405-422, 1992.
312. Dawyber, T., Kannel, W. and Gordon, T., Coffee and cardiovascular disorders: Observations from the Framington study. *New England Journal of Medicine*; 291, 871-874, 1974.
313. Hofer, I., Battig, K., Psychophysiological effects of switching to caffeine tablets or decaffeinated coffee under field conditions. Special Issue: Caffeine research. *Pharmacopsychoecologia*; 7(2), 169-177, 1994.
314. Smith, A., Brockman, P., Flynn, R., Maben, A. and Thomas, M., Investigation of the effects of caffee on alertness and performance during the night and day. *Neuropsychobiology*; 27, 217-223, 1993.
315. Miller, L., Lombardo, T. and Fowler, S. Caffeine and time of day effects on a force discrimination task in humans. *Physiology and Behavior*; 57(6), 1117-1125, 1995.
316. Bruce, M., Scott, N., Lader, M. and Marks, V., The psychopharmacological and electrophysiological effects of a single dose of caffeine in healthy human subjects. *British Journal of Clinical Pharmacology*; 22, 81-87, 1986.
317. Lader, M., Comparison of amphetamine sulphate and caffeine citrate in man. *Psychopharmacologia*; 14, 83-94, 1969.
318. Sawyer, D. A., Julia, H. L., Turin, A. C., Caffeine and human behavior: Arousal, anxiety, and performance effects. *Journal of Behavioral Medicine*; 5(4), 415-439, 1982.
319. Landolt, H. P., Werth, E., Borbely, A. A., Dijk, D. J., Caffeine intake (200 mg) in the morning affects human sleep and EEG power spectra at night. *Brain Research*; 675(1-2), 67-74, 1995.
320. Tharion, W., Kobrick, J., Lieberman, H. and Fine, B., Effects of caffeine and diphenhydramine on auditory evoked cortical potentials. *Perceptual and Motor Skills*; 76, 707-715, 1993.
321. Van Soeren, M., Mohr, T., Kjaer, M. and Graham, T., Acute effects of caffeine ingestion at rest in humans with impaired epinephrine responses. *J Appl Physiol*; 80(3), 999-1005, 1996.
322. Stamler, J., Caggaila, A. and Grandiits, G., Relation of body mass and alcohol, nutrient, fiber and caffeine intkae to blood preussre in the special intervention and usual care groups in the multiple risk factor intervention trial. *Am J Clin Nutr*; 65(1), 338-365, 1997.

323. Del Rio, G., Menozzi, R., Zizzo, G., Avogaro, A., Marrano, P. and Velardo, A., Increased cardiovascular response to caffeine in perimenopausal women before and during estrogen therapy. *Eur J Endocrinol*; 135(5), 598-603, 1996.
324. Wise, K., Bergmann, E., Sherrard, D. and Massey, L., Interactions between dietary calcium and caffeine consumption on caffeine in hypertensive humans. *Am J Hypertens*; 9(3), 223-229, 1996.
325. Pincomb, G. A., Sung, B. H., Sausen, K. P., Lovallo, W. R., and Wilson, M. F., Consistency of cardiovascular response pattern to caffeine across multiple studies using impedance and nuclear cardiography. *Biological Psychology*; 36, 131-138., 1993.
326. Lane, J. and Manus, D., Persistent cardiovascular effects with repested caffeine administration. *Psychosomatic Medicine*; 51, 373-380, 1989.
327. Lotshaw, S., Bradley, R. and Brooks, L., Illustrating caffeine's pharmacological and expectancy effects utilizing a balanced placebo design. *J Drug Educ*; 26(1), 13-24, 1996.
328. Pincomb, G. A., Lovallo, W. R., Passey, R. B., Brackett, D. J., et al., Caffeine enhances the physiological response to occupational stress in medical students. *Health Psychology*; 6(2), 101-112, 1987.
329. Smits, P., Schooten, J. and Thien, T., Cardiovascular effects of two xanthines and the relationship to adenosine antagonism. *Clinical Pharmacological Therapy*; 45, 593-599, 1989.
330. Strickland, T., Myers, H. and Lahey, B., Cardiovascular reactivity with caffeine and stress in black and white normotensive females. *Psychosomatic Medicine*; 51, 381-389, 1989.
331. Rush, C. R., Higgins, S. T., Hughes, J.R., Bickel, W. K., et al., Acute behavioral and cardiac effects of alcohol and caffeine, alone and in combination, in humans. *Behavioural Pharmacology*; 4(6), 562-572, 1993.
332. James, J. E., Richardson, M., Pressor effects of caffeine and cigarette smoking. *British Journal of Clinical Psychology*; 30(3), 276-278, 1991.
333. Nussberger, J., Mooser, V., Maridor, G., Juillerat, L., Waeber, B. and Brunner, H., Caffeine-induced diuresis and atrial natriuretic peptides. *J Cadiovasc Pharmacol*; 15(5), 685-691, 1990.
334. Greenstadt, L., Yang, L., and Shapiro, D., Caffeine, mental stress, and risk for hypertension: A cross-cultural replication. *Psychosomatic Medicine*; 50(1), 15-22, 1988.
335. Hirsch, A., Gervine, E., Nakso, S., Come, P., Silverman, K. and Grossman, W., The effect of caffeine on exercise tolerance and left ventricular function in patinets with coronary heart disease. *Annals of Internal Medicine*; 110, 593-598, 1989.
336. Pennickx, F., Vuysteke, P. and Kerremans, R., Recurrences after highly selective vagotomy in refractory and non-refractory duodenal ulcer disease. *Acta Chirurgica Belgica*; 90, 41-45, 1990.
337. James, J. and Richardson, M., Pressor effects of caffeine and cigarette smoking. *British Journal of Clinical Psychology*; 276-278, 1991.
338. Horne, J. and Reyner, L., Counteracting driver sleepiness: effects of napping caffeine and palcebo. *Psychophysiology*; 33(3), 306-209, 1996.
339. Bonnet, M. and Arand, D., Metabolic rate and the restorative function of sleep. *Physiol Behav*; 59(4-5), 777-782, 1996.
340. Bonnet, M., The effect of varying prophlactic naps on performance, alertness and mood throughout a 52 hour continuous operation. *Sleep*; 14(4), 307-315, 1991.
341. Bonnet, M., Gomez, S., Wirth, O. and Arand, D., The use of caffeine versus prophylatic naps in sustained performance. *Sleep*; *18*(2), 97-104, 1995.

Chapter 13

COFFEE, CAFFEINE AND SERUM CHOLESTEROL

Christopher Gardner, Bonnie Bruce, and Gene A. Spiller

CONTENTS

0-8493-2647-8/98/$0.00+$.50

INTRODUCTION

Daily caffeine consumption is common in many different populations worldwide, thus associations between caffeine and health can have important public health implications. Coffee is one of the two largest sources of caffeine throughout most of the world, the other being tea,[1] and many investigations of caffeine and serum cholesterol have used coffee as a source for caffeine. The relationship between coffee, caffeine, and serum cholesterol has been studied extensively over the past two decades. Reports from both observational and experimental investigations have shown associations between coffee and serum cholesterol which have ranged from being strong and significant to having little or no effect.[2] These conflicting results are likely attributable to confounding associations between coffee consumption, its preparation methods, variability in the chemical composition of different types of coffee beans, the degree of coffee bean roasting, and potential interactions with other dietary factors such as increased saturated fat intake from the addition of dairy products to coffee. The amount of daily coffee consumed and the duration of investigational periods are also important factors that vary among studies. Also, it may be that coffee drinking exerts a differential effect on serum cholesterol levels among diverse population subgroups, e.g., hyper- vs. normolipidemic individuals. When these various factors are taken into consideration, many of the discrepancies between coffee and serum cholesterol studies can be explained, and a consistent pattern emerges. The purpose of this chapter is to provide a current and comprehensive understanding of the relationship between coffee, caffeine, and serum cholesterol levels.

A. Types of Coffee Beans, Chemical Composition, and Methods of Preparation

The world's coffee supply comes primarily from two major types of coffee beans, Arabica (*Coffea arabica*) and Robusta (*Coffea canephora*), which differ in several characteristics as well as caffeine content. Arabica is favored for its finer aroma, flavor, and body, and contains 1% caffeine. Robusta is neutral and contains twice as much caffeine.[1] The ratio of

Arabica/Robusta beans used in different countries ranges from 1.5:1 in Italy, 4:1 to 3:1 in the U.S., and 20:1 in Sweden and Norway.[2] As described in Chapter 6, coffee contains a number of physiologically active components, including caffeine, diterpene alcohols, sterols, hydrocarbons, squalene, and others.

Traditionally, methods of preparing coffee differ distinctively between countries and cultures. Common ways to prepare it include boiling, filtering (sometimes called drip), and espresso. Many of the best publicized studies of coffee and cholesterol emanate from Scandinavian countries where historically boiling has been the conventional method of preparation. Boiled coffee is prepared by boiling coarsely ground coffee in water, which is then consumed without filtering off the grounds. In the U.S. and some European countries, filtered coffee is common. Filtered coffee is prepared by pouring hot, but ideally not boiling, water through a filter (made of paper or other metal, such as gold-mesh) over medium-ground coffee. In countries such as Italy, Spain, and France, and growing in popularity in the U.S., espresso coffee is a preferred choice. Espresso is prepared by forcing water through a metal filter containing finely ground coffee. Italian mocha coffee is also prepared by forcing water through finely ground coffee, but brewing time is slightly longer.

Other methods of preparation include French press coffee (also known as plunger or cafetiere coffee), which is similar to boiled coffee in that it is not filtered. French press is prepared in a special unit where boiling water is poured over ground coffee. Then a metal screen strainer (plunger) is used to move the majority of the grounds to the bottom of the unit. Traditional Greek/Turkish or "mud" coffee is prepared in a special pot called an ibrik by combining very finely ground coffee with water and boiling until foam is produced. It also is an unfiltered coffee.

II. FINDINGS FROM OBSERVATIONAL STUDIES

In one of the earliest key studies, the Tromso Heart study, Thelle et al.[3] cross-sectionally examined the association between coffee consumption and serum cholesterol in 14,581 Norwegian women and men who typically consumed boiled coffee. They found that coffee was a major contributor to variations in levels of serum cholesterol independent of age, body mass index, physical activity, smoking, and alcohol intake; although either weak or no associations were reported for coffee consumption and HDL-cholesterol (HDL-C) and triglycerides (TG). However, in 1987 Thelle et al.[4] reviewed 23 cross-sectional investigations of coffee and serum cholesterol involving 130,000 subjects from eight countries and found inconsistencies in findings among the studies, which they suggested could be largely explained by differences in brewing methods. This led them to conclude that there was insufficient evidence at that juncture to warrant public health concern, although there may be clinical significance for some hyperlipidemic individuals.

A. Relationships Between Caffeine and Serum Cholesterol

Since the Thelle et al.[4] review, several large population studies have investigated the relationship between caffeine intake and serum cholesterol by examining intake of both caffeinated and decaffeinated coffee, tea, and cola beverages.[5-8] In one of the first follow-up studies, Wei et al.[5] evaluated the association between changes in serum cholesterol levels and coffee consumption in 333 women and 1,776 men between 1987 and 1991 (16.7 ± 7.3, mean ± SD, months between visits). They failed to find a relationship between changes in serum cholesterol and decaffeinated coffee, regular tea, decaffeinated tea, or cola, but did find a significant association with coffee intake. Results from the United States Hypertension Detection and Follow-up Study[6] with 9,043 hypertensive women and men showed that coffee intake was significantly associated with serum cholesterol independent of demographic, lifestyle, and physiological factors. However, there were no significant associations between serum cholesterol and caffeinated tea, caffeinated cola beverages, or total caffeine intake. Further, a Finnish study of 4,495 women and 4,744 men also concluded that caffeine was not associated with serum cholesterol levels; however, the reliability of their estimates of caffeine intake was limited.[7] Finally, Curb et al.[8] showed that coffee consumption was associated significantly with serum cholesterol levels among 5,585 Japanese men living in Hawaii, but tea and cola consumption, the other major caffeine contributors, was not.

B. Relationships Between Preparation Methods and Serum Cholesterol

Several epidemiological investigations have examined relationships between serum cholesterol levels and different methods of preparing coffee. Stensvold et al.[9] examined coffee intake and serum cholesterol in 14,859 women and 14,168 men. Intake of boiled coffee was typical in 11 to 49% of the population; filtered coffee was typical in 49 to 87%. After adjusting for several demographic and lifestyle factors, a significant linear increase in serum cholesterol for both men and women was found relative to the amount of boiled coffee consumed. A modest linear increase in serum cholesterol was found among women drinking filtered coffee, but not in men. In a study of 5,704 Finnish women and men,[10] where 24% consumed boiled coffee and 69% consumed paper-filtered coffee, serum cholesterol levels were significantly higher among the group of boiled coffee drinkers in both women (6.22 vs. 5.84 mmol/L [241 vs. 226 mg/dL]) and men (6.37 vs. 6.02 mmol/L [246 vs. 233 mg/dL]). These differences persisted after adjusting for demographic and lifestyle factors including saturated fat intake. Similarly, Lindahl et al.[11] examined serum cholesterol levels in 1,574 middle-aged Swedish women and men, 52% of whom were boiled coffee drinkers, 44.9% were paper-filtered drip-brewed coffee drinkers, and the remaining 3.3% did not drink coffee. Serum cholesterol levels were significantly higher among boiled vs. filtered coffee drinkers and were significant for both moderate coffee drinkers consuming ≤4 cups/day (6.3 vs. 5.8 mmol/L [242 vs. 225 mg/dL]) and for heavy coffee drinkers consuming ≥5 cups/day (6.5 vs. 5.9 mmol/L [252 vs. 227 mg/dL]). Differences persisted after adjusting for the higher fat consumption of the boiled coffee drinkers.

Although boiled coffee has been associated most consistently with elevated serum cholesterol levels, similar associations have been found for other methods of coffee preparation. In a study of 319 Serbian men between the ages of 65 to 84 years,[12] the serum cholesterol levels of subjects who consumed two cups per day of Turkish coffee were 8.2% higher than abstainers. This difference persisted after adjusting for age, smoking, body mass index, and alcohol intake. Salvaggio et al.[2] also reported a significant trend of higher serum cholesterol levels among Italian mocha coffee drinkers who drank either no coffee, 1 to 3, 4 to 5, or >5 cups per day. Among women the corresponding mean levels of serum cholesterol were 5,5. 5,6, 5.7, and 5.7 mmol/L (213, 217, 219, and 221 mg/dL), and among men these levels were 5.7, 5.8, 5.9, and 6.0 mmol/L (221, 225, 227, and 231 mg/dL), respectively. These significant differences persisted after statistically adjusting for demographic and lifestyle factors. However, neither the Serbian nor the Italian study had corresponding dietary intake data to control for confounders such as saturated fat.

Several large observational studies conducted among predominantly paper-filtered or instant coffee drinkers have also reported significant associations between coffee intake and serum cholesterol levels. These findings are in contrast to studies cited above which found a significant association for boiled but not filtered coffee.[9-11] One study in the U.S. investigated the association between changes in serum cholesterol and changes in coffee consumption among 333 women and 1,776 men who were examined at a preventive medical center on two separate occasions between 1987 and 1991.[5] Of the study participants (n=664), 31% reported some change in habitual coffee intake between the first and second clinical exam. It was estimated that for every change of one cup of coffee per day, there was a concomitant change in serum cholesterol levels of 0.05 mmol/L (2 mg/dL).

In another investigation, Davis et al.[6] examined coffee consumption and serum cholesterol levels among 9,043 hypertensive adults from the United States Hypertension Detection and Follow-up Study. The mean serum cholesterol levels among adults consuming 0, 1 to 2, 3 to 4, 5 to 6, 7 to 8 and ≥9 cups of caffeinated coffee per day were significantly higher for those who consumed more coffee, 5.9, 5.9, 6.0, 6.0, 6.1, and 6.1 mmol/L (228, 229, 231, 231, 236, and 235 mg/dL), respectively. The significant association persisted after statistically adjusting for age, race, sex, diuretic status, blood pressure, smoking, relative weight, physical activity, stress, and education level. Neither of the two American studies cited above had any specific information on preparation methods, but it was assumed that the predominant kinds of coffee were paper-filtered and instant coffee. Also, neither of the studies had detailed dietary data, and therefore potential dietary confounders such as saturated fat intake were not adjusted for in the analyses. These observational studies suggest that preparation method may be an important factor in determining whether or not coffee influences serum cholesterol levels. A limitation in many of these studies, though, was lack of control or adjustment for confounding factors such as diet.

III. FINDINGS FROM EXPERIMENTAL STUDIES

The experimental studies cited below have isolated and tested the impact of caffeine, different methods of preparation, and different chemical fractions of coffee beans on serum cholesterol levels over a varied range of time periods.

A. Effect of Caffeine on Serum Lipids

Superko et al.[13] conducted one of the largest clinical investigations which examined the effect of caffeine on serum cholesterol levels using paper-filtered coffee. One hundred eighty-one American men consumed either caffeinated coffee (538 mg caffeine/cup), decaffeinated coffee, or no coffee (~60 men/group). During the study, subjects maintained their habitual levels of coffee consumption, which ranged from 3 to 6 cups/day (average 4.5 cups/day. All subjects first drank caffeinated coffee for two months, at which point mean serum cholesterol was 5.5 mmol/L (213 mg/dL). For the next two months they consumed either caffeinated, decaffeinated, or no coffee. The only result considered to be statistically significant was a slight decrease in LDL-cholesterol (LDL-C) of -0.1 mmol/L (-4 mg/dL) in the caffeinated-coffee group relative to a slight increase in LDL-C of +0.1 mmol/L (5 mg/dL) in the decaffeinated-coffee group.

The failure to find an effect in the American trial above was confirmed in a study conducted in the Netherlands, which also used paper-filtered, drip-brewed coffee.[14] In that 12-week experiment, 23 women and 22 men who habitually drank 4 to 6 cups of coffee per day were assigned to consume 5 cups/day of either caffeinated (417.5 mg caffeine/day) or decaffeinated coffee (15.5 mg caffeine/day) for six weeks, and then switch for another six weeks. The blend of coffee beans was 71% Arabica and 29% Robusta for the caffeinated coffee, and 58% Arabica and 42% Robusta for the decaffeinated coffee. Lipid values at the end of both six-week study periods were almost identical. Total cholesterol was 5.47 vs. 5.48 mmol/L (212 vs. 212 mg/dL), LDL-C was 3.41 vs. 3.40 mmol/L (132 vs. 131 mg/dL), HDL-C was 1.52 vs. 1.52 mmol/L (59 vs. 59 mg/dL), and TG were 1.17 vs. 1.20 mmol/L (104 vs. 106 mg/dL) for the caffeinated vs decaffeinated coffee periods, respectively. Further, a small study of 12 Finnish men also failed to find an effect of caffeinated coffee on serum cholesterol levels.[15] However, the study period was only three weeks which may have been insufficient.

In contrast, the study by Fried et al.,[16] again using paper-filtered coffee, found a modest effect of caffeine on serum cholesterol levels with 100 healthy American men who were assigned randomly to one of four groups. They consumed either 4 cups/day of caffeinated coffee (330 mg caffeine/day), 2 cups/day of caffeinated coffee (165 mg caffeine/day), 4 cups/day of decaffeinated coffee (6 mg caffeine/day), or no coffee for 8 weeks. At the end of the 8-week period, subjects drinking 4 cups/day of caffeinated coffee experienced the most substantial increases in cholesterol levels. Total cholesterol increased by 0.24 mmol/L (9 mg/dL). However, this was attributed to elevations in both LDL-C 0.17 mmol/L (+7 mg/dL) and HDL-C 0.08 mmol/L (+3 mg/dL). Various smaller changes were also observed in the other three groups. When the four groups were compared directly to one another, none of the LDL-C or HDL-C changes was statistically significant.

The results of these studies, when considered together and with the observational studies reviewed above, suggest that any significant effect of coffee on serum cholesterol levels is likely due to something other than caffeine content.

B. Effects of Preparation Methods on Serum Lipids

1. Boiled vs Paper-Filtered Preparation Methods

Several European investigations have compared the effects of boiled vs. filtered coffee on serum cholesterol. In a study with 101 Dutch men and women[17]who typically consumed an average of 5.6 cups/day of filtered coffee, investigators assigned subjects randomly to drink 4 to 6 cups/day for nine weeks of either boiled coffee or filtered coffee, or to abstain from coffee. Results showed that total cholesterol increased significantly in the boiled coffee group (0.52 mmol/L, [20.1 mg/dL]), while there was essentially no change in the other two groups. A similar, although not statistically significant, increase was observed in the boiled coffee group for LDL-C (0.36 mmol/L, [13.9 mg/dL]) when compared to the other two groups. There were no group differences in HDL-C or TG levels. Aro and colleagues[18,19] reported the findings of two separate randomized crossover studies that tested the effects of boiled and paper-filtered coffee in hyperlipidemic adults. In the first investigation,[18] 21 women and 21 men, ages 31 to 60 years, with baseline total cholesterol levels ranging from 6.5 to 10.0 mmol/L (250 to 385 mg/dL) were assigned randomly to consume 8 cups/day for 4 weeks of either boiled coffee, paper-filtered coffee, or tea, which were described only as being of similar blend and degree of roasting. After consuming the boiled coffee, total-cholesterol (8.56 mmol/L, [331 mg/dL]) and LDL-C (6.42 mmol/L [248 mg/dL]) levels were significantly higher than during the periods of paper-filtered coffee consumption (total cholesterol 7.77 mmol/L, [300 mg/dL]; LDL-C 5.75 mmol/L, [222 mg/dL]), and tea consumption (total-C 7.46 mmol/L, [288 mg/dL]); LDL-C 5.52 mmol/L, [213 mg/dL]). There were no significant differences in HDL-C or TG levels.

Their second study[19] examined differences between boiled coffee and paper-filtered coffee for four weeks each with a two-week washout period in between treatment periods in 28 women and 13 men, 23 to 61 years old, with an average baseline total cholesterol of ˜5.5 mmol/L (210 mg/dL). Subjects were instructed to continue to drink their habitual amount of daily coffee, which ranged from 2 to 14 cups, with either boiled or drip coffee. With boiled coffee, both total cholesterol and LDL-C levels were significantly higher (0.32 mmol/L [12 mg/dL]) while HDL-C levels were modestly lower (0.07 mmol/L [3 mg/dL]).

Forde et al.[20] used a more complex study design to examine the effect of boiled coffee vs. paper-filtered coffee vs. coffee abstinence. The investigation involved 33 men with elevated baseline serum cholesterol levels (average 8.7 mmol/L [335 mg/dL]) who apparently were habitual boiled coffee drinkers (implied but not stated). The 10-week study was divided into two 5-week periods. Subjects were assigned to one of four groups: (1) continuation of habitual consumption (control), (2) abstinence from coffee for the full 10 weeks, (3) abstinence from coffee for the first 5-weeks, followed by 5 weeks of paper-filtered coffee consumption, and (4) abstinence from coffee for the first 5 weeks, followed by 5 weeks of boiled coffee consumption.

Among the nine men who continued their habitual coffee intake for the 10 weeks, serum cholesterol levels increased from 8.48 mmol/L (329 mg/dL) to 8.83 mmol/L (341 mg/dL). For the eight men in the second group, after 2.5, 5, 7.5, and 10 weeks, serum cholesterol levels dropped from 8.72 mmol/L (337 mg/dL) to 8.36 mmol/L (323 mg/dL), 7.82 mmol/L (302 mg/dL), 7.71 mmol/L (298 mg/dL) and finally 7.56 mmol/L (292 mg/dL), respectively. After abstaining from coffee consumption for 5 weeks, the eight men in the third group experienced an average decline of 0.91 mmol/L (35 mg/dL) in serum cholesterol, comparable to the five-week drop observed in Group two. This improvement was maintained over the second 5 weeks of the study when the men in Group three drank an average of 7 cups/day of paper-filtered coffee. Among the eight men in Group four, the first 5 weeks of coffee abstention led to an average decrease of 0.88 mmol/L (34 mg/dL), which was strikingly similar to Groups two and three. However, when Group four switched back to 7 cups/day of boiled coffee consumption for the second 5 weeks, the average serum cholesterol level increased by 0.52 mmol/L (20 mg/dL), leaving them close to their baseline levels.

2. *Boiled vs. Boiled and Paper-Filtered Preparation Methods*

In a Norwegian study, Van Dusseldorp et al.[21] randomly assigned 64 women and men to consume either 6 cups/day of boiled coffee, 6 cups/day of boiled coffee that was subsequently also paper-filtered, or to abstain from coffee for 79 days. Boiled coffee intake increased cholesterol levels significantly by 0.55 mmol/L (21 mg/dL), compared to non-significant changes in both of the other groups. Examination of the paper filters used in this study indicated that 88% of the fatty-material present in the boiled coffee was trapped by the paper filter.

Additionally, in a crossover study over two 4-week periods that similarly compared boiled coffee with boiled coffee that was paper-filtered, 20 Finnish women and men consumed an average of 8.3 cups of coffee per day. Total cholesterol, LDL-C, and TG levels were all significantly higher during the boiled coffee period (0.36, 0.33, and 0.26 mmol/L [14,13, and 23 mg/dL], respectively). Examination of the paper filters indicated that 80% of the fatty material present in the boiled coffee was trapped by the paper filter.[22]

3. *Espresso and Mocha Preparation Methods*

To test the effect of espresso and mocha preparation methods on serum cholesterol levels, D'Amicis et al.[23] randomly assigned 84 men to consume 3 cups/day of espresso, mocha, or tea for 6 weeks. Although the amount of a typical espresso (20 to 35 ml) or mocha (40 to 50 ml) serving was considerably less than a typical serving of boiled or paper-filtered coffee used in other studies (100 to 250 ml), the amount of ground coffee per serving (6 g/day) was comparable. After 6 weeks of drinking either espresso or mocha, there were no significant changes from baseline or differences between groups for serum cholesterol or TG levels. The authors concluded that espresso or mocha coffee did not alter serum cholesterol levels. However, it is possible that the dose of 3 cups/day in this study was insufficient to elicit a detectable response in serum cholesterol levels.

IV. LIPID ALTERING FRACTION OF COFFEE

Evidence from the studies above suggest that boiled (i.e., non-filtered) coffee contains a factor that raises serum cholesterol levels, whereas filtered coffee does not appear to induce a significant change in serum cholesterol. There are numerous chemical compounds in coffee that may help explain the effect of boiled coffee on serum cholesterol. Weusten-Van der Wouw et al.[24] attempted to isolate such potential factors through a series of experiments. The first in this series, described above, showed that boiled coffee compared to boiled coffee that was subsequently also paper-filtered had an adverse effect on serum cholesterol levels.[22]

Next, to study further the material that was trapped in the coffee filters,[24] they randomly assigned subjects to consume one of four substances: (1) placebo oil, (2) coffee oil, (3) the non-triglyceride enriched fraction of the coffee oil, and (4) the non-triglyceride depleted fraction of the coffee oil. The amount fed to each group was comparable to that found in 3 g of coffee oil per day. Compared to the placebo oil, the coffee oil significantly raised total cholesterol (1.28 mmol/L [49 mg/dL]) and TG (0.82 mmol/L [73 mg/dL) . The non-triglyceride enriched fraction of the coffee oil also had an effect comparable to the coffee oil (total cholesterol +1.24 mmol/L [+48 mg/dL] and TG +0.75 mmol/dL [+66 mg/dL]), while the non-triglyceride depleted fraction of the coffee oil raised total cholesterol and triglycerides only about half as much as the other substances (total cholesterol [total cholesterol +0.85 mmol/dL {+33 mg/dL}] and TG +0.33 mmol/L [29 mg/dL]) .

Weusten-Van der Wouw et al.[24] then elaborated on these results by manipulating the coffee oil used above, so that the two primary constituents of the non-triglyceride fraction, the diterpenoids cafestol and kahweol, were stripped away. Subjects in this study were assigned randomly to one of three groups: coffee oil, placebo oil, or stripped coffee oil. After four weeks, the original coffee oil again induced increases in serum cholesterol and triglyceride levels in 12 subjects relative to the 15 subjects who received placebo oil, while the stripped coffee oil failed to show any effect.

Their fourth study[24] was conducted with a select group of three subjects. A highly purified mixture of cafestol and kahweol was dissolved in placebo oil (sunflower oil and palm oil, 3:2 ratio) to a concentration equivalent to that in the coffee oil. Three particularly well-informed subjects (including two of the scientists themselves) then received three weeks of placebo oil, followed by six weeks of the purified mixture, followed by another five weeks of the placebo oil. The cafestol and kahweol mixture significantly increased total cholesterol by 1.7 mmol/L (66 mg/dL) and TG by 1.8 mmol/L (159 mg/dL), while decreasing HDL-C by 0.3 mmol/L (12 mg/dL).

To identify further which substance, cafestol or kahweol, or both, was inducing changes in serum cholesterol, the investigators attempted, but failed due to technical limitations, to separate the two chemical compounds. Alternatively, they compared coffee oil from Arabica vs. Robusta coffee beans. Arabica beans contain both cafestol and kahweol, while Robusta beans contain cafestol, but almost no kahweol. The investigators found that Arabica and Robusta oils both increased serum cholesterol and triglyceride levels comparably. They thus concluded that cafestol is, and kahweol might be, a serum cholesterol raising factor.

Coffee oil lipid extracts from Arabica vs. Robusta beans were also compared in a Norwegian study conducted by van Rooij et al.[25] In this experiment, 36 adults were assigned randomly to three groups of six women and six men each. For six weeks they took two daily supplements that contained either peanut oil (control), Arabica coffee oil, or Robusta coffee oil. The amount of coffee oil was comparable to that of drinking 1.0 to 2.9 L of coffee per day. Compared to the control group, total cholesterol levels increased in the Arabica group by 1.07 mmol/L (41 mg/dL), and in the Robusta group by 0.45 mmol/L, (17 mg/dL), although the differences were not statistically significant. Also, there were no statistically significant differences between the two coffee oil groups in levels of LDL-C or HDL-C. However, relative to the control group, TG levels increased in the Arabica group (by 0.75 mmol/L [66 mg/dL]), and in the Robusta group (by 0.08 mmol/L [7 mg/dL]), with the differences between the two groups being significant. Similarly, in a small crossover study with six women and five men, assigned randomly to either 2 g/day of Arabica oil or Robusta oil (equivalent to 1 to 2 L coffee day) for three weeks, Mensink et al.[26] failed to find statistically significant differences between the two oils.

Finally, a recently published crossover study of coffee oil lipid extracts by Urgert et al.[27] compared the effects of ~60 mg/day of cafestol with a mixture of 60 mg/day of cafestol plus ~50 mg/day of kahweol. These doses were comparable to consuming 10 to 20 cups of boiled Turkish or French-press coffee. In 10 healthy men, 18 days of cafestol alone resulted in significant increases in total cholesterol (0.79 mmol/L [31 mg/dL]), LDL-C (0.57 mmol/L [22 mg/dL]), and TG (0.65 mmol/L [58 mg/dL]), relative to baseline. Compared to cafestol alone, the cafestol/kahweol mixture resulted in additional increases in total cholesterol (0.23 mmol/L [9 mg/dL), LDL-C (0.23 mmol/L [9 mg/dL]), and TG (0.09 mmol/L [8 mg/dL]), but none was significant. The authors concluded that cafestol, not kahweol, is the primary cholesterol raising factor found in boiled coffee. However, the findings of these latter two studies[26,27] should be interpreted cautiously because they were both conducted over short time periods and involved small numbers of subjects. Urgert et al.[28] also studied the amounts of cafestol and kahweol present in both the oil droplets and the floating fines (the very small particles of coffee grounds) by measuring the amount of coffee ground fines in 11 types of coffee. Turkish coffee (made from finely ground coffee beans) had the highest content of fines, 5 g/L of coffee, while paper-filtered drip-brewed coffee (made typically from medium ground coffee beans) had the lowest content, 0.1 g/L of coffee. These investigators then randomly assigned eight women and six men to consume either 8 g of coffee ground fines per day or to a control group. After 21 days, total cholesterol and TG levels were significantly higher among the group that received the coffee fines, 0.65 mmol/L, (25 mg/dL) and 0.30 mmol/L (27 mg/dL), respectively. Neither LDL-C nor HDL-C were reported in this study.

In summary, these investigations suggest that the diterpenoid alcohol content of coffee, primarily cafestol and kahweol, is the cholesterol raising fraction. It can be present in either oil droplets or floating fines found predominantly in boiled coffee. Studies have shown that the use of a filter in coffee preparation can trap most of the diterpenoid material and the fines, thereby producing coffee without these cholesterol raising factors.

V. INFLUENCE OF CAFFEINE/COFFEE DOSE

Whether or not the magnitude of coffee's effects (boiled coffee, in particular) on serum cholesterol levels is proportional to the amount consumed (dose) is an important question that has not yet been addressed adequately by current published reports. It remains unclear if there are any threshold or plateau effects. With few exceptions, existing studies have used doses of four or more cups of coffee per day, with little variability within each investigation. Subjects in one study had maintained their habitual levels of coffee intake, which varied from 2 to 14 cups/day, rather than any specific amount.[19] Across their range of intake, it appeared that there was a proportional relationship between the amount of coffee consumed and the magnitude of the increase in serum cholesterol. However, closer examination revealed that there was no clear "dose response" among the majority of subjects who consumed 2 to 8 cups/day. One subject, though, who consumed 14 cups/day did experience the most dramatic increase in cholesterol levels of the entire group, but an additional confounder in this study was the lack of control or assessment for cream added to coffee by subjects. Further, when this subject was excluded from the analysis, there was little remaining evidence to support a dose response. More study is needed to determine if any dose-response effects exist.

VI. TIME INTERVAL FOR EFFECTS ON SERUM CHOLESTEROL

The full effect of changes in coffee consumption on serum cholesterol does not occur as quickly as it does to changes in dietary fat intake. Typically, when a stable high-saturated fat diet is replaced with a stable low-saturated fat diet, the maximum changes in serum lipid levels are achieved in two to four weeks.[29,30] The serum lipid response to changes in coffee consumption does not appear to reach its full effect until after four weeks or more.

In a study described above, subjects consumed either boiled or filtered coffee for 79 days, and serum levels of cholesterol were measured eight times.[21] The maximum increase of ~0.5 mmol/L (20 mg/dL) observed in the boiled coffee group was not reached until approximately four weeks into the study, after which the higher cholesterol level was maintained for the remainder of the study. Also described previously, another investigation with men who were apparently boiled coffee drinkers was conducted over a 10-week period with cholesterol measured every 2.5 weeks.[20] In the group that abstained from coffee for the entire 10-week period, serum cholesterol levels continued to drop; there was no apparent plateau reached. Since the study ended at 10 weeks, it is not certain what the ultimate extent of change would have been if it had continued beyond that time. One more example comes from the four-week study of boiled vs. boiled and then filtered coffee among 20 Finnish adults, predominantly women.[22] Serum cholesterol levels were measured at weeks three and four. At week three, differences in serum cholesterol were not statistically significant between the two groups, but at week four it was higher in the boiled coffee group. Since the study ended at four weeks, it is unknown here too whether an even greater difference would have been seen over a longer period of time.

These studies suggest that at least four weeks are needed before maximum changes in serum cholesterol levels, resulting from coffee consumption or cessation, are likely to be achieved.

VII. EFFECTS OF CAFFEINE/COFFEE IN POPULATION SUBGROUPS

Serum cholesterol responses to coffee or caffeine consumption in subgroups of the population may differ. For example, women may respond differently than men. The majority of clinical studies reviewed here have included both women and men;[14,15,17-19,21,22,25,26] however, inconsistent gender differences have been reported.[2,8,9,31] A few of the investigators have commented that results were similar for both groups, but none has presented findings separately by gender; although this was probably due to insufficient sample sizes which did not allow for stratified analyses. Thus, although it has been implied that women and men respond similarly, direct evidence is lacking. Further, few investigators have conducted studies with hypercholesterolemic populations,[18,20] although some have included individuals with modestly elevated serum cholesterol levels.[17,19,22] Hypercholesterolemic individuals may respond to changes in coffee consumption in a manner different than normocholesterolemics, and this needs to be studied.

A striking observation among these clinical trials is that, prior to participation, the vast majority of subjects had consumed paper-filtered coffee. The only notable exceptions were the hypercholesterolemic Norwegian men in the study by Forde et al.,[20] who apparently had been habitual boiled coffee drinkers, and the normocholesterolemic Italian men in the study by D'Amicis et al.[23] who had typically consumed espresso and mocha coffees. The study by Forde et al.[20] provides evidence that abstaining from boiled coffee or switching from boiled to paper-filtered coffee will improve serum cholesterol levels in hypercholesterolemic men. At least five other studies found that when habitual paper-filtered coffee drinkers consumed boiled coffee, serum lipids were affected adversely.[17-19,21,22] However, none of the studies included populations of habitual boiled coffee drinkers with normal serum cholesterol levels. Thus, it is unknown whether this population subgroup would benefit from either abstaining from boiled coffee or from switching to other types of coffee, such as paper-filtered. In addition to these few examples, there may be other groups including those of varying ages and ethnicities that have not been represented adequately in studies of coffee, caffeine, and serum cholesterol.

VIII. SUMMARY

The accumulated scientific evidence of the relationships between coffee, caffeine, and serum cholesterol allows for several conclusions to be drawn, while some important issues remain either equivocal or unaddressed. The links involve a number of factors, including the chemical composition of coffee beans, its preparation method, the amount of daily consumption, and specific characteristics of coffee drinkers. Coffee contains hundreds of chemical compounds, caffeine being perhaps the best recognized and studied. Although caffeine has several well-established effects on the human body, numerous studies have shown that it has little or no effect on serum cholesterol levels.

In recent studies, at least two coffee oil lipid extracts have been shown to be cholesterol-raising factors: cafestol and kahweol. The content of cafestol and kahweol in coffee differs depending on the method of coffee preparation and the type of coffee bean. Current evidence indicates that filtering removes the majority of the coffee oil lipid extracts, including the currently recognized cholesterol raising factors, and that filtered coffee does not induce significant changes in serum cholesterol. In contrast, boiled (i.e., unfiltered) coffee retains these factors. Boiled coffee, a method of preparation common in Scandinavian countries, has a well-demonstrated adverse effect on serum cholesterol. Intakes of five or more cups per day have been shown to increase cholesterol levels by 0.5 to 1.0 mmol/L (20 to 40 mg/dL) in men and women as compared to a similar number of cups per day of filtered coffee, tea, or to coffee abstinence. These strong and reproducible findings are sufficient to warrant public health recommendations for consumers of boiled coffee to switch to other types, such as filtered coffee. In many Scandinavian countries, this transition has already occurred for large segments of the population.[10]

Despite the large number of investigations that have been conducted, several important questions remain unanswered. Presently, it is unknown if there are threshold or plateau effects of coffee on serum cholesterol. Most studies have examined the impact of drinking four cups or more per day of boiled coffee. However, whether consuming less or considerably more than that would induce changes in serum cholesterol proportional to the amount of intake is unknown. Further, it is inconclusive whether cafestol and/or kahweol act alone or together, or are the sole responsible factors which elicit differential responses in serum cholesterol between boiled and filtered coffee. The two major types of coffee beans, Arabica and Robusta, both contain cafestol and kahweol, although in different proportions, and either type of coffee bean has been shown to increase serum cholesterol levels depending on the method of preparation.

Additional issues remain in question regarding methods of coffee preparation other than boiling or filtering. French press, Turkish/Greek, and espresso and mocha coffees are not filtered coffees, and therefore may contain the cholesterol-raising factors, but there is insufficient evidence currently to reach any solid conclusions. Finally, although it appears that men and women with either normal or elevated cholesterol levels respond similarly to coffee intake, this does not exclude the possibility that there are individuals with specific characteristics that respond differently. Additional studies into these areas will provide greater understanding of the effects of coffee on serum cholesterol.

TABLE 1

Summary of Clinical Trials on Coffee Consumption and Serum Cholesterol Levels

Author/ year nationality	Coffee type/ preparation type/ coffee chemical	Caffeine content (mg/day)	Coffee bean/ brand used	Cups or amount/ day	Study design/ duration	Subject # and characteristics age (years) TC (mmo/L)	Main results/conclusions	Comments
Caffeine Studies								
Superko[13] 1991 US	1: Caffeinated 2: Decaffeinated 3: Abstinence	1: 415-830 2: na 3: 0	1: Arabica[a] 2: Robusta[a]	1: 3-6 2: 3-6 3: 0	Parallel 2 months	181 M, healthy Age: 46±11 Baseline TC: ~5.5	Only significant result was higher LDL-C with decaf. 3-6 cups/day of caffeinated coffee have no adverse effect on TC.	
van Dusseldorp[14] 1990 Netherlands	1: Caffeinated 2: Decaffeinated	1: 417.5 2: 15.5	1: 71% Arabica 29% Robusta 2: 58% Arabica 42% Robusta	5	Crossover 6 wks/Rx	22 F, 23 M, healthy Ages: 25-45 Baseline TC: ~5.6	No significant differences between caffeinated and decaffeinated group. In healthy adults, replacing regular coffee with decaf has no effect on TC.	
Aro[15] 1985 Finnish	1: Instant coffee 2: Instant tea 3: Rosehips "tea" (caffeine-free)	1: 520 2: 200 3: 0	1: Nescafe Gold 2: Nescafe/Nestea 3: Lipton Ltd.	8	Crossover 3 wks/Rx	6 F, 6 M, healthy Ages: 33-35 Baseline TC: ~5.5	No differences between groups in TC, HDL_2-C, HDL_3-C, or TG. Caffeine does not exert an important effect on serum lipids.	Small study, of short duration
Fried[16] 1992 U.S.	1: Caffeinated, high 2: Caffeinated, low 3: Decaffeinated 4: Abstinence	1: 331 2: 166 3: 6 4: 0	na	1: 4 2: 2 3: 4 4: 0	Parallel 8 weeks	100 M, healthy Ages: 20-60 Baseline TC: 5.2	The only significant difference was an increase of 0.25 mmol/L in TC for the caffeinated group (4 cups/day)	The significant increase in TC was due to small changes in both LDL-C and HDL-C.

							relative to abstainers. Conclusion: Modest effect of 4 cups/day, no effect of 2 cups/day.	
Coffee Brewing/Preparation Studies								
Bak[17] 1989 Netherlands	1: Paper-filtered 2: Boiled 3: Abstinence	1: 375-563 2: 353-529 3: 0	na	1: 4-6 2: 4-6 3: 0	Parallel 9 weeks	47 F, 54 M Age: 26±4 (SD) Baseline TC: ~5.1	TC was 0.48 mmol/L higher among boiled coffee group vs. filtered. Boiled, but not filtered coffee, raises TC.	There was a substantial but not significant increase in LDL-C, but essentially no change in HDL-C.
Aro[18] 1987 Finnish	1: Boiled 2: Paper-filtered 3: Tea	na	Similar blend and roasting	8	Crossover 4 wks/Rx (2-wk run-in)	21 F, 21 M, HC Ages: 31-60 Baseline TC: 6.5-10.0	TC and LDL-C higher with boiled coffee vs. paper-filtered or tea. Cholesterol raising fraction found in boiled, but not paper-filtered coffee.	Changes not detectable at 2-weeks.
Aro[19] 1990 Finland	1: Boiled 2: Paper-filtered	na	na	2-14 (habitual)	Crossover 4 wks/Rx (2-wk washout)	28 F, 13 M, healthy Ages: 23-61 Baseline TC: ~5.5	Boiled coffee had adverse effect on TC (+0.32 mmol/L), LDL-C (+0.32 mmol/L), and HDL-C (-0.07 mmol/L) Boiled coffee adversely affects serum lipids relative to paper-filtered coffee.	Relatively short study. Effect may have been larger if study had been longer.
Forde[20] 1985 Norwegian	1: Habit./Habit. 2: Abstain/Abstain 3: Abstain/Filter 4: Abstain/Boiled	na	na	Not clear (perhaps 1 L/day)	Parallel 10-weeks (2-phases) I: 5-weeks II: 5-weeks	32 M, HC Age: na Baseline TC: ~8.7	At 10-weeks, TC was: highest for habitual drinkers (group 1), lowest for continued abstainers (group 2), much improved for abstainers who switched	Cholesterol levels appeared to still be dropping after 10 weeks in the continued abstainers (group 2)

TABLE 1 (continued)

Summary of Clinical Trials on Coffee Consumption and Serum Cholesterol Levels

Author/ year nationality	Coffee type/ preparation type/ coffee chemical	Caffeine content (mg/day)	Coffee bean/ brand used	Cups or amount/ day	Study design/ duration	Subject # and characteristics age (years) TC (mmol/L)	Main results/conclusions	Comments
							to paper-filtered for the last 5-weeks (group 3), and improved but then got worse for the men who abstained and then switched to boiled coffee for the last 5-weeks (group 4)	
van Dusseldorp[21] 1991 Netherlands	1: Boiled 2: Boiled & Paper-filtered 3: Tea	1: 860 2: 887 3: na	Roodemerk Douse Egberts	6	Parallel 79 days	31 F, 33 M Ages: 17-57 Baseline TC: 5.2	TC & LDL-C higher with boiled coffee than with either boiled and filtered or tea. No difference for HDL-C or TG. Paper filters remove the cholesterol raising factor from boiled coffee.	88% of lipid material found trapped by paper filter.
Ahola[22] 1991 Finnish	1: Boiled 2: Boiled & paper-filtered	na	na	6	Crossover 4 wks/Rx	18 F, 2 M Age: 45±8 (SD) Baseline TC: ~5.6	Serum lipids higher with boiled coffee (TC +0.36, LDL-C +0.33, HDL-C ns, TG +0.26 mmol/L) Filtering boiled coffee removes the cholesterol raising factors.	Changes detectable at 4 weeks, but not after 3 weeks. 80% of lipid material from boiled coffee found trapped by paper-filter.

D'Amicis[23] 1996 Italian	1: Espresso 2: Mocha 3: Tea	na	Arabica	1: 3.1 2: 2.8 3: 0	Parallel 6-weeks	84 M, healthy Age: 27±2.1 (SD) Baseline TC: ~4.7	No differences found in TC, LDL-C, HDL-C or TG between any of the groups. Italian coffee does not adversely affect serum lipids.	Dose of coffee was relatively small. Instead of using end-of-study serum lipids, the ave. of weekly measures was used
Coffee bean component studies								
Weusten-van der Wouw[24] 1994 Netherlands	1: Placebo oil 2: Coffee oil 3: Coffee oil, non-TG enriched 4: Coffee oil, non-TG depleted	na	Arabica: Robusta (88:12 w/w)	1: 3 g 2: 3 g 3: 3 g 4: 0.75 g	Parallel 4 weeks	32 F, 31 M (~16/Rx) Age: 22.2 ±2.8 (SD) Baseline TC: 4.5 ±0.5	TC and TG significantly elevated in all groups relative to placebo/control. Non-TG enriched fraction similar to coffee oil, with smaller response to non-TG depleted fraction. Cholesterol elevating fraction located primarily .in non-TG enriched fraction.	
same as above	1: Placebo oil 2: Coffee oil 3: Coffee oil without kahweol and cafestol	na	same as above	2g/d (all Rx)	Parallel 4 weeks	23 F, 20 M Age: 21.8±1.9 (SD) Baseline TC: 4.6±0.7	TC and TG significantly elevated in coffee oil group relative to placebo/control. Coffee oil stripped of kahweol and cafestol had virtually no effect on lipids. Cholesterol raising fraction found in kahweol and/or cafestol.	
same as above	1: Placebo oil 2: Kahweol and	na	1 & 3: sunflower:palm	2 g/ (all Rx)	Control-test-control	3 M Age: 49.3±7.6	TC increased 1.4-2.3 mmol/L, and TG	

TABLE 1 (continued)

Summary of Clinical Trials on Coffee Consumption and Serum Cholesterol Levels

Author/ year nationality	Coffee type/ preparation type/ coffee chemical	Caffeine content (mg/day)	Coffee bean/ brand used	Cups or amount/ day	Study design/ duration	Subject # and characteristics age (years) TC (mmo/L)	Main results/conclusions	Comments
	Cafestol 3: Placebo oil		oil (3:2) 2: Kahweol:Cafestol (45:55, w/w) in placebo oil	(5 capsules/d)	3 wks-6 wks-5 wks	(SD) Baseline TC: 5.1±0.5	increased 1.2-3.0 mmol/L during test period with concentrated kahweol and cafestol Cholesterol raising fraction found in kahweol and/or cafestol.	
same as above	1: Arabica oil 2: Robusta oil	na	1: Arabica 2: Robusta	2 g/day, both Rx	Cross-over 3 wks/Rx	11 F & M Age: na Baseline TC: na	Strikingly similar changes in TC, and TG with either Arabica or Robusta oil Cafestol is, and kahweol may be, a cholesterol raising factor.	Carry-over effect reported in liver enzymes
van Rooij[25] 1995 Netherlands	1: Peanut oil 2: Arabica oil 3: Robusta oil	na	1: 2: Arabica 3: Robusta	2 g/day coffee oil or placebo oil	Parallel 6 weeks	18 F, 18 M Ages: 19-64 Baseline TC: 5.1 the two.	TG were higher with Arabica vs. Robusta. TC, LDL-C and HDL-C were not significantly different between elevated AST values.	8 in the Arabica group had to stop early because of elevated AST values
Mensink[26] 1995 Netherlands	1: Diterpenes from Arabica beans 2: Diterpenes from Robusta beans	na	1: Arabica 2: Robusta	2 g/day coffee oil or placebo oil	Crossover 3 weeks/Rx	6 F, 5 M, healthy Ages: 20-26 Baseline TC: 4.9	None of the Arabica vs. Robusta differences were significant.	Arabica oil: 72 mg/d cafestol 53 mg/d kahweol Robusta oil: 59 mg/d cafestol

								2 mg/d kahweol
Urgert[27] 1997 Netherlands	1: Cafestol 2: Cafestol & Kahweol	na	na	1: ~60mg Cafestol/d 2: ~60mg Cafestol plus ~50 mg Kahweol/d	Crossover 14d run-in 18d Rx 48d wash-out 14d run-in 18d Rx 49d follow-up	10 M, healthy Ages: 24±4 (SD) Baseline TC: 4.8±0.9	Cafestol alone raised TC, LDL-C and TG significantly. Additional increases were observed with cafestol and kahweol combined, but the	Short study duration. Kahweol alone not tested directly vs cafestol alone.
								additional increases
were								
							not statistically significant. Cholesterol raising factor is primarily cafestol.	
Urgert[28] 1995 Netherlands	1: Coffee fines 2: Control	na	1: Arabica	8 g/day fines extracted from boiled coffee	Parallel 3 weeks	8 F, 6 M, healthy Ages: 24 ± 3 (SD) Baseline TC: ~4.7	TC higher in group consuming coffee fines vs. control. Floating fines can contribute to serum cholesterol response.	Extreme dose (equivalent to 4 L/day boiled coffee) Short duration

na = not available; TC = total cholesterol, TG = triglyceride; HDL-C = HDL-cholesterol; LDL-C = LDL-cholesterol; HC = Hypercholesterolemic; Rx = Treatment group; Habit. = Habitual; serum lipids = TC, LDL-C, HDL-C, TG; ns = not significant

[a]From source other than original article: press release, Stanford University Medical Center, November 9, 1989.

REFERENCES

1. Spiller, G. A., *The methylxanthine beverages and foods: Chemistry, consumption and health effects,* Chapter 6, Alan R. Liss, Inc., New York, 1984
2. Salvaggio, A., Periti, M., Miano, L., Quaglia, G., Marzorati, D., Coffee and cholesterol, an Italian study, *Am J Epidemiol.,* 134, 149, 1991
3. Thelle, D. S., Heyden, S., Fodor, J. G., Coffee and cholesterol in epidemiological and experimental studies, *Atherosclerosis,* 67, 97, 1987
4. Thelle, D. S., Arnesen, E., Forde, O. H., The Tromso Heart Study: Does coffee raise serum cholesterol? *N Engl J Med,* 308, 1454, 1983
5. Wei, M., Macera, C. A., Hornung, C. A., Blair, S. N., The impact of changes in coffee consumption on serum cholesterol, J Clin Epidemiol., 48, 1189, 1995
6. Davis, B. R., Curb, J. D., Borhani, N. O., Prineas, R. J., Molteni, A., Coffee consumption and serum cholesterol in the Hypertension Detection and Follow-Up Program, *Am J Epidemiol.,* 128, 124, 1988
7. Tuomilehto, J., Tanskanen, A., Pietinen, P., Aro, A., Salonen, J. T., Happonen, P., Nissinen, A., Puska, P., Coffee consumption is correlated with serum cholesterol in middle-aged Finnish men and women, *J Epidemiol Community Health,* 41, 237, 1987
8. Curb, J. D., Reed, D. M., Kautz J. A., Yano K., Coffee, caffeine, and serum cholesterol in Japanese men in Hawaii, *Am J Epidemiol.,* 123, 655, 1986
9. Stensvold, I., Tverdal, A., Foss, O. P., The effect of coffee on blood lipids and blood pressure: Results from a Norwegian cross-sectional study, men and women, 40-42 years, *J Clin Epidemiol.,* 42, 877, 1989
10. Pietinen, P., Aro, A., Tuomilehto, J., Uusitalo, U., Korhonen, H., Consumption of boiled coffee is correlated with serum cholesterol in Finland, *Intl J Epidemiol.,* 19, 586, 1990
11. Lindahl, B., Johansson, I., Huhtasaari, F., Hallmans, G., Asplund, K., Coffee drinking and blood cholesterol - effects of brewing method, food intake and life style. *J Internal Medicine,* 230, 299, 1991
12. Jansen, D. F., Nedeljkovic, S., Feskens, E. J. M., Ostojic, M. C., Grujic, M. Z., Bloemberg, B. P. M., Kromhout D., Coffee consumption, alcohol use, and cigarette smoking as determinants of serum total and HDL cholesterol in two Serbian cohorts of the Seven Countries Study. *Arterioscler Thromb Vasc Biol.,* 15, 1793, 1995
13. Superko, H. R., Bortz, W. Jr., Williams, P. T., Albers, J. J., Wood, P. D., Caffeinated and decaffeinated coffee effects on plasma lipoprotein cholesterol, apolipoproteins, and lipase activity: A controlled, randomized trial, *Am J Clin Nutr,* 54, 599, 1991
14. van Dusseldorp, M., Katan, M. B., Demacker, P. N. M., Effect of decaffeinated versus regular coffee on serum lipoproteins: A 12-week double blind trial, *Am J Epidemiol.,* 132, 33, 1990
15. Aro, A., Kostiainen, E., Huttunen, J. K., Seppala, E., Vapaatalo, H., Effects of coffee and tea on lipoproteins and prostanoids, *Atherosclerosis,* 57, 123, 1985
16. Fried, R. E., Levine, D. M., Kwiterovich, P. O., Diamond, E. L., Wilder, L. B., Moy, T. F., Pearson, T.A., The effect of filtered-coffee consumption on plasma lipid levels: Results of a randomized clinical trial, *JAMA,* 267, 811, 1992
17. Bak, A. A. A., Grobbee, D.E., The effect on serum cholesterol levels of coffee brewed by filtering or boiling, *N Engl J Med,* 321, 1432, 1989
18. Aro, A., Tuomilehto, J., Kostiainen, E., Uusitalo, U., Pietinen, P., Boiled coffee increases serum low density lipoprotein concentration, *Metabolism,* 36, 1027, 1987

19. Aro, A., Teirila, J., Gref, C-G., Dose-dependent effect on serum cholesterol and apoprotein B concentrations by consumption of boiled, non-filtered coffee, *Atherosclerosis*, 83, 257, 1990
20. Forde, O. H., Knutsen, S.F., Arnesen, E., Thelle, D. S., The Tromso heart study: Coffee consumption and serum lipid concentrations in men with hypercholesterolemia: A randomized intervention study, *Br Med J*, 290, 893, 1985
21. van Dusseldorp, M., Katan, M. B., van Vliet, T., Demacker, P. N. M., Stalenhoef, A. F. H., Cholesterol-raising factor from boiled coffee does not pass a paper filter, *Arterioscler Thromb.*, 11, 586, 1991
22. Ahola, I., Jauhiainen, M., Aro, A., The hypercholesterolemic factor in boiled coffee is retained by a paper filter, *J Int Med*, 230, 293, 1991
23. D'Amicis, A., Scaccini, C., Tomassi, G., Anaclerio, M., Stornelli, R., Bernini, A., Italian style brewed coffee: Effect on serum cholesterol in young men. *Intl J Epidemiol.*, 25, 513, 1996
24. Weusten-van der Wouw, M. P. M. E., Katan, M. B., Viani, R., Huggett, A. C., Liardon, R., Lund-Larsen, P. G., Thelle, D. S., Ahola, I., Aro, A., Meyboom, S., Beynen, A. C., Identity of the cholesterol-raising factor from boiled coffee and its effects on liver function enzymes. *J Lipid Res.*, 35, 721, 1994
25. van Rooij, J., van der Stegen, G. H. D., Schoemaker, R.C., Kroon, C., Burggraaf, J., Hollaar, L., Vroon, T. F. F. P., Smelt, A. H. M., Cohen, A.F., A placebo-controlled parallel study of the effect of two types of coffee oil on serum lipids and transaminases: Identification of chemical substances involved in the cholesterol-raising effect of coffee, *Am J Clin Nutr*, 61, 1277, 1995
26. Mensink, R. P., Lebbink, W. J., Lobbezoo, I. E., Weusten-van der Wouw, M. P. M. E., Zock, P. L., Katan, M. B., Diterpene composition of oils from Arabica and Robusta coffee beans and their effects on serum lipids in man, *J Int Med*, 237, 543, 1995
27. Urgert, R., Essed, N., van der Weg, G., Kosmeijer-Schuil, T. G., Katan, M. B., Separate effects of the coffee diterpenes cafestol and kahweol on serum lipids and liver aminotransferases, *Am J Clin Nutr*, 65, 519, 1997
28. Urgert, R., Schulz, A. G. M., Katan, M. B., Effects of cafestol and kahweol from coffee grounds on serum lipids and serum liver enzymes in humans, *Am J Clin Nutr*, 61, 149, 1995
29. Mensink, R. P., Katan, M. B., Effect of a diet enriched with monounsaturated or polyunsaturated fatty acids on levels of low-density and high-density lipoprotein cholesterol in healthy women, *N Engl J Med*, 321, 436, 1989
30. Becker, N., Illingsworth, R., Alaupovic, P., Connor, W. E., Sundberg, E. E., Effects of saturated, monounsaturated, and *w*-6 polyunsaturated fatty acids on plasma lipids, lipoproteins and apoproteins in humans, *Am J Clin Nutr*, 37, 355, 1983
31. Pietinen, P., Geboers, J., Kesteloot, H., Coffee consumption and serum cholesterol: An epidemiological study in Belgium, *Intl J Epidemiol*, 17, 98, 1988

Chapter 14

Coffee, Tea, Methylxanthines, Human Cancer, and Fibrocystic Breast Disease

Gene A. Spiller and Bonnie Bruce

CONTENTS

0-8493-2647-8/98/$0.00+$.50

I. INTRODUCTION

Over the past 30 years a large number of observational investigations have examined associations between coffee, tea, and other methylxanthine-containing products and human cancers. A few studies have examined the association between these products and benign breast disease. As we review results of epidemiological studies on any caffeine-containing product, we need to remember that it is difficult to isolate the effect of caffeine from that of the hundreds of other compounds present in coffee or tea, compounds that may have a positive or negative impact on the effect of caffeine or other methylxanthines. Additionally, coffee is prepared with different varieties of beans and even more importantly, it can be prepared in a variety of ways, from Italian espresso, to boiled or filtered coffees. To confound results even more, there are various degrees of roasting. Further, as heavy coffee drinking is often associated with other lifestyle behaviors, statistical analyses to isolate coffee as a causative factor is often problematic. For tea, there are hundreds of varieties of *Camellia sinensis* teas, which are usually not discussed in published reports.

Considering the large volume of research that has been done over the past three decades, only selected studies will be reviewed or mentioned chronologically. At the end of the chapter, in addition to our conclusions, we will report the opinions of some recent reviewers of this topic.

II. PANCREATIC CANCER

Although earlier work had showed a positive association between coffee consumption and pancreatic cancer rates across countries,[2] it was the much-publicized case-control study of MacMahon et al.[3] in 1981 that attracted widespread attention to the question of a possible link. In that study, which was designed primarily to investigate the role of smoking and alcohol in pancreatic cancer, 369 pancreatic cancer patients prior to diagnosis and 644 hospital controls reported their typical daily coffee and tea consumption. Unexpectedly, the authors found a significantly increased risk of pancreatic cancer associated with coffee consumption (overall relative risk 1.8, 95% confidence limits, 1.0 to 3.0), although a dose–response relation was evident only in women. An inverse association with tea drinking was found, although it was not significant. Serious questions have been raised about that study, in particular, relative to the selection of control subjects.[4] Of the 644 controls, 39% had had gastroenterologic conditions that might have caused them to avoid coffee, thereby artificially inflating differences with pancreatic cancer patients. Further, because the authors were interested initially in studying smoking and tobacco, they also excluded from the controls individuals with diseases known to be related to those factors and, in so doing, may have excluded heavy coffee drinkers as well. In later correspondence,[5] the authors replied that although the association of coffee with pancreatic cancer was greatest when cases were compared to controls with gastrointestinal diseases, it held up across subgroups of control patients.

That study by MacMahon et al.[3] in 1981, the investigations by Linn and Kessler[6] in 1981 that had earlier reported finding a relation between decaffeinated coffee and pancreatic cancer in women only, and Kessler[7] in 1981 who had reported that regular coffee was not found to be a risk factor for the disease, prompted several investigators elsewhere to examine existing data for a possible relation between coffee and pancreatic cancer. In 1982, Goldstein[8] reviewed coffee consumption histories of 91 patients with pancreatic cancer, 45 prostatic cancer patients, and 48 breast cancer patients and found no significant differences in the proportion of coffee drinkers between the pancreatic cancer and other cancer patients. in 1981, Jick and Dinan[9] reported on a matched case-control study in which pancreatic cancer cases from different countries were individually matched on age, sex, hospital or country, and year of admission to two hospital control groups, one with cancer, the other admitted for an acute medical condition or for surgery for a benign condition. They successfully matched 78 case–control pairs in the series using cancer controls and 83 pairs in the series using non-cancer controls. No association was found for drinkers of 1 to 5 cups daily or for ≥6 cups daily when compared to non-drinkers. On the other hand, in 1981, Nomura et al.,[10] examining data from their 13–year prospective study of 8,000 Hawaiian Japanese men, found a modest but significant increase in rates associated with increasing coffee consumption. The dose trend was not entirely consistent, however, because men who drank three to four cups of coffee per day had rates similar to nondrinkers. The authors noted too that other potential confounding variables were not taken into account in their analysis.

A few years later in 1983, Whittemore and colleagues[11] analyzed data on 50,000 former male students who had attended Harvard University between 1916 and 1950. In a 16 to 50 year follow-up, they compared coffee and tea drinking practices of 126 men in the college cohort, who had subsequently died of pancreatic cancer, with those of 504 surviving classmates. The relative risk associated with collegiate coffee drinking was 1.1, compared with non-drinkers. Tea consumption during college was associated with a significantly decreased risk of pancreatic cancer.

In a population study in 1981, Cuckle and Kinlen[12] correlated coffee consumption patterns for 16 countries with pancreatic cancer mortality rates in those countries a decade or more later and found significant positive associations in both males and females. However, when Japan alone was excluded, the correlation coefficients became much smaller and non-significant. In 1982, Bernarde and Weiss[13] then plotted per capita coffee consumption patterns for the U.S. from 1950 to 1982, together with pancreatic cancer incidence rates and found a rise and fall in coffee rates that was followed approximately 10 years later by a rise and fall in pancreatic cancer rates. However, major inconsistencies in the patterns for specific race and sex groups led the authors to conclude that any association between coffee and cancer of the pancreas was probably noncausal. The same paper reported on a correlation study of per capita coffee consumption across 13 countries in 1960 and age-adjusted pancreatic cancer rates in 1967. Although the resultant correlation coefficient of 0.59 was statistically significant, the authors noted that it was "not impressive", and an examination of the scattergram showed that one or two countries, again including Japan, were largely responsible for the observed results.

In 1986 in a cohort of Japanese men, Nomura et al.[14] failed to find an association of coffee with pancreatic cancer, whereas a large prospective study of Seventh Day Adventists in the U.S. in 1988 by Mills et al.[15] found increased risk for pancreatic cancer for recent but not past coffee consumption. In another Japanese study in 1989, Hirayama[16] found a suggestion of an association with coffee in Japanese men. In 1989, Clavel et al.[17] in France also found a significant association of pancreatic cancer and coffee drinking while in 1990, Farrow and Davis[18] in the U.S., analyzing data from 16,713 subjects, failed to find an association for coffee as did Jain et al. [19] and Ghardirian et al. [20] in 1991 in two case-control studies in Canada. Finally, in 1996, Nish[21] conducted a community-based case-control study in Hokkaido, Japan, with 141 pancreatic cancer patients and 282 controls matched for sex, age, and place of residence. They concluded that the lowest relative risks were found among "occasional" drinkers.

III. BLADDER AND RENAL CANCER

In an early study in 1971, Cole[22] found an association between coffee drinking and lower urinary tract cancer based on a case-control study of 445 cancer patients (345 men, 100 women) and 451 population controls who were matched for age and sex. The analyses had controlled for cigarette smoking and occupation; however, there was no consistent dose response relation, and the summary risks were significant only in women, not men. Using data from the same study, in a subsequent paper in 1974 Schmauz and Cole[23] compared the coffee drinking habits of patients with renal pelvis and urethra cancers to those with bladder cancer and with controls. In that analysis, significantly elevated risks for all sites were found only for drinking ≥7 cups of coffee daily, and only 2 of the 18 male cases of renal pelvis and ureter cancer were in that high exposure category. However, cigarette smoking was not controlled for and, probably due to small numbers, data for women were not reported. In 1974, Simon and colleagues[24] later conducted another similar study, this time confined to 135 white women with lower urinary tract cancer and 390 female hospital-based controls who were matched to the cases on age, urban-rural residence, and time (~2 years) of diagnosis. Although women who drank ≥1 cups of coffee daily had a relative risk of lower urinary tract cancer of 2.1 compared to nondrinkers (95% confidence limits, 1.1 to 4.3), there was no dose-response relationship with usual coffee consumption or with "cups-years" and cancer. Results were similar for caffeinated, decaffeinated, regular, and instant coffees. The authors concluded that any association between coffee consumption and lower urinary tract cancer was probably non-causal. Following Cole's first report,[22] in 1971 Fraumeni et al.[25] examined data on coffee drinking for 493 bladder cancer patients and 527 controls interviewed in New Orleans between 1958 and 1964. They also concluded that any association between coffee and bladder cancer was likely non-causal.

Results from a number of other case-control studies published between 1973 and 1980[26-30] and one international correlation paper[31] were subsequently reported. Most provided only weak support for an association between coffee drinking and bladder cancer or contradicted the findings of the earlier investigations. Evidence for a weak positive association between coffee and bladder cancer was reported by Hartge[32] in 1983 from a national multicenter case-control study, based on 2,982 new cases of the disease and 5,782 population-based controls.[32] The overall relative risk of bladder cancer associated with coffee drinking was 1.4, but there was no clear dose-response relationship, and heavy consumption (>49 cups/week) was related to an increased risk in men but not women. Results were essentially the same when the analysis was confined to caffeine-containing coffee, whereas there appeared to be no relation between the disease and tea consumption. Variation in relative risks across the 10 geographic areas they studied was impressive, e.g., ranging from 0.3 to 3.2 for drinking vs. never drinking coffee in males, although the authors reported that the geographic variation observed was similar to what would be expected by normal change.

Early on, Shennan[33] in 1973 and later Armstrong and Doll[34] in 1975 found strong positive correlations between international kidney cancer rates and coffee consumption. However, in a matched case-control study

(202 cases, 394 controls) of renal adenocarcinoma, Wynder et al.[35] in 1974 failed to find a significant association between daily coffee consumption and the disease in males or females, while controlling for level of smoking, although numbers were small in some categories. In another matched case-control study, Armstrong et al.[36] in 1976 also found no association between coffee and adenocarcinoma of the renal parenchyma (106 cases) or carcinoma of the renal pelvis (33 cases). For renal parenchymal cancer, the relative risk associated with daily coffee drinking was 1.15 (95% confidence limits, 0.51 to 2.65), and for renal pelvic cancer it was 0.11 (0.0 to 0.8), the latter suggesting a decreased risk, although based on small numbers. Further, the authors found no marked differences between cases and controls in tea drinking habits or in those who had ever consumed chocolate beverages. McLaughlin et al.'s population-based case-control study of cancer of the renal pelvis in the Minneapolis-St. Paul area also failed to find a statistically significant association with coffee drinking.[37] However, in females, the relative risk of the disease associated with tea drinking was 4.1 and statistically significant. In men, however, no such relation was observed.

In 1988, Kantor and colleagues[38] studied the epidemiology of squamous cell carcinoma and bladder adenocarcinoma and found a significant trend with the amount of coffee consumed; however, their findings were based on small numbers. In a population-based case-control investigation of the correlation between analgesics, cigarette smoking, and other risk factors and cancer of the renal pelvis and ureter, Ross et al.[39] in 1989 interviewed 187 residents of Los Angeles County who had been diagnosed with cancer of the renal pelvis and ureter over a four-year period, and individually matched them to controls by sex, age, race, and neighborhood. While they identified cigarette smoking as the major risk factor for cancer of the renal pelvis and ureter followed by heavy use of over-the-counter analgesics, heavy coffee drinkers (≥7 cups/day) showed a 1.8-fold increase in risk compared to nondrinkers. Although risk tended to increase with increasing consumption, this result was not statistically significant, and risk associated with heavy coffee consumption was reduced to 1.3 after results were adjusted for smoking.

Further, a case-control study in Turkey of 194 bladder cancer patients and the same number of age- and sex-matched hospital controls was carried out by Akdas et al.[40] in 1990 to estimate the role of various factors in the etiology of bladder cancer. In a country where smoking is widespread, cigarette smoking appeared to be the most significant cause of this cancer, followed by alcohol intake, by Turkish coffee consumption and artificial sweeteners. However, coffee drinking and alcohol were found to be promoting factors when results were adjusted for smoking. In 1992, Kunze[41] in Germany then studied lifestyle and occupational risk factors for bladder cancer in a hospital-based, case-control study of 531 male and

144 females with matched pairs. Multivariate logistic regression analyses showed coffee to be a significant contributor to the risk of bladder cancer in men after accounting for the effects of tobacco smoking, occupational exposure, and history of bladder infection.

IV. NON-HODGKIN'S LYMPHOMA

In northern Italy in 1994, Tavani and co-workers[42] examined coffee consumption and risk of non-Hodgkin's lymphoma in a case-control study. They interviewed 429 patients with histologically confirmed non-Hodgkin's lymphoma and 1,157 controls who had been hospitalized for acute, non-neoplastic, non-immunological, non-digestive tract diseases. They reported no association between non-Hodgkin's lymphoma and consumption of regular or decaffeinated coffee and tea consumption, while cola beverages were associated with a borderline risk.

V. OVARIAN CANCER

In his international correlational study in 1970, Stocks[2] showed a positive association between coffee consumption and ovarian cancer mortality rates. In Greece in 1981, Trichopoulos et al.[43] interviewed 92 women with epithelial ovarian tumors and 105 hospital-based controls and also showed a positive association and a relative risk of 2.2 associated with drinking ≥2 cups of coffee per day compared to drinking no coffee. This group also found a statistically significant dose-response relation for life-long total number of cups consumed, but women who drank ≤1 cup per day were not at increased risk. In 1982, Hartge et al.[44] attempted to test the association in a U.S. investigation using data from a case-control study of 158 women with epithelial ovarian tumors and 187 hospital-based controls who were frequency-matched to cases on age, race, and hospital. Although the authors reported a relative risk of 1.3 in women who drank any coffee compared to nondrinkers and noted that it indicated "an apparently greater risk of ovarian cancer among women who drink coffee than among those who do not", the confidence interval for the relative risk was 0.8 to 2.2, which was clearly consistent with no effect, and their data, as they acknowledged, demonstrated no dose-response.

Recently, Polychronopoulou[45] examined tobacco, ethanol, and coffee as risk factors for ovarian cancer in Greek women in a hospital-based case-control study with data collected from 1989 to 1991. Cases were 189 women who were residents of Greater Athens and less than 75 years old with histologically confirmed common malignant epithelial tumors of the ovary. Controls were female residents of Greater Athens, less than 75 years old, who had never had cancer or an ovary removed. They found no association with coffee, tobacco, and moderate alcohol intake.

IV. BREAST CANCER

Over a decade ago in 1985, Lubin et al.[46] in Israel studied 818 newly diagnosed breast cancer patients between 1975 and 1978 for possible correlations between total methylxanthine intake from coffee, tea, colas, chocolate, and cocoa beverages and breast cancer. When these cases were compared to matched surgical and neighborhood controls, they failed to find any significant associations. In 1985, Rosenberg and colleagues[47] in the U.S. evaluated the relation of *recent* coffee consumption with breast cancer in various Eastern hospitals. They compared 2,651 women with breast cancer to 1,501 controls free from cancer and 385 controls with cancer at other sites. Consumption of coffee, tea, or methylxanthine beverages was found not to influence the incidence of breast cancer. Further, in their 1986 case control study, Katsouyanni and co-workers[48] collected data from 120 patients and matched controls residing in Athens, Greece, and also failed to find a relationship with coffee consumption. In 1986, La Vecchia et al.[49] in Italy then compared 616 women with breast cancer and 616 controls free from cancer and also failed to find an association between coffee and breast cancer. In 1988, Rohan and McMichael[50] in Adelaide, South Australia, then examined the association between methylxanthine intake and breast cancer in a case-control study of 451 cases with one control matched to each case for age. In the postmenopausal subjects, they found a significant association between breast cancer and total methylxanthine intake or caffeine intake. In premenopausal women, they found a greater risk at high levels of intake.

In 1990, Vatten et al.[51] in Norway subsequently reviewed data on breast cancer risk from a cohort of 14,593 women with 152 cases of breast cancer during a follow up of 12 years on subjects who were between 35 and 51 years old at the beginning of the study and between 46 and 63 years at the end. They reported no overall statistically significant correlation between breast cancer and coffee consumption, but when body mass index was taken into account, lean women who consumed ≥5 cups per day had a lower risk than women who drank two cups or less. In obese women, however, there was a positive correlation between coffee intake and breast cancer. In a 1993 study, though, Folsom and associates[52] failed to find an association between caffeine and postmenopausal breast cancer in 34,388 women in the Iowa Women's Health Study, with a median caffeine intake of 212 mg/day in women who developed breast cancer and 201 mg/day for women who did not; and in Denmark, Ewertz[53] studied

2,445 women with breast cancer and did not find any association with coffee drinking.

Finally, the very recent report (1996) from the Rancho Bernardo study by Ferrini and Barrett-Connor[54] suggested associations between caffeine and sex steroid levels in postmenopausal women. This included a positive relationship between caffeine intake and plasma estrone levels and sex hormone-binding globulin and an inverse association with endogenous androgens. The authors hypothesized that caffeine may have mediated a possible decrease in breast cancer risk, thus favoring a protective effect, by the increase in sex hormone binding protein levels that may have resulted in decreased bioavailability of estradiol and testosterone.

VII. GASTRIC CANCER

In an investigation of 110 patients with gastric adenocarcinoma in Piraeus, Greece, in 1985, Trichopoulos[55] found no association with either coffee or tea and gastric cancer. Subsequently, in 1986, Heilbrun and associates[56] reported on black tea consumption and cancer risk in Japanese men living in Hawaii and found no significant differences in risk for tea. In Englandin 1988, Kinlen and associates[57] then studied 151 men from a cohort of 14,085 men who had died from gastric cancer. The trend with increasing tea consumption was significantly associated with death from gastric cancer from 0-3 cups per day to 7-9 cups per day, whereas in 1990 Demerir and co-workers[58] in Turkey found no association with tea drinking in 100 cases and 100 controls. Between 1977 and 1991, Memik et al.[59] studied 252 Turkish patients with gastric carcinoma, mostly from a low socio-economic population, and compared them with 609 age and gender matched controls and failed to find an association between coffee consumption and gastric cancer. In their review of data from 354 cases of gastric adenocarcinoma in Spain, Agudo and associates[60] in 1992 also failed to find a relationship between coffee or tea drinking and gastric cancer. Moreover, in 1993, Hansson et al.[61] in Sweden found no association of gastric cancer to coffee consumption in 330 patients compared to 669 controls.

Recently, in 1995, Yu and associates[62] in Shanghai examined the relationship between green tea consumption and gastric cancer in 711 cases compared to the same number of controls, and found green tea to have a strong protective effect. In 1996, Goldbohm and co-workers[63] in the Netherlands, on the other hand, reviewed data from 62,572 women and 58,279 men, and their results indicated that tea drinking did not appear to be a related factor.

VIII. COLORECTAL CANCER

In 1986, Heilbrun and colleagues[56] in Hawaii found a relationship between black tea consumption and higher risk of rectal cancer in men. In 1985, Tajima and Tominaga[64] in Japan carried out a study with only 42 cases and also showed that black tea drinkers had a higher risk of colon cancer; however, the results were not statistically significant. Subsequently, in a large Belgium study in 1988, Tuyns and associates[65] examined tea and coffee consumption and showed a significant trend for both colon and rectal cancer with increased consumption. Further, two studies conducted in the U.S., one by Phillips and Snowdon in 1985,[66] and one by Slatterty and associates in 1990,[67] also showed positive associations between high levels of coffee intake and colorectal cancer.

In contrast, a lowered risk for high coffee consumption reached significance for colon cancer in the case-control studies in 1988 by Tuyns et al.[65] in Belgium of 453 patients, in 1989 by Rosenberg and co-workers[68] in the U.S. of 717 patients, and in 1989 by La Vecchia and colleagues[69] in Italy of 445 patients. Moreover, in 1990, Kato and associates[70] in Japan found a protective effect of green tea. In Italy in 1992, La Vecchia et al.[71] studied 673 cases of colon cancer and 406 of rectal cancer, compared to 6,147 controls, and found that about 17% of controls consumed tea compared to about 20% of the colon cancer patients and 21.2% of rectal cancer patients. In 1994, Baron et al.[72] in Sweden found a significant reduction in rectal cancer for tea drinkers but no significant associations with colon cancer in 352 colon cancer cases and 217 rectal cancer cases.

A 1993 review by La Vecchia[73] concluded that there were many inconsistencies in the results of the association between coffee and colorectal cancers. For tea, in 1997 Kohlmeier and associates[74] after an in-depth review of tea studies concluded that there appeared to be some protective effect of green tea on colon cancer, while they found that the data for black tea was not clear since some studies showed no association and others found increased risk with regular use.

IX. PROSTATE CANCER

In an investigation of caffeine-containing products in 1993, Slattery et al.[75] reported on alcohol, coffee, tea, caffeine, and theobromine intake and the risk of prostate cancer in a Utah study. Data were gathered from a population-based sample of 362 newly diagnosed cases of prostate cancer and 685 age-matched controls. The Utah population was comprised predominantly of members of the Church of Jesus Christ Latter-Day Saints. The researchers found that pack-years of cigarettes smoked and consumption of alcohol, coffee, tea, and caffeine were not associated with prostate cancer risk, but found some possible correlation with increased theobromine consumption and concluded that more studies are needed for the possible role of large amounts of theobromine in cancer risk.

X. OVERALL RISK OF CANCER

Two decades ago in 1979 Heyden et al.[76] in an Evans County, Georgia, prospective investigation examined heavy coffee consumption relative to overall cancer mortality. In a comparison of 74 patients who died of cancer with 74 patients matched on sex, age, and race who died of cardiovascular disease, and 74 healthy survivors, also matched on sex, age, and race, they failed to find an association between relatively heavy coffee consumption (≥5 cups/day) and cancer.

About a decade later in 1988, in their study of gastric cancer, Kinlen and associates[57] analyzed data from 14,085 men in London for overall cancer risk. They found that frequent tea consumption was associated with increased risk of cancer, and that for men drinking less than 6 cups a day the risk was lower than expected. A year later, in the People's Republic of Mongolia, Dorzhgotov et al.[77] compared 1,263 cases of cancer to 2,526 healthy controls to identify potential risk factors for the five most common cancers in that region: esophagus, stomach, lungs, liver, and cervix or uterus. Consumption of large amounts of hot tea was one of the factors that correlated with risk for stomach cancer. Hot tea is often salted in this region and consumed very hot, thus suggesting a correlation between the high temperature of the beverage rather than with the tea. In a different line of evidence in their prospective study in 1991, Grossarth-Maticek et al.[78] analyzed data from cola drinkers in the U.K. and found that heavy consumption of cola drinks may prevent cancer but promote coronary heart disease.

In 1992, La Vecchia et al.[71] also studied the relationship between tea consumption and cancer from a series of case control studies carried out between 1983 and 1990, using cases with histologically confirmed cancers which included the following: 119 of the oral cavity and pharynx, 294 of the esophagus, 564 of the stomach, 673 of the colon, 406 of the rectum, 258 of the liver, 41 of the gallbladder, 303 of the pancreas, 149 of the larynx, 2,860 of the breast, 567 of the endometrium, 742 of the ovary, 107 of the prostate, 365 of the bladder, 147 of the kidney, and 120 of the thyroid, and compared them to a total of 6,147 controls who had been admitted to the hospital for acute non-cancer-related conditions. All estimates of relative risk for tea consumption were close to unity, confirming that there was no significant relationship between tea consumption and cancer risk. In 1993, Klatsky and associates[79] also confirmed the absence of a relationship between tea and cancer in analyses of health examination data between 1978 and 1985 from 128,934 individuals.

The large prospective study of Norwegian men and women conducted by Stensvold and colleagues[80] in 1994 examined the relationship between coffee drinking and cancer incidence in a 10-year follow-up of 21,735 men and 21,230 women aged 35 to 54 years. No association was found between coffee consumption and overall cancer risk. A negative association was found with cancer of the buccal cavity and pharynx and with malignant melanoma in women. No significant associations were found between coffee drinking and incidence of cancer of the pancreas or the bladder.

A very recent report by Zheng et al.[81] in 1996 investigated tea consumption and cancer incidence in the prospective Iowa Women's Health Study of 35,369 postmenopausal women. At eight years, 2,936 incident non-skin cancer cases were determined. Regular tea consumption was related to a slight, but not statistically significant, *reduced* incidence of all cancers combined. Inverse associations with increasing frequency of tea drinking were seen for cancers of the digestive tract and the urinary tract in women who drank ≥2 cups of tea per day, compared with those who never or occasionally drank tea. No appreciable association between tea drinking and melanoma, non-Hodgkin's lymphoma, or cancers of the pancreas, lung, breast, uterine corpus, or ovary were found.

The consumption of black tea and the subsequent risk of stomach, colorectal, lung, and breast cancers was investigated by Goldbohm[82] in 1996 in the Netherlands Cohort Study on Diet and Cancer among 58,279 men and 62,573 women aged 55 to 69 years. During 4.3 years of follow-up, 200 stomach cancers, 650 colorectal cancers, 764 lung cancers, and 650 breast cancers were diagnosed. Tea was not consumed by 13% of the subjects in the cohort, whereas 37%, 34%, and 16% consumed 1 to 2, 3 to 4, and 5 or more cups of tea per day, respectively. No association between tea consumption and risk of colorectal cancer was observed. Goldbohm concluded that black tea did not protect against four of the major cancers in humans but also that it was not leading to increased risk.

XI. BENIGN BREAST DISEASE

In 1979 two reports by Minton et al.,[83,84] both based on the same groups of women, described impressive improvement in benign breast disease among women who eliminated caffeine and other methylxanthine-containing products from their diet for periods ranging from one to six months. The reports received considerable attention in medical publications and especially in the lay press. The clinical implications were viewed as potentially important, because benign breast disease is common, in many cases requires biopsy to rule out malignancy, and because certain benign lesions are associated with a twofold or greater risk of breast cancer. However, there were serious flaws[85] in the studies. The observations were essentially uncontrolled, data were based on very small numbers of women, and it was inadequately presented to support some of the researchers' claims. Similar concerns apply to a subsequent paper in 1996 from the same group[86] that reached similar conclusions, although that report had been based on a larger group of women. Several subsequent studies have investigated the relationship between methylxanthines and benign breast disease. With one or two exceptions, those studies have examined the role of caffeine and other methylxanthines in the etiology of benign breast disease rather than in its treatment, and thus their results may not be comparable to the earlier work of Minton et al.[83,84]

In 1981, Lawson et al.,[87] for example, compared a group of 210 women hospitalized for fibrocystic disease with 241 women who had breast cancer and were drawn from two ongoing studies in different countries. They matched each case to three female control patients on age, current smoking habits, country, and study. Recent coffee and tea consumption in cases and controls were compared and were shown to have a modest positive association with "hot beverage consumption" for both fibrocystic disease and breast cancer, but there was no dose-response relationship. The risk of fibrocystic disease associated with heavy consumption of hot beverages (7+ cups per day) vs. none was elevated but not statistically significant.

About the same time in 1981, Marshall and co-workers[88] compared daily coffee and tea consumption by 323 women with benign breast disease and 1,458 controls admitted to a hospital between 1957 and 1965. Using the number of cups consumed per day for analysis, these authors found no relationship between benign breast disease and coffee, a nonsignificant reduction in risk associated with tea consumption, and also found no relationship when both beverages were combined. However, their control group included, among other diagnoses, women with gastrointestinal diseases who might have voluntarily reduced coffee consumption in response to those conditions. If anything, though, this would have tended to inflate artificially the relative risk although no elevated risks were demonstrated.

In 1982, Ernster and colleagues[89] attempted to replicate the study by Minton et al.[84] showing that methylxanthine abstention had a beneficial role in the *treatment* of benign breast disease. In their investigation, 158 women who presented with a breast concern were randomly assigned either to a group that was encouraged to abstain from methylxanthine-containing foods and beverages for a four-month period or to a group that received no dietary recommendations, but was also asked to return in four months. Although a statistically significant reduction in clinically palpable breast findings was associated with the methylxanthine-free diet, the absolute reduction in breast nodularity was minor and was probably of little clinical significance.

A few years later in 1984, Boyle[90] compared 634 women with fibrocystic disease with 1,066 female controls hospitalized for a variety of diagnostic conditions, and found a clear and significant dose response relationship with fibrocystic disease and amount of caffeine consumed daily. The relative increase was particularly high among women with benign breast conditions which were most related to increased risk of breast cancer, namely those with higher ductal atypia scores, atypical lobular hyperplasia, and sclerosing adenosis with papillomatosis or papillary hyperplasia.

In 1986, Parazzini[91] conducted a clinical trial in Italy with 192 women with fibrocystic breast disease, but found no benefit of coffee elimination. However, in a 1989 study of caffeine restriction as initial treatment for breast pain, Russell[92] studied 138 fibrocystic breast disease patients and showed that caffeine restriction was an effective means of alleviating breast pain associated with fibrocystic disease. More recently, in 1990, Bullough and associates[93] in New York found that 46% of the 102 women they studied showed some level of fibrocystic breast disease, but a significant association with the disease was found only when all methylxanthine-containing beverages rather than a single one (e.g., coffee) were taken into account.

XII. HOT TEAS AND MATÉ AND ESOPHAGEAL CANCER

The habitual drinking of tea, coffee, and maté when extremely hot has been shown to cause damage to the upper digestive tract that later may lead to cancer. This damage is most likely related to the temperature of the beverage rather than to caffeine or other constituents of the beverage. In 1993, Dhar and co-workers[94] thus studied the distribution of cancers in the valley of Cashmere in India because drinking boiling hot, salted tea was common there. They reviewed the records at the Department of Oncology of the Institute of Medical Science for 1986-88 for patients with cancer who were valley residents. Cancer of the esophagus was the most frequent type in both sexes, accounting for 42.9% of all types of cancer in the valley, which was very different from other regions of India where oropharyngeal cancer was the most common form. Dhar attributed this preponderance of esophageal cancer to the common practice of drinking boiling hot salted tea. In another investigation of hot beverages, maté, an ancient Brazilian caffeinated drink (Chapter 8), was studied because it has been shown to be associated with esophageal cancer. Shimada et al.[95] in their 1986 investigation of maté and esophageal cancer related the increased mortality prevalence of this cancer with very hot maté-tea drinking that was common in that region.

XIII. SUMMARY AND CONCLUSION

Contradictory findings among published reports of relationships between caffeine, coffee, tea, and cancer result in part from the complexity of coffee and tea and the diversity of these beverages. Studies often have not distinguished between preparation methods, sources of the beverages (e.g., type of coffee beans), intake itself is self-reported and amounts are idiosyncratic. It is unknown whether these factors play any influential role in the relationship of caffeine-containing beverages to cancer. Further, that heavy coffee drinking may often be associated with lifestyle habits or situations that may increase disease risk such as smoking, altered eating patterns, inactivity, severe over- or under-weight likely also contributes to inconsistent findings, notwithstanding attempts by some investigators to control for them. For coffee, the presence of contaminants such as ochratoxin A, a nephrogenic and nephrocarcinogic mycotoxin found in improperly stored green coffee beans, may be a factor to be considered.

It appears useful to summarize opinions published in some recent reviews. Lubin,[96] who in 1990 reviewed specifically the consumption of methylxanthine-containing beverages (tea, coffee, and chocolate) and the risk of breast cancer, had concluded that there appeared to be no evidence of an association, and although various methodologies were employed and diverse populations studied, results were consistently negative. With regard to pancreatic cancer and coffee, the association which in the early 1980s had stimulated a plethora of studies on that topic, Gold[97] concluded in 1995 that coffee consumption had little, if any, association with pancreatic cancer. In 1996, Nishi and co-workers[21] in a meta analyses of studies published between 1981 and 1993 concluded that "it appears that small amounts of coffee might prevent pancreas cancer, while large amounts might cause the disease". In a 1993 review of tea and cancer, Yang and Wang[98] reported that some studies had shown a protective effect of tea consumption against certain types of cancers, while other studies had indicated an opposite effect. They concluded that since many laboratory studies had demonstrated inhibitory effects of polyphenols in tea against tumor formation and growth, tea may have a protective effect, but cautioned that the effect of tea on cancer was likely related to the causative factors of the specific cancer. Therefore, a protective effect observed for a certain cancer with a specific population may not be observable with a cancer of a different etiology.

The data presented here has provided a chronological picture of the evolution and current state of the possible positive or negative association of some methylxanthine-containing products and various types of cancer. Perhaps the best conclusion at this time is an extension to tea and other methylxanthine-containing products of the statement by Stavric[99] who in 1990 wrote that certain controversial issues about the effect of coffee on human health remains unresolved. Future work should focus on types and methods of preparation of teas, roasting and preparation methods for coffees, and consider the whole beverage rather than caffeine or other methylxanthine per se. Meanwhile it appears that both tea and coffee and other methylxanthine-containing products may be safe and may even be protective for certain cancers when consumed in moderation.

ACKNOWLEDGMENT

The authors wish to acknowledge the contribution of Virginia Ernster of the University of California, San Francisco, whose reviews of selected studies have been made an integral part of this chapter.

REFERENCES

1. Ernster, V. L., Epidemiologic studies of caffeine and human health, in *The Methylxanthine Beverages and Food*, Spiller, G. A., Ed., Alan R. Liss, Inc., New York, 1984, Chapter 16.
2. Stocks, P., Cancer mortality in relation to national consumption of cigarettes, said fuel, tea and coffee, *Br J Cancer*, 24, 215, 1970.
3. MacMahon, B., Yen, S., Trichopoulos, D., Wamn, K., Nardi, G., Coffee and cancer of the pancreas, *N Engl J Med*, 304, 630, 1981.
4. Feinstein, A.R., Horwitz, R. I., Spitzer, W. O., Battista, R. N., Coffee and pancreatic cancer: The problems of etiologic science and epidemiologic case-control research, *JAMA*, 246, 957, 1981.
5. MacMahon, B., Yen, S., Trichopoulos, D., Wamn, K., Nardi, G., Coffee and cancer of the pancreas, *N Engl J Med*, 304, 1605, 1981.
6. Lin, R. S., Kessler, I. I., A multifactorial model for pancreatic cancer in man: Epidemiologic evidence, *JAMA* 245, 147, 1981.
7. Kessler, I. I., Coffee and cancer of the pancreas, *N Engl J Med*, 304, 1605, 1981.
8. Goldstein, H. R., No association found between coffee and cancer of the pancreas, *N Engl J Med*, 306, 997,1982.
9. Jick, H., Dinan, B. J., Coffee and pancreatic cancer, *Lancet*, ii, 92, 1981.
10. Nomura, A., Stemmerman, G. N., Heilbrun, L. K., Coffee and pancreatic cancer, *Lancet*, ii, 415, 1981.
11. Whittemore, A. S., Paffenbarger, R. S., Jr., Anderson, K., Halpern, J., Early precursors of pancreatic cancer in college men, *J Chronic Dis*, 36, 251,1983.
12. Cuckle, H. S., Kinlen, W., Coffee and cancer of the pancreas, *Br J Cancer*, 44, 760,1981.
13. Bernarde, M. A., Weiss ,W., Coffee consumption and pancreatic cancer: Temporal and spatial correlation, *Br Med J*, 284, 400, 1982.
14. Nomura, A., Heilbrun, L. K., Stemmermann, G. N., Prospective study of coffee consumption and the risk of cancer, *J Natl Cancer Inst*, 76, 587, 1986.
15. Mills, P. K., Beeson, W. L., Abbey, D. E., et al., Dietary habits and past medical history as related to fatal pancreas cancer risk among Adventists, *Cancer*, 61, 2578, 1988.
16. Hirayama, T., Epidemiology of pancreatic cancer in Japan, *Jpn J Clin Oncol*, 19, 208, 1989.
17. Clavel, F., Benhamou, E., Auquier, A., Tarayre, M., Flamant, R., Coffee, alcohol, smoking and cancer of the pancreas: a case-control study, *Int J Cancer*, 43, 17, 1989.

18. Farrow, C. C., Davis, S., Diet and the risk of pancreatic cancer in men, *Am J Epidemiol*, 132, 423, 1990.
19. Jain, M., Gowe, G. R., St. Louis, P., Miller, A. B., Coffee and alcohol as determinants of risk of pancreas cancer: a case-control study from Toronto, *Int J Cancer*, 47, 384, 1991.
20. Gharidian, P., Simard, A., Baillargeon, J., Tobacco, alcohol, and coffee and cancer of the pancreas. A population-based, case-control study in Quebec, Canada, *Cancer*, 67, 2664, 1991.
21. Nishi, M., Ohba, S., Hirata, K., Miyake, H., Dose-response relationship between coffee and the risk of pancreas cancer, *Jpn J Clin Oncol*, 26, 42, 1996.
22. Cole, P, Coffee-drinking and cancer of the lower urinary tract, *Lancet*, i, 1335, 1971.
23. Schmauz, R., Cole, P., Epidemiology of cancer of the renal pelvis and ureter, *JNCI*, 52, 1431, 1974.
24. Simon, D., Yen, S., Cole, P., Coffee drinking and cancer of the lower urinary tract, *JNCI*, 54, 587, 1975.
25. Fraumeni, J. F., Scotto, J., Dunham, L. J., Coffee-drinking and bladder cancer, *Lancet*, ii, 1204, 1971.
26. Bross, I. D., Tidings, J., Another look at coffee drinking and cancer of the urinary bladder, *Prev Med*, 2, 445, 1973.
27. Wynder, E. L., Goldsmith, R., The epidemiology of bladder cancer–A second look, *Cancer*, 40, 1246, 1977.
28. Mettlin, C., Graham, S., Dietary risk factors in human bladder cancer, *Am J Epidemiol*, 110, 255, 1979.
29. Morgan, R. W., Jain, M. G., Bladder cancer: Smoking, beverages and artificial sweeteners, *Can Med Assoc J*, 111, 1067, 1974.
30. Howe, G. R., Burch, J. D., Miller, A. B., Cook, G. M., Estere, J., Tobacco use, occupation, coffee, various nutrients, and bladder cancer, *JNCI*, 64, 701,1980.
31. Morrison, A. S., Geographic and time trends of coffee imports and bladder cancer, *Eur J Cancer Clin Oncol*, 14, 51, 1978.
32. Hartge, P., Hoover, R., West, D. W., Lyon, J. L., Coffee drinking and risk of bladder cancer, *JNCI*, 70, 1021, 1983.
33. Shennan, D. H., Renal carcinoma and coffee consumption in 16 countries, *Br J Cancer*, 28, 473, 1973.
34. Armstrong, B., Doll, R., Environmental factors and cancer incidence and mortality in different countries, with special reference to dietary practices, *Int J Cancer*, 15, 617, 1975.
35. Wynder, E. L., Mabuchi, K., Whitmore, W. F., Epidemiology of adenocarcinoma of the kidney, *JNCI*, 53, 1619, 1974.
36. Armstrong, B., Garrod, A., Doll, R., A retrospective study of renal cancer with special reference to coffee and animal protein consumption, *Br J Cancer* 33, 127, 1976.
37. McLaughlin, J. K., Blot, W. J., Mandel, J. S., Schuman, L. M., Mehl, E. S., Fraumeni, J. F., Jr., Etiology of cancer of the renal pelvis, *JNCI*, 71, 287, 1983.
38. Kantor, A. F., Hartge, P., Hoover, R. N., Fraumeni, J. F., Jr., Epidemiological characteristics of squamous cell carcinoma and adenocarcinoma of the bladder, *Cancer Res*, 48, 3853, 1988.
39. Ross, R. K., Paganini-Hill, A., Landolph, J., Gerkins, V., Henderson, B. E., Analgesics, cigarette smoking, and other risk factors for cancer of the renal pelvis and ureter, *Cancer Res*, 49, 1045, 1989.
40. Akdas, A., Kirkali, Z., Bilir, N. Epidemiological case-control study on the etiology of bladder cancer in Turkey. *Eur Urol*, 17, 23, 1990.

41. Kunze, E., Chang-Claude, J., Frentzel-Beyme, R., Life style and occupational risk factors for bladder cancer in Germany: A case-control study, *Cancer*, 69, 1776, 1992.
42. Tavani, A., Coffee consumption and risk of non-Hodgkin's lymphoma, *Eur J Cancer Prev*, 3, 351, 1994.
43. Trichopoulos ,D., Papapostolou, M., Polychronopoulou, A., Coffee and ovarian cancer, *Int J Cancer*, 28, 691,1981.
44. Hartge, P., Lesher, L. P., McGowan, L., Hoover, R., Coffee and ovarian cancer, *IntJ Cancer*, 30, 531, 1982.
45. Polychronopoulou, A., Reproductive variables, tobacco, ethanol, coffee and somatometry as risk factors for ovarian cancer, *Int J Cancer*, 55, 402, 1993.
46. Lubin, F., Ron, E., Wax, Y., Modan, B., Coffee and methylxanthines and breast cancer, *J Natl Cancer Inst*, 74, 569, 1985.
47. Katsouyanni, K., Trichopoulos, D., Boyle, P., Xirouchaki, E., Trichopoulou, A., Lisseos, B., Vasilaros, S., MacMahon, B., Diet and breast cancer: A case-control study in Greece, *Int J Cancer*, 38, 815, 1986.
48. Rosenberg, L., Miller, D. R., Helmrich, S. P., Kaufman, D. W., Schottenfeld, D., Stolley, P. D., Shapiro, S., Breast cancer and the consumption of coffee, *Am J Epidemiol*, 122, 391, 1985.
49. La Vecchia, C., Talamini, R., Decarli, A., Francheschi, S., Parazzini, F., Tognoni, G., Coffee consumption and the risk of breast cancer, *Surgery*, 100, 477, 1986.
50. Rohan, T. E., McMichael, A. J., Methylxanthines and breast cancer, *Int J Cancer*, 41, 390, 1988.
51. Vatten, L. J., Solvoll, K., Løken, E. B., Coffee consumption and the risk of breast cancer. A prospective study of 14,593 Norwegian women, *Br J Cancer*, 62, 267, 1990.
52. Folsom, A. R., McKenzie, D. R., Bisgard, K. M., Kushi, L. H., Sellers, T. A., No association between caffeine intake and postmenopausal breast cancer incidence in the Iowa Women's Health Study, *Am J Epidemiol*, 138, 380, 1993.
53. Ewertz, M., Breast cancer in Denmark. Incidence, risk factors, and characteristics of survival, *Acta Oncol*, 32, 595, 1993.
54. Ferrini, R. L., Barrett-Connor, E., Caffeine intake and endogenous sex steroid levels in postmenopausal women: The Rancho Bernardo study, *Am J Epidemiol*, 144, 642, 1996.
55. Trichopoulos, D., Ouranos, G., Day, N. E., Tzonou, A., Manousos, O., Papadimitriou, C., Trichopoulos, A., Diet and cancer of the stomach: A case-control study in Greece, *Int J Cancer*, 36, 291, 1985.
56. Heilbrun, L. K., Nomura, A., Stemmermann, G. N., Black tea consumption and cancer risk: A prospective study, *Br J Cancer*, 54, 677, 1986.
57. Kinlen, L. J., Tea consumption and cancer, *Br J Cancer*, 58, 397,1988.
58. Demerir, T., Icli, F., Uzunalimoglu, O., Kucuk, O., Diet and stomach cancer incidence. A case-control study in Turkey, *Cancer*, 2, 169, 1991.
59. Memik, F., Nak, S. G., Gulten, M., Ozturk, M., Gastric carcinoma in Northwestern Turkey: Epidemiologic characteristics, *J Environ Pathol Oncol*, 11, 335, 1992.
60. Agudo, A., Gonzalez, C. A., Marcos, G., Sanz, M., Saigi, E., Verge, J., Boleda, M., Ortega, J., Consumption of alcohol, coffee, and tobacco, and gastric cancer in Spain, *Cancer Causes Control*, 3, 137, 1992.
61. Hansson, L. E., Nyrén, O., Bergström, R., Wolk, A., Lindgren, A., et al, Diet and risk of gastric cancer. A population-based case-control study in Sweden, *Int J Cancer*, 55, 181, 1993.
62. Yu, G., Hsieh, C., Wang, L., Yu, S., Li, X., et al, Green-tea consumption of risk of stomach cancer: A population-based case-control study in Shanghai, China, *Cancer Causes Control*, 6, 532, 1995.

63. Goldbohm, R. A. Consumption of black tea and cancer risk: a prospective cohort study, *J Natl Cancer Inst*, 88, 93, 1996.
64. Tajima, K., Tominaga, S., Dietary habits and gastro-intestinal cancers: A comparative case-control study of stomach and large intestinal cancers in Nagoya, Japan, *Jpn J Cancer Res*, 76, 705, 1985.
65. Tuyns, A. J., Kaaks, R., Haelterman, M., Colorectal cancer and the consumption of foods: A case-control study in Belgium, *Nutr Cancer*, 11, 189, 1988.
66. Phillips, R. L., Snowdon, D. A., Dietary relationships with fatal colorectal cancer among Seventh-day Adventists, *J Natl Cancer Inst*, 74, 307, 1985.
67. Slattery, M. L., West, D. W., Robinson, L. M., et al., Tobacco, alcohol, coffee, and caffeine as risk factors for colon cancer in a low-risk population, *Epidemiology*, 1, 141, 1990.
68. Rosenberg, L., Werler, M. M., Palmer, J. R., et al., The risks of cancers of the colon and rectum in relation to coffee consumption, *Am J Epidemiol*, 130, 895, 1989.
69. La Vecchia, C., Ferraroni, M., Negri, E., et al., Coffee consumption and digestive tract cancers, *Cancer Res*, 49, 1049, 1989.
70. Kato, I., Tominaga, S., Matsuura, A., Yoshii, Y., Shirai, M., et al, A comparative case-control study of colorectal cancer and adenoma, *Jpn J Cancer Res*, 81, 1101, 1990.
71. La Vecchia, C., Negri, E., Franceschi, S., D'Avanzo, B., Boyle, P., Tea consumption and cancer risk, *Nutr Cancer*, 17, 27, 1992.
72. Baron, J. A., Gerhardsson de Verdier, M., Ekbom, A., Coffee, tea, tobacco, and cancer of the large bowel, *Cancer Epidemiol Biomed Prev*, 3, 565, 1994.
73. La Vecchia, C., Coffee and cancer epidemiology, in *Caffeine, Coffee, and Health*, Garattini, S., Ed., Raven Press, Ltd., New York, 1993, chap. 15.
74. Kohlmeier, L., Weterings, K. G. C., Steck, S., Kok, F. J., Tea and cancer prevention: An evaluation of the epidemiologic literature, *Nutr Cancer*, 27, 1, 1997.
75. Slattery, M. L., West, D. W., Smoking, alcohol, coffee, tea, caffeine, and theobromine: risk of prostate cancer in Utah, *Cancer Causes Control*, 4, 559, 1993.
76. Heyden, S., Tyroler, H. A., Heiss, G., Hames, C. G., Bartel, A., Coffee consumption and mortality: Total mortality, stroke mortality, and coronary heart disease mortality, *Arch Intern Med*, 138, 1472, 1978.
77. Dorzhgotov, B., Risk factors in the manifestations of the 5 principal forms of cancer in the People's Republic of Mongolia, *Sante Publique (Bucur)*, 32, 361, 1989.
78. Grossarth-Maticek, R., Eysenck, H. J., Coca-Cola, cancers, and coronaries: personality and stress as mediating factors, *Psychol Rep*, 68, 1083, 1991.
79. Klatsky, A. L., Armstrong, M. A., Friedman, G. D., Coffee, tea and mortality, *Ann Epidemiol*, 3, 375, 1993.
80. Stensvold, I., Coffee and cancer: a prospective study of 43,000 Norwegian men and women, *Cancer Causes Control*, 5, 401, 1994.
81. Zheng, W., Tea consumption and cancer incidence in a prospective cohort study of postmenopausal women, *Am J Epidemiol*, 144, 175, 1996.
82. Goldbohm, R. A., Consumption of black tea and cancer risk: a prospective cohort study, *J Natl Cancer Inst*, 88, 93, 1996.
83. Minton, J. P., Foecking, M. K., Webster, D. J. T., Matthews, R. H., Caffeine, cyclic nucleotides, and breast disease, *Surgery*, 86, 105, 1979.
84. Minton, J. P., Foecking, M. K., Webster, D. J. T., Matthews, R. H., Response of fibrocystic disease to caffeine withdrawal and correlation of cyclic nucleotides with breast disease, *Am J Obstet Gynecol*, 135, 157, 1979.
85. Heyden, S., Coffee and fibrocystic breast disease, *Surgery*, 88, 741, 1980.
86. Minton, J. P., Abou-Issa, H., Reiehes, N., Roseman, J. M., Clinical and biochemical studies on methylxanthine-related fibrocystic breast disease, *Surgery*, 90, 299, 1981.

87. Lawson, D. H., Jick, H., Rothman, K. J., Coffee and tea consumption and breast disease, *Surgery*, 90, 801, 1981.
88. Marshall, J., Graham, S., Swanson, M., Caffeine consumption and benign breast disease: A case-control comparison, *Am J Public Health*, 72, 610, 1982.
89. Ernster, V. L., Mason, L., Goodson, W. H., III, Sickles, E. A., Sacks, S. T., Selvin, S., Dupuy, M. E., Hawkinson, J., Hunt, T. K., Effects of caffeine-free diet on benign breast disease: A randomized trial, *Surgery*, 91, 263, 1982.
90. Boyle, C. A., Berkowitz, G. S., LiVolsi, V. A., Ort, S., Merino, J. J., White, C., Kelsey, J. L., Caffeine consumption and fibro cystic breast disease in a case control epidemiologic study, *J Natl Cancer Inst*, 72, 1015, 1984.
91. Parazzini, F., La Vecchia, C., Riundi, R., Pampallona, S., Regallo, M., Scanni, A., Methylxanthine alcohol-free diet and fibrocystic breast disease: A factorial clinical trial, *Surgery*, 99, 576, 1986.
92. Russell, L. C., Caffeine restriction as initial treatment for breast pain, *Nurse Pract.*, 14, 36, 1989.
93. Bullough, B., Hindi-Alexander, M., Fetopuh, S., Methylxanthines and fibrocystic breast disease: study of correlations, *Nurse Pract*, 15, 43, 1990.
94. Dhar, G. M., Shah, G. N., Naheed, B., Hafiza, Epidemiological trend in the distribution of cancer in Kashmir Valley, *J Epidemiol Community Health*, 47, 290, 1993.
95. Shimada, A., Etiological approach to the eating habits and the cancer mortality of Brazilian people, *Gan No Rinsho*, 32, 631, 1986.
96. Lubin, F., Consumption of methylxanthine-containing beverages and the risk of breast cancer, *Cancer Lett*, 53, 81, 1990.
97. Gold, E. B., Epidemiology of and risk factors for pancreatic cancer, *Surg Clin North Am*, 75, 819, 1995.
98. Yang, C. S., Wang, Z. Y., Tea and cancer, *J Natl Cancer Inst*, 85, 1038, 1993.
99. Stavric, B., An update on research with coffee/caffeine (1989-1990), *Food Chem Toxicol*, 30, 533, 1992.

Chapter 15

Caffeine, Calcium, and Bone Health

Bonnie Bruce and Gene A. Spiller

CONTENTS

I. INTRODUCTION

Osteoporosis is an age-related disorder estimated to affect twice as many women as men.[1] Characterized by loss of bone mass over a lifetime, it accounts for more than one million fractures annually with one of every five American women over 65 years old having one or more fractured bones.[2-3] With the elderly projected to represent 25% of the population by 2030, the consequences of bone loss are a significant public health problem.

A number of dietary and nondietary variables have been proposed as risk factors for osteoporosis. Among dietary factors, the relation between caffeine intake and bone health has been studied extensively. Although proof that caffeine adversely affects calcium metabolism and is detrimen-

0-8493-2647-8/98/$0.00+$.50

tal to bone health is still lacking, several lines of evidence support the notion that it is an important factor (Table 1). The purpose of this chapter is to present the evidence from human studies on the relations among caffeine intake, perturbations in calcium balance, bone loss, and osteoporosis in women.

II. IMPACT OF CAFFEINE ON CALCIUM METABOLISM

One of the earliest observational investigations to find a positive association between caffeine and calcium balance was Daniell's[4] case control study. He documented that large amounts of caffeine (more than 4 cups coffee per day) were associated with hypercalcuria in a group of 311 postmenopausal osteoporotic subjects, but his findings did not persist after controlling for weight and smoking. In Heaney and Recker's[5] correlational study with 170 premenopausal nuns (mean 40 years), caffeine intake from coffee, tea, and cola was associated with both increased urinary and intestinal calcium losses, although significance did not persist when adjusted for calcium intake. More recently, in a northern European study, Hasling et al.[6] examined the relation between selected dietary constituents and calcium balance in 85 postmenopausal osteoporotic women. Multivariate analyses showed that the only dietary constituent having a statistically significant impact on calcium metabolism was coffee. However, the authors suggested that while a high coffee intake in excess of 4 to 5 cups/day could induce physiologically significant hypercalcuria, low to moderate intakes of 1 to 2 cups/day would not be significant.

Direct experimental studies to date have yielded mixed results with the majority of positive findings emanating from Massey's lab. In a blinded, randomized, crossover study, Massey and colleagues[7] demonstrated a significant increase in acute urinary calcium loss in healthy young females (mean 25 years) that were fed 150 to 300 mg caffeine loads, consisting of caffeine added to decaffeinated coffee, decaffeinated tea, or herbal tea. In this same study, they additionally compared the women who had a habitually low caffeine intake (13 to 85 mg/d) with those who consumed 230 to 435 mg/d and found that there was no adaptation to caffeine-induced hypercalcuria. In a similar trial, but with younger adolescent females,[8] they also documented an acute negative impact from caffeine loading on calcium excretion.

Massey and Opryszek[9] elaborated further by showing that habitual caffeine consumption induced chronic hypercalcuria in young women (mean 24 years) after an oral caffeine challenge where they were fed either 300 mg of caffeine tablets per day or 6 mg caffeine per kilogram lean body mass (LBM) per day (range 274 to 325 mg/caffeine) mixed with decaffeinated coffee or tea when compared to a week of abstinence. Additionally, they[10] studied a mixed group of 37 premenopausal, perimenopausal, and postmenopausal women (30 to 78 years old) and found that those who habitually consumed 200 mg caffeine/d and had a low dietary calcium intake of less than 600 mg/d (estimated from 6-d diet records) experienced increased bone turnover.

On the other hand, when Barger-Lux et al.[11] fed an oral caffeine load of about 6 mg/kg of LBM mixed with decaffeinated coffee crystals in a blinded, randomized crossover study to 16 healthy premenopausal women (median age 30 years) who had habitual calcium intakes of 600 mg/d or more (estimated from food frequency data), they failed to show significant effects of caffeine on urinary or fecal calcium excretion against a placebo. Smith et al.[12] extended these findings to caffeinated carbonated beverages in a small sample of healthy premenopausal women (mean age not reported) and demonstrated that a diet high in nonalcoholic carbonated beverages did not appear to adversely affect serum or urinary measures of calcium metabolism. Finally, Lloyd and his colleagues[13] in a recent cross-sectional study that compared urinary calcium excretion in lacto-ovo vegetarian vs. nonvegetarian women (mean age 35 years) reported that in both groups, both of which had adequate calcium intakes (mean 870 mg/d), there was a positive association between caffeine intake (estimated from a 3-d dietary record) and urinary calcium excretion.

III. CAFFEINE INTAKE, BONE MASS, AND OSTEOPOROSIS

Several longitudinal epidemiological studies have reported significant positive findings between caffeine intake and bone density or risk of fracture. Data from the Nurses' Health Study,[14] a prospective cohort investigation of nurses from 11 states, found a strong positive association between women who consumed more than 192 mg of caffeine/d (estimated from food frequency data) and risk of hip fractures, after adjustment for weight, menopausal status, hormone use, alcohol, calcium intake, and smoking. The finding was most evident in women with a high coffee intake (> 4 cups/d) who had a threefold increase in hip fracture risk when compared to women who seldom/never drank coffee.

The 12-year report from the Framingham Study,[15] a long-term prospective investigation of cardiovascular disease, of 1,817 women found that after controlling for weight, alcohol, smoking, and estrogen use, caffeine intake equivalent to 2 or more cups of coffee per day (estimated from self-report and imputed caffeine values) was associated with a significantly increased hip fracture risk in women less than 65 years old.

In the Massachusetts Women's Health Study, a population-based cross-sectional investigation of women, Hernandiz-Avila and colleagues[16] also found an inverse linear association with caffeine intake (estimated from

TABLE 1

Chronological Summary of Studies on Caffeine and Bone Health

Ref.	Subject	Design	Outcome variable(s)	Source of caffeine data	Findings
4 (1976)	Postmenopausal women (60-69 y) N=571	Observational	Urinary mineral excretion, bone mass	Self report	No association between calcium excretion or bone mass in abstainers and coffee drinkers with similar smoking habits and degree of obesity.
5 (1982)	Premenopausal women (mean 40 y) N=170	Observational	Urinary mineral excretion	Duplicate analyzed samples of coffee, tea, cola	Caffeine inversely related to calcium intake and balance, but did not hold up after stratification for calcium intake.
22 (1983)	Pre-, peri-, and postmenopausal women (mean 44 y) N=48	Observational	Changes in radial bone mass	Not reported	No significant relationships between bone mass and caffeine.
7 (1984)	Premenopausal women (mean 25 y) N=12	Blinded, randomized cross over	Urinary mineral excretion	Oral caffeine load added to decaffeinated coffee, tea, or herbal tea	Significantly increased calcium excretion with caffeine loads of 150 mg and 300 mg.
18 (1985)	Postmenopausal women (mean 66 y) N=912	Observational	Bone mineral content of radius, ulna, Os calcis	24-hour diet recall and food frequency data	Inverse relationship between bone mineral content of distal radius and ulna and high caffeine intake.
25 (1988)	Postmenopausal women (mean 75 y) N=513	Observational	Risk of hip fracture	24-hour diet recall	No association between risk of hip fracture and caffeine intake.

8 (1988)	Premenopausal females (mean 16) N=9	Controlled cross over	Urinary mineral excretion	Oral caffeine loads added to non-caffeinated carbonated beverage (3 mg/kgm body weight)	Significantly increased calcium excretion in females.
23 (1988)	Premenopausal women (40-50 y) N=183	Observational	Bone mineral content of L2 and L4 and forearm	Self report	No overall association between bone mineral content or coffee intake.
10 (1989)	Pre-, peri-, and postmenopausal women (mean 60 y) N=37	Experimental (design not described)	Measures of calcium metabolism	Not reported	Fasting ultrafilterable calcium increased and serum bone alkaline phosphatase isoenzyme levels decreased, but only in those with calcium intakes < 600mg/d.
12 (1989)	Premenopausal young women (mean age not given) N=8	Randomized cross over	Measures of calcium metabolism	1.4 L diet coke fed daily	No effect on calcium metabolism in women consuming 800 mg calcium/d.
11 (1990)	Premenopausal women (mean 29 y) N=16	Double blind, placebo, controlled cross over	Serum and urinary measures of calcium metabolism	Oral caffeine load added to decaf coffee (400 mg)	Failed to show any significant effect of caffeine.
9 (1990)	Premenopausal women (mean 24 y) N=17	Randomized cross over	Urinary mineral excretion	Oral caffeine loads added to decaffeinated coffee or tea	Calcium excretion increased significantly after caffeine challenges with no adaptation to caffeine-induced excretion after one week.
	Premenopausal women (mean 29 y) N=101	Observational	Calcaneal bone density	Self report of daily intake of cups of coffee	Failed to show effect after adjustment for smoking and found insignificant decline with consumption of > 2 cups/d.

TABLE 1 (continued)

Chronological Summary of Studies on Caffeine and Bone Health

Ref.	Subject	Design	Outcome variable(s)	Source of caffeine data	Findings
15 (1990)	Peri- and postmenopausal women (50-84 y) N=1817	Observational	Hip fracture	Self report of coffee and tea intake	Caffeine intake equivalent to 2 or more cups/day (estimated from self-report and imputed caffeine values) was associated with a significantly increased hip fracture risk in women less than 65 years old.
24 (1990)	Perimenopausal women (mean 51 y) N=124	Observational	Serum and urinary measures of calcium metabolism, bone mass of radius lumbar spine, and hip	3-day diet records and food frequency data	No association between caffeine intake and bone mineral in axial or appendicular skeleton.
14 (1991)	Pre- and perimenopausal women (34-59 y) N=84,484	Observational	Forearm and hip fractures	Food frequency data	Reported that only coffee among caffeine sources was the significant predictor of hip fracture, although no association between caffeine intake and forearm fracture found.
13 (1991)	Premenopausal women (mean 35 y) N=64	Observational	Measures of calcium metabolism and bone mass	Three-day diet records	No association between bone density and caffeine intake, although caffeine was found to have significant negative effect on calcium metabolism.
19 (1992)	Pre-, peri- and postmenopausal women (est. 30-75 y) N=209	Observational	Serum and urinary measures of calcium	Seven-day diet record	Among the oldest women with impaired calcium balance a high caffeine intake may predispose to cortical bone loss. However, effects were age and site specific and after

			metabolism, bone mass		adjusting for age, caffeine was not correlated with bone metabolism, hormone, or other dietary or musculoskeletal variable.
6 (1992)	Postmenopausal women (mean 66 y) N=85	Observational	Calcium metabolism and bone mineralization	Four-day diet records	Of dietary constituents studied, only caffeine negatively impacted calcium and bone metabolism.
27 (1992)	Postmenopausal women (mean 66 y) N=85	Observational	Bone mass	24-hour diet recall and diet history	In association with caffeine intake a lower bone mineral content was shown bivariately, but not multivariately, however, there was no relationship between coffee and fracture risk
26 (1992)	Peri- and postmenopausal women (mean 74 y) N=533	Observational	Risk of hip and wrist fracture	Food frequency data	Caffeine intake unrelated to hip or wrist fracture.
16 (1993)	Pre- and perimenopausal women (mean 53 y) N=281	Observational	Bone density	Food frequency data	Caffeine intake inversely associated with bone density, independent of dietary anthropometric and hormonal factors.
17 (1994)	Postmenopausal women (mean 73 y) N=980	Observational	Bone density at hip and lumbar spine	Self report of lifetime caffeinated coffee intake	Increasing lifetime caffeinated coffee intake significantly inversely associated with bone mineral at hip and spine in subjects who did not report drinking at least one glass of milk a day between 20-50 years of age.
20 (1994)	Postmenopausal women (mean 61 y) N=205	Randomized clinical trial of vitamin D and bone loss	Bone density of spine and total body, biochemical and urinary measures	Food frequency data	Caffeine did not have adverse effect in subjects with adequate calcium intakes near or above 800 mg/d, although daily caffeine intake ≥2-3 servings of brewed coffee may accelerate bone loss from the spine and total body in women with a low calcium intake.

food frequency data) and bone density in 281 pre- and perimenopausal women (mean age 53) that was independent of dietary, anthropometric, and hormonal variables.

Further, in 980 postmenopausal women (mean 73 years old) from the Rancho Bernardo Study, a population-based study of an upper middle class community, Barrett-Connor et al.[17] demonstrated a significant graded positive association between lifetime intake of 2 cups coffee/day (obtained by self report questionnaire) and worsening of bone mineral density at both the hip and spine in subjects who did not report drinking at least one glass of milk on a daily basis between 20 and 50 years of age. These effects also persisted after controlling for putative modifying factors such as age, weight, parity, smoking, alcohol, estrogen, thiazides, calcium supplements, exercise, and years postmenopausal.

Finally, Yano et al.[18] reported a significant negative association between forearm bone mineral content and current caffeine intake among a group of elderly Japanese-American women living in Hawaii, after controlling for intake of milk, calcium, and vitamin D.

Other cohort studies have suggested that the existence of inverse associations between bone mass and women consuming high amounts of caffeine may relate to specific factors. In an age-stratified random sample of white women (range 30 to 60+ years), Cooper et al.[19] reported that among the oldest women with impaired calcium balance a high caffeine intake appeared to predispose to cortical bone loss from the proximal femur. They suggested that the effects were age and site specific, and after adjusting for age and caffeine consumption, were not correlated with bone metabolism, hormone, or other dietary or musculoskeletal variable.

In their study of 205 healthy, nonsmoking postmenopausal women (mean 60 years), which evaluated vitamin D and bone loss, Harris and Dawson-Hughes[20] reported that a daily caffeine intake of 2 to 3 servings of brewed coffee accelerated bone loss from the spine and total body in women with a low calcium intake, but in subjects with adequate calcium intakes near or above 800 mg/d, caffeine did not have adverse effects. Lastly, the Study of Osteoporotic Fractures Research Group's[21] multicenter, prospective investigation of 9704 ambulatory women, 65 years and older, showed that caffeine intake was significantly correlated with lower bone mass, but that among factors that influenced bone mass of elderly women, age, weight, muscle strength, and hormone use were most important.

In contrast, other investigations have shown no overall association between bone and caffeine intake. In addition to studying calcium balance, Daniell[4] had also assessed metacarpal cortical area relative to caffeine intake and did find a greater prevalence of lower bone mass in women, 60 to 69 years old, consuming more than 4 cups of coffee per day, but significance disappeared after stratification by weight and smoking. Eliel[22] looked at longitudinal changes prospectively in radial bone mass in a mixed group of pre-, peri-, and postmenopausal women (24 to 60 years old), and similarly did not demonstrate an effect of caffeine consumption on rate of bone loss while taking into account milk intake and physical activity, although their data also included men. These authors concluded that if caffeine does have an effect on rate of bone loss in normal subjects, its magnitude was insufficient and undetectable by longitudinal measurements. The study by Picard and colleagues[23] with 40- to 50-year-old premenopausal women also failed to find a significant relationship between caffeine intake and bone mineral, as did Slemenda et al.[24] in their study with 84 peri- and postmenopausal women, which did not show caffeine intake to be a predictor of bone mineral in the axial or appendicular skeleton. Although Holbrook et al.'s[25] 14-year follow up of Framingham subjects indicated that women with hip fracture had higher caffeine intakes than those without hip fracture, their results were not significant, which was probably due to failure to consider confounding variables such as weight. In their case control study of 433 postmenopausal women (mean 70 years old) with hip and wrist fractures, Krieger and colleagues[26] also failed to find an association between caffeine and fracture risk in their subjects. Finally, a European prospective cohort study[27] of older adults (76 years old), which evaluated the relationship between caffeine intake, bone mineral, and fracture risk while controlling for smoking, weight, physical activity, and other putative modifying factors found no relationship between coffee consumption and fracture risk, and in their multivariate models coffee was not a significant risk factor for osteoporosis.

IV. SUMMARY

Collectively, the literature shows a trend indicating that a lifetime pattern of high caffeine intake in women contributes to a negative impact on calcium and bone metabolism and is correlated with bone loss or fracture risk, particularly when there is a low calcium intake. Both experimental and observational studies have demonstrated that the calciuretic effect of caffeine, if sustained chronically, induces a biologically significant impact on calcium balance. However, when caffeine is consumed in small to moderate amounts, defined as 1 to 2 cups of coffee per day in some studies and is accompanied by an adequate calcium intake (at least 600 mg), it may not have significant physiological effects. Although epidemiological and experimental studies have failed to indicate consistently that caffeine is a significant factor in incidence of bone fracture, the well-known pharmacologic effects of caffeine have raised important questions about its role in calcium balance and the metabolic consequences associated with caffeine.

In spite of this reasonable scientific evidence, there is a considerable amount of conflicting data. This is due conceivably to uncontrolled known and postulated putative modifying factors associated with calcium balance and bone mass which may have been responsible for attenuating any effects. Some studies have not stratified for tobacco, which often accompanies caffeine intake, alcohol consumption, hormone use, or body weight, all of which have been reported to affect calcium or bone metabolism. Menopausal status has not been considered consistently or, alternatively, mixed age groups of women have been used. Thus, results could have been modulated by differential effects of caffeine at different stages of a woman's lifespan. Moreover, the use of small sample sizes which reduces the power necessary to reveal moderate changes, varying research designs, and methodological differences among studies also contributes to the confusion.

Additionally, latent confounding factors concerning measurement of caffeine are prevalent. Although in some studies coffee is used as the dependent variable due to its putative use or as a surrogate for caffeine, the complex nature of coffee itself is overlooked. Coffee varies widely in caffeine content and other constituents, depending on the kind of coffee bean and the brewing method (see Chapter 6). Further, consumption of other sources of caffeine, i.e., teas, colas, other beverages fortified with caffeine, and many pharmacological agents, are not specified clearly in all studies. The heterogeneous nature of coffee and different sources of caffeine suggest that errors in quantification of caffeine intake could mitigate true associations. Furthermore, the amounts consumed are typically self-reported and idiomatic, and when measured cross-sectionally, may not be reflective of cumulative exposure. It is hoped that future studies will clarify the role of caffeine vs. whole caffeinated beverages and ensure that intake is reported accurately.

In summary, the current literature indicates that the state of our knowledge is incomplete to permit firm conclusions about the direct relationship between caffeine intake, calcium balance, and hence risk of fracture. Additional characterization will provide greater understanding of the long term effects of differing levels of caffeine on bone health in women. Longitudinal investigations which control for putative modifying variables are needed to help resolve current inconsistencies between caffeine consumption and the severity of its long term impact on calcium and bone metabolism. This in turn will help address issues related to risk of fracture in old age. Assuming there is a link between caffeine and, ultimately, bone fracture, its impact on the huge toll it is predicted to extort in suffering and health care costs in our aging population could be substantially affected.

REFERENCES

1. Wolinsky, I., Klimis-Tavantzis, D., eds., *Nutritional Concerns of Women*, CRC Press Inc., Boca Raton, 1996, 54.
2. Spencer, H., Dramer, L., NIH Consensus Conference: Osteoporosis. Factors contributing to osteoporosis, *Journal of Nutrition*, 116, 316, 1986.
3. Heaney, R., Bone mass, nutrition and other lifestyle factors, *American Journal of Medicine*, 95, 29S, 1993.
4. Daniell, H., Osteoporosis and the slender smoker: vertebral compression fractures and loss of metacarpal cortex in relation to postmenopausal cigarette smoking and lack of obesity, *Archives of Internal Medicine*, 136, 298, 1976.
5. Heany, R. P., Recker, R. R., Effects of nitrogen, phosphorus, and caffeine on calcium balance in women, *Journal of Laboratory Clinical Medicine*, 99, 46, 1982.
6. Hasling, C., Sondergaard, K., Charles, P., Mosekilde, L., Calcium metabolism in postmenopausal osteoporotic women is determined by dietary calcium and coffee intake, *Journal of Nutrition*, 122, 1119, 1992.
7. Massey, L. K., Wise, K. J., The effect of dietary caffeine on urinary excretion of calcium, magnesium, sodium and potassium in healthy young females, *Nutrition Research*, 4, 43, 1984.
8. Massey, L. K., Hollingberry, P. W., Acute effects of dietary caffeine and sucrose on urinary mineral excretion of healthy adolescents, *Nutrition Research*, 8, 1005, 1988.
9. Massey, L. K., Opryszek, M. S., No effects of adaptation to dietary caffeine on calcium excretion in young women, *Nutrition Research*, 10, 741, 1990.
10. Massey, L. K., Sherrard, D. J., Bergman, E. A., Dietary caffeine lower ultrafiltrable calcium levels in women consuming low dietary calcium, *Journal of Bone and Mineral Research*, 4(Sup 1), 249(Abstract), 1989.
11. Barger-Lux, M. J., Heaney, R. P., Stegman, M. R., Effects of moderate caffeine intake on the calcium economy of premenopausal women, *American Journal of Clinical Nutrition*, 52, 722, 1990.
12. Smith, S., Swain, J., Brown, E. M., Wyshak, G., Albright, T., Ravnikar, V. A., Schiff, I., A preliminary report of the short-term effect of carbonated beverage consumption on calcium metabolism in normal women, *Archives of Internal Medicine*, 149, 2517, 1989.
13. Lloyd, T., Schaeffer, J., Walker, M., Demers, L., Urinary hormonal concentrations and spinal bone densities of premenopausal vegetarian and nonvegetarian women, *American Journal of Clinical Nutrition*, 54, 1005, 1991.
14. Hernandez-Avila, M., Colditz, G. A., Stampfer, M. J., Rosner, B., Speizer, F. E., Willett, W. C., Caffeine, moderate alcohol intake, and risk of fractures of the hip and forearm in middle-aged women, *American Journal of Clinical Nutrition*, 54, 157, 1991.
15. Kiel, D. P., Felson, D. T., Hannan, M. T., Anderson, J. J., Wilson, P. W. F., Caffeine and the risk of hip fracture: the framingham study, *American Journal of Epidemiology*, 132, 675, 1990.
16. Hernandez-Avila, M., Stampfer, M. J., Ravnikar, V. A., Willett, W. C., Schiff, I., Francis, M., Longscope, C., McKinlay, S. M., Caffeine and other predictors of bone density among pre- and perimenopausal women, *Epidemiology*, 4, 128, 1993.
17. Barrett-Connor, E., Change, J. C., Edelstein, S. L., Coffee-associated osteoporosis offset by daily milk consumption: the Rancho Bernardo Study, *Journal of the American Medical Association*, 271, 280, 1994.

18. Yano, K., Heilbrun, L. K., Wasnich, R. D., Hankin, J. H., Vogel, J. M., The relationship between diet and bone mineral content of multiple skeletal sites in elderly Japanese-American men and women living in Hawaii, *American Journal of Clinical Nutrition*, 42, 877, 1985.
19. Cooper, C., Atkinson, E. J., Wahner, H. W., OFallon, W. M., Riggs, B. L., Judd, H. L., Melton, L. J., Is caffeine consumption a risk factor for osteoporosis?, *Journal of Bone and Mineral Research*, 7, 465, 1992.
20. Harris, S. S., Dawson-Hughes, B., Caffeine and bone loss in healthy post-menopausal women, *American Journal of Clinical Nutrition*, 60, 573, 1994.
21. Bauer, D. C., Browner, W. S., Cauley, J. A., Orwoll, E. S., Scott, J. C., Black, D. M., Tao, J. L., Cummings, S. R., Factors associated with appendicular bone mass in older women. The study of osteoporotic fractures research group, University of California, San Francisco., *Annals of Internal Medicine*, 118, 741, 1993.
22. Eliel, L. P., Smith, L. C., Ivey, J. L., Baylink, D. J., Longitudinal changes in radial bone mass — dietary caffeine, milk, and activity, *Calcified Tissue International*, 35, 669 (Abstract), 1983.
23. Picard, D., Ste-Marie, L. G., Coutu, D., Carrier, L., Chartrand, R., Lepage, R., Fugere, P., Damour, P., Premenopausal bone mineral content relates to height, weight, and calcium intake during early adulthood, *Bone and Mineral Research*, 4, 299, 1988.
24. Slemenda, C. W., Siu, L. H., Longscope, C., Wellman, H., Johnston, C., Predictors of bone mass in perimenopausal women: a prospective study of clinical data using photon absorptiometry, *Annals of Internal Medicine*, 112, 96, 1990.
25. Holbrook, T. L., Barrett-Connor, E., Wingard, D. L., Dietary calcium and risk of hip fracture: 14 year prospective population study, *Lancet*, 2, 1046, 1988.
26. Kreiger, N., Gross, A., Hunter, G., Dietary factors and fracture in postmenopausal women: a case-control study, *International Journal of Epidemiology*, 21, 953, 1992.
27. Johansson, C., Mellstrom, D., Lerner, U., Osterberg, T., Coffee drinking: a minor risk factor for bone loss and fractures, *Age and Ageing*, 21, 20, 1992.

Chapter 16

CAFFEINE AND REPRODUCTION

Myron Winick

CONTENTS

There has been some question whether caffeine, even in large doses, has any adverse effect on the outcome of pregnancy. In 1980, the Food and Drug Administration advised pregnant women to limit their intake of caffeine. These recommendations were based almost exclusively on animal experiments. The recommendations were also nonspecific, i.e., nothing was said about how much caffeine was safe during pregnancy, nor was any mention made of when during pregnancy caffeine was most detrimental to the fetus. During the past 17 years, a great deal of evidence has accumulated about the role of caffeine during pregnancy in human populations. Although the results of these studies have not been entirely

0-8493-2647-8/98/$0.00+$.50

consistent, the preponderance of evidence suggests that caffeine, especially in large doses, may have adverse effects on several outcomes of pregnancy. This evidence will be examined in the following way:

1. The animal data upon which the F.D.A. based its recommendation and animal evidence gathered subsequently.
2. Human data divided into specific problems that occur during the reproductive cycle in which caffeine might be implicated.

   These would include:

   a) The ability to conceive

   b) Congenital malformations

   c) Spontaneous abortions (SAB)

   d) Retarded fetal growth

   e) Premature labor

   f) Changes in fetal physiology

   g) Lasting effects on the offspring

I. ANIMAL DATA

Before discussing the animal data it is important to note that caffeine is metabolized differently in experimental animals than it is in humans. This is particularly so in the rat, which is the most common experimental model used. Therefore results in animals, either positive or negative, cannot be directly applied to humans. However, since caffeine itself and some of its metabolites are present in both the animal experiments and during human exposure, an adverse effect of caffeine in an animal model should be verified or excluded in the human.

Caffeine and almost all of its metabolites cross the placenta and diffuse into virtually all fetal tissues.[1,2] Caffeine has been shown to produce chromosomal damage in mammalian cells.[3] There is an increase in fetal mortality and morbidity when pregnant rats are fed caffeine in increasing doses.[4]

Thus, it is clear that, in animals, there are enough data to implicate caffeine ingestion by the mother in poor pregnancy outcome, including spontaneous abortion, congenital malformations, fetal growth retardation, and residual effects in the newborn. These data have made human studies extremely important. Fortunately many human studies have been carried out in the past 17 years, since the F.D.A. warning was put in place. Unfortunately these studies have not always produced consistent results. However, I believe that a pattern is emerging which is implicating caffeine, at least in doses above 300 mg per day (3 cups of coffee per day) in several types of poor pregnancy outcomes.

II. STUDIES IN HUMAN POPULATIONS

A. The Ability to Conceive

There have been a number of studies that have strongly suggested that ingestion of caffeine, particularly in doses of 300 mg per day and above, is associated with an increased risk of infertility.[5-7] The data suggest that both male and female fertility may be affected. In women, the timing of events during the menstrual cycle may be disturbed. In men, sperm motility may be reduced. Although caffeine consumption is certainly not a major cause of infertility, I believe the evidence is strong enough to advise couples having difficulty in conceiving to refrain from consuming caffeine while they are trying to become pregnant.

B. Congenital Malformations

Although a few animal studies have shown an increase in the number of congenital malformations among the offspring of dams fed high doses of caffeine during pregnancy, the preponderance of animal evidence finds no significant increase in such malformations. In human populations there are no studies which have shown any correlation between maternal caffeine intake, even at the highest doses studied, and congenital abnormalities of the fetus.

C. Spontaneous Abortions (SAB)

In 1993, two articles appeared in the December 22 issue of the *Journal of the American Medical Association* describing studies carried out to examine whether an association exits between caffeine intake during pregnancy and the incidence of SAB.[8,9] The articles reach different conclusions. In the study by Mills et al., the conclusion was that moderate intake of caffeine during pregnancy (150 to 300 mg per day) had no effect on the incidence of SAB. By contrast, the study by Infante-Rivard et al. concludes that ingestion of 300 mg or more of caffeine per day results in three times the risk of SAB than in non-consumers of caffeine. Ingestion of 150 to 300 mg of caffeine per day doubles the risk of SAB. In an editorial in the same issue of the *Journal*, Brenda Eskenazi discusses the discrepancies.[10] She notes that in the first study mentioned, there were not enough women consuming 300 mg or more per day to reach any conclusions. Also, the populations studied were very different. In the study showing no effect of caffeine the women were from a higher socioeconomic class, better educated, and more health conscious. In addition, the total number of women studied was much lower. In the study showing a direct correlation between caffeine and SAB, there was a clear dose response. The greater the intake of caffeine, above 150 mg per day, the higher the risk for SAB. From these and other studies, the evidence suggests that at levels of intake of 300 mg per day or above, caffeine increases the risk for SAB about three times. At levels of 150 to 300 mg per day, the risk in some women for SAB is doubled. Although more studies are needed to confirm these results, I believe the existing data are strong enough to warrant counseling women contemplating pregnancy to limit their caffeine intake to less than 150 mg per day.

D. Retarded Fetal Growth

There is some debate whether caffeine consumption during pregnancy can affect fetal growth and thereby lower birth weight. Most studies indicate that there is a small but significant effect that increases as the quantity of ingested caffeine increases.[11] For example, one study found that women who consumed more than 300 mg per day of caffeine had a relative risk of 4.6 of giving birth to a low birth weight infant, and the mean birth weight of their infants was 105 grams lower than that of nonconsumers of caffeine.[11]

Smoking increases the effect of caffeine on intrauterine growth.[12] Smokers usually consume more caffeine than nonsmokers but their blood caffeine levels are lower than in women who do not smoke. This apparent discrepancy can be explained by the fact that smoking increases caffeine metabolism *in vivo*. In this study,[12] although moderate caffeine intake in nonsmokers had little effect on birth weight, the same intake in smokers resulted in significant fetal growth retardation and a lower birth weight. These data suggest that there is an interaction between maternal smoking and maternal caffeine consumption which affects fetal growth and birth weight. They also suggest that the offending substance may be a metabolite of caffeine rather than caffeine itself. Finally, the data reinforce other reasons for stopping smoking before or during pregnancy, particularly if the woman consumes moderate amounts of caffeine.

E. Premature Labor

The lower birth weight of infants of mothers who consume 300 mg or more of caffeine per day is due entirely to retarded fetal growth. There is no evidence that premature labor and delivery are associated with caffeine during pregnancy.

F. Physiologic Changes in the Fetus

There is evidence that at least two physiologic functions of the fetus may be disturbed by maternal consumption of high doses of caffeine during pregnancy. Fetuses of mothers consuming more than 500 mg of caffeine per day spent less time in active sleep and more time in arousal than fetuses of mothers consuming 200 mg of caffeine per day.[13] In another study, women who consumed any caffeine during pregnancy were compared with those who consumed little or no caffeine. Of the newborns of the women consuming caffeine, 25% had cardiac tachyarrhythmia, compared with only 2% of the newborns of the women who did not consume caffeine.[14] These two studies demonstrate that caffeine or one or more of its metabolites can affect fetal physiology. The significance of these physiological changes, if any, is unknown.

G. Long-Term Changes in the Offspring

There is no evidence that maternal consumption of caffeine, even in relatively large amounts, has any long-term effects on the offspring. However, it must be remembered that such studies are very difficult to carry out in human populations. Therefore, in my judgment, the lack of evidence linking maternal caffeine consumption with long-term consequences to the offspring does not mean that such an association does not exist.

III. SUMMARY

In summary, maternal consumption of caffeine, particularly in doses of 300 mg or more per day, can result in both male and female infertility, an increase in spontaneous abortions, fetal growth retardation, particularly in women who smoke, and physiological changes in the fetus and newborn. In addition, even though no long-term changes in the offspring have been described, they cannot be entirely ruled out. There appears to be a dose response effect. The more caffeine consumed, the greater the effect. The effects of caffeine on the fetus seem to be greatest at intake levels of 300 mg or more per day. Therefore, I believe that pregnant women should be cautioned to consume less than 300 mg of caffeine per day.

REFERENCES

1. Yesair D.W., Branfman A.R., Callahan M.M. Human disposition and some biochemical aspects of methylxanthines. In: Spiller G.A., ed. *The Methylxanthine Beverages and Foods: Chemistry,Consumption and Health Effects.* New York, Alan R. Liss, 1984, 215-233.
2. Mirkin B.L., Singh S., Placental transfer of pharmacologically active molecules. In: Mirkin B.L., ed., *Perinatal Pharmacology and Theraputics.* New York, Academic Press, 1976, 1-69.
3. Kihlman B.A., *Caffeine and Chromosomes.* Amsterdam: Elsevier,1977.
4. Dlugosz L., Braken M. S., Reproductive effects of caffeine: a review and theoretical analysis. *Epidemiol. Rev.,* 1992,14, 83100.
5. Wilcox A., Weinberg C.,Baird D., Caffeinated beverages and decreased fertility. *Lancet,* 1988, 2, 1453-1456.
6. Joesoes M.R., Beral V., Rolfs R.T., Aral S.O. Are caffeinated beverages risk factors for delayed conception? *Lancet,* 1990, 1, 136-137.
7. Olsen J., Cigarette smoking, tea and coffee drinking and subfecundity. *Am. J Epidemiol.,* 1991, 133, 734-739.
8. Enfante-Rivard C., Fernandez A., Gauthier R., David M., Bivard G.E., Fetal loss associated with caffeine intake before and during pregnancy. *JAMA,* 1993, 270, 24, 2940-2943.
9. Mills J.L., Holmes L.B., Aarons J.H., et al., Moderate caffeine use and the risk of spontaneous abortion and intrauterine growth retardation. *JAMA,* 1993, 269, 593-597.
10. Eskenazi B., Caffeine during pregnancy: Grounds for concern? *JAMA,* 1993, 270, 24, 2973-2974.
11. Effect of caffeine on pregnancy outcome. *Nutr. Res. Newsletter,* 1996, 15, 11-12, 120.
12. Cook D.G.,Peacock J., Feyerabend C., et al., *BMJ,* 313, 7069, 1358-1363.
13. Devoe LD., Murray C., Youssif A., Arnaud M., *Am. J Ob. Gyn.,* 1993, 168, 4, 1105-1113.
14. Hadeed A., Siegel S., Newborn cardiac arrythmias associated with maternal caffeine use during pregnancy. *Clin. Pediatr.,* 1993, 32, 1, 45-48.

Appendix 1

Caffeine Content of Some Cola Beverages*

Gene A. Spiller

Beverage Name	Caffeine Content (mg/12 fl oz)[a]
Cherry Coca-Cola®	46
Diet Cherry, Coca-Cola®	46
Cherry Cola Slice®	48
Diet Cherry Cola Slice®	41
Cherry RC®	12
Coca-Cola®	46
Diet Coke®, Coca-Cola®	46
Coca-Cola Classic®	46
Dr. Pepper®	41
Diet Dr. Pepper®	41
Mr. Pibb®	40
Pepsi Cola®	38
Diet Pepsi®	36
Pepsi Lite®	36
RC Cola®	18
Diet Rite Cola®	48
7UP Gold®	46
Diet 7UP Gold®	46
Tab®	46
Diet cola, aspartame sweetened	50
Diet soda, sodium saccharin sweetened	39

From *Agriculture Handbook* No. 8 and cola industry data.

[a] The following cola beverages contain 0 mg caffeine: Caffeine-free Coca-Cola®, Caffeine-free Diet Coke®, Caffeine-free Diet Rite Cola®, Caffeine-free Dr. Pepper®.

*See Chapter 3 for caffeine content of tea, Chapter 7 for caffeine content of chocolate foods/beverages, and Chapter 13 for caffeine content of coffee.

0-8493-2647-8/98/$0.00+$.50

Index

C

D

E

K

L

M

Q

R

S

V

W